Craniofacial Surgery for the Facial Plastic Surgeon

Editors

LISA M. MORRIS
SHERARD A. TATUM

FACIAL PLASTIC SURGERY CLINICS OF NORTH AMERICA

www.facialplastic.theclinics.com

Consulting Editor
J. REGAN THOMAS

November 2016 • Volume 24 • Number 4

ELSEVIER

1600 John F. Kennedy Boulevard • Suite 1800 • Philadelphia, Pennsylvania, 19103-2899

http://www.theclinics.com

FACIAL PLASTIC SURGERY CLINICS OF NORTH AMERICA Volume 24, Number 4
November 2016 ISSN 1064-7406, ISBN-13: 978-0-323-47682-9

Editor: Jessica McCool
Developmental Editor: Alison Swety

Facial Plastic Surgery Clinics of North America (ISSN 1064-7406) is published quarterly by Elsevier Inc., 360 Park Avenue South, New York, NY 10010-1710. Months of issue are February, May, August, and November. Business and Editorial Offices: 1600 John F. Kennedy Blvd., Suite 1800, Philadelphia, PA 19103-2899. Periodicals postage paid at New York, NY, and additional mailing offices. Subscription prices are $390.00 per year (US individuals), $575.00 per year (US institutions), $445.00 per year (Canadian individuals), $716.00 per year (Canadian institutions), $535.00 per year (foreign individuals), $716.00 per year (foreign institutions), $100.00 per year (US students), and $255.00 per year (foreign students). Foreign air speed delivery is included in all *Clinics* subscription prices. All prices are subject to change without notice. POSTMASTER: Send address changes to *Facial Plastic Surgery Clinics*, Elsevier Health Sciences Division, Subscription Customer Service, 3251 Riverport Lane, Maryland Heights, MO 63043. **Customer service: 1-800-654-2452 (US and Canada); 1-314-447-8871 (outside US and Canada); Fax: 314-447-8029; E-mail: journalscustomerservice-usa@elsevier.com (for print support); journalsonline support-usa@elsevier.com (for online support).**

Reprints. For copies of 100 or more of articles in this publication, please contact the Commercial Reprints Department, Elsevier Inc., 360 Park Avenue South, New York, NY 10010-1710. Tel.: 212-633-3874; Fax: 212-633-3820; E-mail: reprints@elsevier.com.

Facial Plastic Surgery Clinics of North America is covered in *MEDLINE/PubMed* (*Index Medicus*).

Contributors

CONSULTING EDITOR

J. REGAN THOMAS, MD, FACS
Professor and Chairman, Department of
Otolaryngology, University of Illinois at
Chicago, Chicago, Illinois

EDITORS

LISA M. MORRIS, MD
Craniofacial/Facial Plastic and Reconstructive
Surgery, Craniofacial Foundation of Utah, Salt
Lake City, Utah

SHERARD A. TATUM, MD, FACS, FAAP
Professor of Otolaryngology and Pediatrics,
Cleft and Craniofacial Center, Division of Facial
Plastic Surgery, Upstate Medical University,
Syracuse, New York

AUTHORS

DANIEL ALAM, MD
Professor of Surgery, University of Hawaii,
John A. Burns School of Medicine, Honolulu,
Hawaii

YASEEN ALI, MD
Fellow, Facial Plastic and Reconstructive
Surgery, Queens Medical Center, Honolulu,
Hawaii

AMIT D. BHRANY, MD
Clinical Associate Professor, University of
Washington, Seattle, Washington

ADITI A. BHUSKUTE, MD
Resident, Department of Otolaryngology-Head
and Neck Surgery, UC Davis Medical Center,
Sacramento, California

RANDALL A. BLY, MD
Acting Assistant Professor, Pediatric
Otolaryngology, Seattle Children's Hospital,
University of Washington, Seattle, Washington

LAUREN A. BOHM, MD
Assistant Professor, Children's ENT and Facial
Plastic Surgery, Children's Hospitals and
Clinics of Minnesota; Department of
Otolaryngology, University of Minnesota,

Minneapolis, Minnesota; Division of Pediatric
Otolaryngology, University of Michigan, Ann
Arbor, Michigan

KATHLEYN A. BRANDSTETTER, MD
Resident, Department of Otolaryngology-Head
and Neck Surgery, Medical University of South
Carolina, Charleston, South Carolina

TIFFANY CHEN, MD
Albany Medical Center; St Peter's Hospital;
Stratton VA Medical Center, Albany,
New York

DANIEL COVENTRY, BSc
Medical Student, Oxford University School of
Medicine, Oxford, United Kingdom

ASHLEY M. DAO, MD
Otolaryngology Resident, Emory University
School of Medicine, Atlanta, Georgia

JOSHUA C. DEMKE, MD
Associate Professor, Division of Facial Plastic
and Reconstructive Surgery, Department of
Otolaryngology-Head and Neck Surgery;
Co-Chair, West Texas Craniofacial Center of
Excellence, Texas Tech University Health
Sciences Center, Lubbock, Texas

CELESTE GARY, MD
Division of Facial Plastic and Reconstructive Surgery, Department of Otolaryngology, University of California Davis, Sacramento, California

STEVEN L. GOUDY, MD
Associate Professor; Chief, Division of Pediatric Otolaryngology, Emory University School of Medicine, Children's Healthcare of Atlanta, Atlanta, Georgia

LISA E. ISHII, MD, MHS
Associate Professor, Facial Plastic & Reconstructive Surgery, Department of Otolaryngology-Head & Neck Surgery, Johns Hopkins School of Medicine, Baltimore, Maryland

CHRISTOPHER KLEM, MD
Assistant Professor of Surgery, University of Hawaii, John A Burns School of Medicine, Honolulu, Hawaii

ANN W. KUMMER, PhD, CCC-SLP, ASHA-F
Senior Director, Division of Speech-Language Pathology, Cincinnati Children's Hospital Medical Center, Professor of Otolaryngology, Professor of Clinical Pediatrics, University of Cincinnati College of Medicine, Cincinnati, Ohio

JEREMY D. MEIER, MD
Assistant Professor of Surgery, Division of Otolaryngology, University of Utah School of Medicine, Salt Lake City, Utah

JILL M. MERROW, MA, CCC-SLP
Speech-Language Pathologist, State University of New York (SUNY) Upstate Medical Center, Syracuse, New York

DAVID M. MIRSKY, MD
Director, Pediatric Neuroradiology Fellowship, Assistant Professor of Radiology, Children's Hospital Colorado, University of Colorado School of Medicine, Aurora, Colorado

LISA M. MORRIS, MD
Craniofacial/Facial Plastic and Reconstructive Surgery, Craniofacial Foundation of Utah, Salt Lake City, Utah

HARLAN R. MUNTZ, MD
Professor of Surgery, Division of Otolaryngology, University of Utah School of Medicine, Salt Lake City, Utah

CRAIG S. MURAKAMI, MD
Clinical Professor, Virginia Mason Medical Center, University of Washington, Seattle, Washington

LASZLO NAGY, MD
Associate Professor, Pediatric Neurosurgery, Department of Pediatrics; Co-Chair, West Texas Craniofacial Center of Excellence, Texas Tech University Health Sciences Center, Lubbock, Texas

KRISHNA G. PATEL, MD, PhD
Associate Professor, Department of Otolaryngology-Head and Neck Surgery, Medical University of South Carolina, Charleston, South Carolina

BRIANNE ROBY, MD
Assistant Professor, Children's ENT and Facial Plastic Surgery, Children's Hospitals and Clinics of Minnesota; Department of Otolaryngology, University of Minnesota, Minneapolis, Minnesota

HOWARD M. SAAL, MD, FAAP, FACMG
Professor, Division of Human Genetics, Department of Pediatrics, Cincinnati Children's Hospital Medical Center, University of Cincinnati College of Medicine, Cincinnati, Ohio

JAMES D. SIDMAN, MD
Professor, Children's ENT and Facial Plastic Surgery, Children's Hospitals and Clinics of Minnesota; Department of Otolaryngology, University of Minnesota, Minneapolis, Minnesota

KATHLEEN C.Y. SIE, MD
Richard and Francine Loeb Endowed Chair in Childhood Communication Research, Seattle Children's Hospital, Professor, University of Washington, Seattle, Washington

KEIMUN A. SLAUGHTER, MD
Albany Medical Center, Albany, New York; New England Laser and Cosmetic Surgery Center; Williams Center Plastic Surgery Specialists, Latham, New York; St Peter's Hospital, Albany Memorial Hospital; Stratton VA Medical Center, Albany, New York

SVEN-OLRIK STREUBEL, MD, MBA
Pediatric Otolaryngology and
Craniomaxillofacial Surgery, Associate
Professor, Department of Otolaryngology,
Children's Hospital Colorado, University of
Colorado School of Medicine, Aurora,
Colorado

JONATHAN M. SYKES, MD
Division of Facial Plastic and Reconstructive
Surgery, Department of Otolaryngology,
University of California Davis, Sacramento,
California

TRAVIS T. TOLLEFSON, MD, MPH, FACS
Professor and Director, Facial Plastic and
Reconstructive Surgery, Department of
Otolaryngology-Head and Neck Surgery,
UC Davis Medical Center, Sacramento,
California

JAMES C. WANG, MD, PhD
Research Assistant Professor, Department of
Otolaryngology-Head and Neck Surgery,
Texas Tech University Health Sciences Center,
Lubbock, Texas; Resident Physician,
Department of Otolaryngology-Head and Neck
Surgery, University of Cincinnati, Cincinnati,
Ohio

EDWIN WILLIAMS III, MD
Albany Medical Center, Albany, New York; New
England Laser and Cosmetic Surgery Center;
Williams Center Plastic Surgery Specialists,
Latham, New York; St Peter's Hospital, Albany
Memorial Hospital, Albany, New York

RYAN WINTERS, MD, FAAP
Facial Plastic & Reconstructive Surgeon,
Surgery Service Line, Sunrise Health System
and Sunrise Children's Hospital, Las Vegas,
Nevada

Contents

There are thousands of craniofacial disorders, each with a different etiology. All cases of orofacial clefts have an underlying genetic cause, ranging from multifactorial with an underlying genetic predisposition to chromosomal and single-gene etiologies. More than 50% of cases of Pierre Robin sequence are syndromic and 25% of craniosynostoses are syndromic. Clinical genetics evaluation is important for each patient with a craniofacial condition to make a proper diagnosis, counsel the family, and assist in management. This is an overview of the major components of the clinical genetics evaluation with a review of many syndromes associated with craniofacial disorders.

This article reviews the presentation of children with craniofacial anomalies by the most common sites of airway obstruction. Major craniofacial anomalies may be categorized into those with midface hypoplasia, mandible hypoplasia, combined midface and mandible hypoplasia, and midline deformities. Algorithms of airway interventions are provided to guide the initial management of these complex patients.

 Video content accompanies this article at http://www.facialplastic.theclinics.com.

The instinctual drive to gain nourishment can become complicated by structural differences, physiologic instability and environmental influences. Infants with craniofacial anomalies may experience significant feeding and swallowing difficulties related to the type and severity of the anomalies present as well as social-emotional interactions with caregivers. Typical outcome measures and feeding goals are discussed. Details regarding clinical and instrumental evaluation, including fiberoptic endoscopic evaluation of swallowing and modified barium swallow study, as well as management techniques are reported.

 Video content accompanies this article at http://www.facialplastic.theclinics.com.

Children with craniofacial anomalies often demonstrate disorders of speech and/or resonance. Anomalies that affect speech and resonance are most commonly caused by clefts of the primary palate and secondary palate. This article discusses how speech-language pathologists evaluate the effects of dental and occlusal anomalies on speech production and the effects of velopharyngeal insufficiency on speech sound production and resonance. How to estimate the size of a velopharyngeal opening based on speech characteristics is illustrated. Nasometry, nasopharyngoscopy, and low-tech tools are discussed as adjunct methods to aid in the evaluation, treatment planning, and measurement of outcomes.

 Video content accompanies this article at http://www.facialplastic.theclinics.com.

Cleft lip and palate are the fourth most common congenital birth defect. Management requires multidisciplinary care owing to the complexity of these clefts on midface growth, dentition, Eustachian tube function, and lip and nasal cosmesis. Repair requires planning, but can be performed systematically to reduce variability of outcomes. The use of primary rhinoplasty at the time of cleft lip repair can improve nose symmetry and reduce nasal deformity. Use of nasoalveolar molding ranging from lip taping to the use of preoperative infant orthopedics has played an important role in improving functional and cosmetic results of cleft lip repair.

Repair of the cleft palate intends to establish the division between the oral and nasal cavity, thereby improving feeding, speech, and eustachian tube dysfunction all while minimizing the negative impact on maxillary growth. Before palate repair candidacy, timing and surgical method of repair is dependent on comorbid conditions, particularly cardiac disease, mandibular length, and palate width. Additionally, management of the alveolar cleft and the indications for gingivoperiosteoplasty versus secondary alveolar bone grafting is a controversial topic that weighs the risks and benefits of potentially sparing the patient an additional surgery against iatrogenic restriction of facial growth and malocclusion.

Velopharyngeal dysfunction (VPD) can significantly impair a child's quality of life and may have lasting consequences if inadequately treated. This article reviews the workup and management options for patients with VPD. An accurate perceptual speech analysis, nasometry, and nasal endoscopy are helpful to appropriately evaluate patients with VPD. Treatment options include nonsurgical management with speech therapy or a speech bulb and surgical approaches including double-opposing Z-plasty, sphincter pharyngoplasty, pharyngeal flap, or posterior wall augmentation.

 Video content accompanies this article at http://www.facialplastic.theclinics.com.

Intermediate and definitive cleft rhinoplasties are a challenging part of definitive cleft care. The anatomy of the cleft nose is severely affected by the structural deficits associated with congenital orofacial clefting. A comprehensive understanding of the related anatomy is crucial for understanding how to improve the appearance and function in patients with secondary cleft nasal deformities. Timing of intermediate and definitive rhinoplasty should be carefully considered. A thorough understanding of advanced rhinoplasty techniques is an important part of providing adequate care for patients with these deformities.

complicated conditions. Tessier's classification is reviewed in detail, and a separate discussion of hypertelorism (increased distance between the bony orbits) follows, focusing on orbital hypertelorism in the setting of craniofacial clefts.

Keimun A. Slaughter, Tiffany Chen, and Edwin Williams III

Classification of vascular lesions based on the biological behavior has greatly facilitated more accurate diagnoses, optimally defined treatment plans, and better outcomes. Treatment of vascular lesions has taken a more conservative surgical approach with reliance on select medical treatment options, which has greatly reduced morbidity and mortality resulting from extensive surgery. A multidisciplinary approach involving multiple surgical and pediatric subspecialties has led to advancement in both understanding and ideal treatment strategies of these lesions.

Lisa E. Ishii

Facial nerve paralysis, although uncommon in the pediatric population, occurs from several causes, including congenital deformities, infection, trauma, and neoplasms. Similar to the adult population, management of facial nerve disorders in children includes treatment for eye exposure, nasal obstruction/deviation, smile asymmetry, drooling, lack of labial function, and synkinesis. Free tissue transfer dynamic restoration is the preferred method for smile restoration in this population, with outcomes exceeding those of similar procedures in adults.

Randall A. Bly, Amit D. Bhrany, Craig S. Murakami, and Kathleen C.Y. Sie

Microtia reconstruction is a challenging endeavor that has seen significant technique evolution. It is important to educate patients and their families to determine the best hearing rehabilitation and ear reconstructive options. Microtia is often associated with aural atresia, hearing loss, and craniofacial syndromes. Optimal care is provided by multiple disciplines, including a reconstructive surgeon, an otologic surgeon, an audiologist, and a craniofacial pediatrician. Microtia management includes observation, prosthetic ear, autologous cartilage reconstruction, or alloplastic implant placement. Hearing management options are observation, bone conduction sound processor, or atresiaplasty with and without hearing aids. Appropriate counseling should be done to manage expectations.

Daniel Alam, Yaseen Ali, Christopher Klem, and Daniel Coventry

Orbito-malar reconstruction after oncological resection represents one of the most challenging facial reconstructive procedures. Until the last few decades, rehabilitation was typically prosthesis based with a limited role for surgery. The advent of microsurgical techniques allowed large-volume tissue reconstitution from a distant donor site, revolutionizing the potential approaches to these defects. The authors report a novel surgery-based algorithm and a classification scheme for complete midface reconstruction with a foundation in the Gillies principles of like-to-like reconstruction and with a significant role of computer-aided virtual planning. With this approach, the authors have been able to achieve significantly better patient outcomes.

Craniomaxillofacial Trauma 605

Sven-Olrik Streubel and David M. Mirsky

Facial trauma causes significant morbidity in the United States. With injuries varying widely, the clinical benefits of antibiotics use in facial fracture treatment are not easily determined. The pediatric population is more predisposed to craniofacial trauma secondary to their increased cranial mass to body ratio. All patients with traumatic injury should be assessed according to the Advanced Trauma Life Support protocol. This article discusses the types and prevalence of injuries and approaches to management.

FACIAL PLASTIC SURGERY CLINICS OF NORTH AMERICA

THE CLINICS ARE AVAILABLE ONLINE!
Access your subscription at:
www.theclinics.com

Preface
Craniofacial Surgery for the Facial Plastic Surgeon

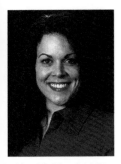

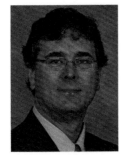

Lisa M. Morris, MD   Sherard A. Tatum, MD, FACS, FAAP

Editors

The care and management of patients with craniofacial anomalies is one of the most challenging, and often the most rewarding, aspects of facial plastic and reconstructive surgery. Due to the complexity of the craniofacial skeleton, patients often have a constellation of associated problems, both aesthetic and functional. Management of these patients may begin as early as infancy and often continues into adulthood, requiring a coordinated, multidisciplinary approach.

In this issue of the *Facial Plastic Surgery Clinics of North America*, we start off with an in-depth review on the evaluation and treatment of children with craniofacial anomalies, beginning with genetics, airway management, feeding, and speech evaluation. Multiple articles are dedicated to the comprehensive surgical management for cleft lip and/or palate disorders. Insightful articles on the diagnosis of and treatment for the more common craniofacial disorders, including craniofacial microsomia, craniosynostosis, facial clefts, hypertelorism, vascular lesions, and facial nerve abnormalities, are offered. Finally, acquired disorders of the craniofacial skeleton are discussed, including the management of facial trauma as well as complex midface microsurgical reconstruction.

It has been an honor to serve as guest editors for this issue and a pleasure working with the distinguished authors who are dedicated to advancing the field of craniofacial surgery. We hope that you not only find these articles insightful and enjoyable to read but also are able to apply what you learn to your own practice, offering exemplary care to patients with craniofacial anomalies.

Lisa M. Morris, MD
Craniofacial Foundation of Utah
5089 South 900 East, Suite 100
Salt Lake City, UT 84117, USA

Sherard A. Tatum, MD, FACS, FAAP
Cleft and Craniofacial Center
Division of Facial Plastic Surgery
Upstate Medical University
750 East Adams Street
Syracuse, NY 13210, USA

E-mail addresses:
Dr.Lisa.Morris@gmail.com (L.M. Morris)
tatums@upstate.edu (S.A. Tatum)

Facial Plast Surg Clin N Am 24 (2016) xiii
http://dx.doi.org/10.1016/j.fsc.2016.08.001
1064-7406/16/© 2016 Published by Elsevier Inc.

Genetic Evaluation for Craniofacial Conditions

Howard M. Saal, MD

KEYWORDS

- Genetic evaluation • Genetic counseling • Family history • Teratogens • Dysmorphology
- Genetic testing • Cleft lip • Cleft palate

KEY POINTS

- Every child born with a craniofacial disorder should be evaluated by a clinical geneticist.
- Many craniofacial disorders have a genetic etiology, and large variety of genetic testing is available for testing affected individual and family members.
- Although many genetic disorders are common, many patients present with rare or unique conditions requiring specialized genetics evaluations and tests.
- All children with craniofacial disorders should be managed by an interdisciplinary craniofacial or cleft team.

INTRODUCTION

Congenital anomalies and disorders are those conditions that are present at birth and that require some level of medical intervention. These conditions occur in approximately 3% to 5% of all live births.[1] Craniofacial conditions, including orofacial clefts, craniosynostoses, the mandibulofacial dysostoses, and craniofacial macrosomia, are among the most common birth congenital anomalies. Many of these conditions have a genetic etiology (chromosomal, single-gene disorders, or epigenetic mutation) or may be caused by teratogens. Because of this, it is important for each child born with a craniofacial condition to be evaluated and followed by a medical geneticist. The American Cleft Palate-Craniofacial Association in their Standards for Cleft Palate and Craniofacial Teams states, "The Team also must demonstrate access to refer to a neurosurgeon, an ophthalmologist, a radiologist, and a geneticist."[2] The role of the medical geneticist is to assist in making a diagnosis of any known genetic disorder or syndrome, assist families and craniofacial team members in understanding the natural history of any syndrome, and ensure that additional medical evaluations and interventions are performed as indicated. There are thousands of different causes for craniofacial conditions. Identifying the etiologies is important for understanding the cause of a particular condition and influencing the management of a particular disorder. Also, craniofacial conditions are chronic conditions and follow-up evaluations with a medical geneticist should be encouraged.

THE GENETICS EVALUATION

The purpose of the genetics evaluation is to

- Make a diagnosis
- Characterize natural history
- Establish appropriate follow-up evaluations and testing
- Determine recurrence risk and potential genetic testing for family
- Provide genetic counseling for family

Disclosure: Dr H.M. Saal is a member of the Medical Advisory Board and the Speakers Bureau for Alexion Pharmaceuticals.
Division of Human Genetics, Department of Pediatrics, Cincinnati Children's Hospital Medical Center, University of Cincinnati College of Medicine, 3333 Burnet Avenue, MLC 4006, Cincinnati, OH 45229, USA
E-mail address: Howard.Saal@cchmc.org

facialplastic.theclinics.com

Ideally, the genetics evaluation should be performed as early as possible, often soon after birth. Given the technical advances in prenatal diagnosis, prenatal genetic evaluation has become a common occurrence. The genetics evaluation differs from the typical medical evaluation with greater emphasis on prenatal and family histories.

Prenatal Evaluation

Congenital craniofacial conditions begin in utero. Therefore, obtaining a comprehensive pregnancy history is essential to understanding etiology, especially with regard to teratogen exposure, maternal illness, and prenatal testing. Teratogens are substances that interfere with normal embryologic and fetal development. Teratogens include medications and drugs, high-dose radiation, viruses, and maternal illnesses.

Maternal illnesses that are known to cause craniofacial anomalies are diabetes and maternal phenylketonuria. Women with diabetes, both type 1 diabetes mellitus and type 2 diabetes mellitus, have least a 2-fold risk for having a child with birth defects, the greatest risks associated with type 1 diabetes mellitus.[3] The major birth defects are renal, vertebral, brain, and craniofacial anomalies. Craniofacial anomalies include cleft lip, cleft palate (CP), and Pierre Robin sequence (PRS). In my institution, maternal diabetes is among the most common causes of cleft lip with or without CP (CLP) and CP. Women who have phenylketonuria are unable to properly metabolize the amino acid phenylalanine. If an affected woman does not follow a phenylalanine-restricted diet, the elevated levels of the metabolites of phenylalanine can cause multiple anomalies, including microcephaly, ear anomalies, congenital heart defects, and CP.[4] Maternal hyperthyroidism and Graves disease have been associated with neonatal craniosynostosis.[5]

Prenatal testing is commonly performed, especially fetal ultrasound. Ultrasound is performed in midtrimester in most pregnancies in the United States. Cleft lip can be identified with routine ultrasound in approximately 75% of cases[6] and diagnosis approaches 100% with high-resolution ultrasound.[7] It is more difficult to diagnose CP by ultrasound; however, micrognathia and PRS can be diagnosed prenatally.[8] For more complex cases, especially with those with multiple anomalies, fetal MRI scans are performed at several high-risk centers and can be useful for assessing severity of fetal structural and brain anomalies and have a direct impact on pregnancy management (**Fig. 1**).[9]

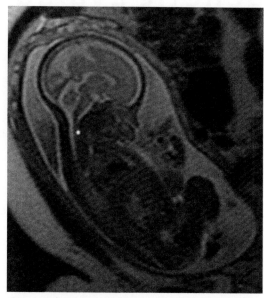

Fig. 1. Fetal MRI scan demonstrating severe micrognathia in a fetus with PRS.

If fetal anomalies are suspected, prenatal genetic testing should be considered. Invasive testing includes amniocentesis, which can be performed from 14 weeks' gestation to term, and chorionic villus sampling can be performed at 12 weeks' gestation. These procedures are usually

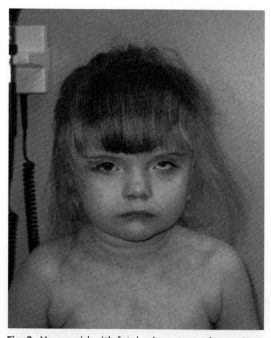

Fig. 2. Young girl with fetal valproate syndrome. Note the short nose, long philtrum, and up-slanting palpebral fissures.

performed to obtain chromosome analysis, chromosomal microarray, fluorescence in situ hybridization (FISH), or single-gene sequencing analysis.

Teratogens

Teratogens are those exogenous substances or physical agents, which, if there is fetal exposure, can cause birth defects. Many teratogens cause craniofacial anomalies. These include but are not limited to

- Physical agents – amniotic bands, radiation
- Infectious agents
- Medications
- Maternal illnesses
- Tobacco

Box 1
Clinical genetics history for the evaluation for craniofacial conditions

History of present illness

- Gestational age
- Type of delivery and complications
- Birth parameters: weight, length, and head circumference
- Other congenital anomalies or major illnesses
- Neonatal complications
- Early feeding and growth

Pregnancy history

- Maternal illnesses
- Maternal medications
- Exposure to other substance (alcohol, cigarettes, and history of substance abuse)
- Prenatal genetic testing (maternal screening tests, ultrasounds, and fetal chromosome or genetic testing)

Past medical history

- Major illnesses
- Hospitalizations
- Surgeries
- Feeding, nutrition, and growth
- Prior medical specialty evaluations

Comprehensive review of systems

- Ten-system review
- Overall health assessment

Developmental history

- Early developmental milestones
- Therapeutic interventions (early intervention, speech, physical, and occupational therapies)
- School performance
- Developmental and neuropsychological evaluations

Family history

- Four-generation pedigree
- Birth defects
- Pregnancy losses (miscarriages and stillbirths)
- Infant, childhood, and early adult deaths
- Infertility
- Consanguinity

- Alcohol
- Toluene (solvent for glues and spray paints)
- Cocaine

Alcohol is a commonly used and potent teratogen. Exposed children are at risk for many serious birth defects, the most common being developmental delay and intellectual disability.[10] Fetal alcohol syndrome and fetal alcohol spectrum disorder are associated with a large number of birth defects. Dysmorphic facial features are common as are microcephaly, brain anomalies, holoprosencephaly, limb anomalies, short stature, and behavior disorders. Craniofacial anomalies include CLP, CP, and PRS.[11,12]

Isotretinoin is a medication prescribed for cystic acne. Although this is an extremely effective medication for treatment of acne, it is a potent teratogen. Isotretinoin can cause multiple anomalies, including microcephaly, brain anomalies, microtia, absent auditory canal, hearing loss, and congenital heart defects.[13]

Valproic acid is an anticonvulsant with significant teratogenicity. This medication causes neural tube defects in approximately 1% of children exposed in utero. Other reported findings include facial dysmorphism, microcephaly, developmental delay and cognitive impairment, CP, and metopic craniosynostosis (**Fig. 2**).[14,15] Diphenyl hydantoin is another anticonvulsant that is teratogenic. It is associated with short stature, developmental disabilities, distal digital and nail hypoplasia, and craniofacial anomalies, including CLP and CP.[16]

Methotrexate is used to treat malignancies, autoimmune disorders, molar pregnancies, and tubal pregnancies. It acts as a folic acid antagonist and interferes with nucleic acid synthesis (thymidine) and, therefore, is highly cytotoxic. Because of this, methotrexate is a potent teratogen and can cause multiple birth defects, including CLP, CP, craniosynostosis, digital anomalies, microcephaly, brain anomalies, and developmental disabilities.[17]

Cigarette smoking, in addition to causing intrauterine growth restriction, can also cause birth defects. There is an association between cigarette smoking and gastroschisis.[18] Cigarettes have also been shown to cause CLP and CP. It is estimated that 6.1% of oral clefts can be attributed to smoking during pregnancy.[19–21] In addition, several genes have been identified, which have been associated with risk for CLP in women who smoke during pregnancy.[22]

Medical History

Obtaining a comprehensive history is essential for genetic diagnosis. Data should include birth history, including length of gestation, birth weight, length, and head circumference. Any

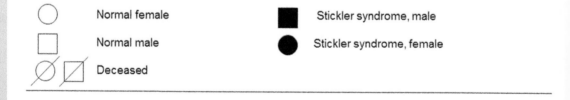

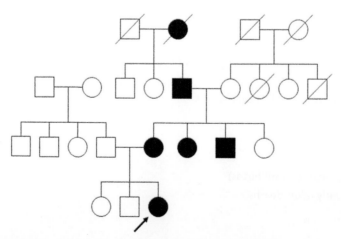

Fig. 3. Four-generation pedigree in a family with an autosomal dominant disorder, in this case Stickler syndrome.

Box 2
Craniofacial genetics physical examination

- Growth parameters – including z scores and growth trends on standardized charts
  - Height
  - Weight
  - Head circumference
  - Arm span
  - Upper to lower segment ratios (for disproportionate short stature)
- Skin
  - Birth marks
  - Hemangiomas
  - Hyperpigmented or hypopigmented macules
  - Hair – alopecia, texture, or hypertrichosis
  - Nails – missing nails or dysplastic nails
- Head/craniofacial
  - Cranial shape – evidence of craniosynostosis, ridging of sutures, or plagiocephaly
  - Fontanelles
  - Inner canthal, interpupillary, and outer canthal distances (hypertelorism and hypotelorism)
  - Facial asymmetry
  - Palpebral fissures – length and epicanthic folds
  - Ear position – low set and posteriorly rotated
  - Ear shape, microtia, and anotia
  - External auditory canal (stenosis and atresia)
  - Preauricular skin tags or fistulae (ear pits)
  - Eye examination – red reflex, iris colobomas, epibulbar dermoids, extraocular movements, nystagmus, and ptosis
  - Nose – short, anteverted nares, shape of nasal tip, and flat or prominent nasal bridge
  - Upper lip – clefting, unilateral, bilateral, and midline
  - Lower lip – clefting and lip pits
  - Palate – clefting (V-shaped or U-shaped), bifid uvula, and SMCP
  - Dentition – abnormally shaped teeth and missing teeth
  - Tongue – lobulations, microglossia or macroglossia, and asymmetry
  - Oral synechiae
  - Mandible – micrognathia, asymmetry, and ankylosis
- Neck
  - Masses
  - Torticollis
  - Branchial clefts or cysts
- Chest
  - Symmetry
  - Chest size and shape
  - Lung auscultation
  - Intercostal and subcostal retractions
  - Pectus deformities

- Cardiovascular
  - Heart murmurs
  - Pulses (upper and lower extremities)
- Abdomen
  - Organomegaly
  - Masses
  - Bowel sounds
- Genitalia — male
  - Penis size
  - Hypospadias
  - Testes – cryptorchidism and testicular size
- Genitalia – female
  - Labial adhesions and fusion
  - Vaginal discharge
- Musculoskeletal
  - Limb deformities
  - Brachydactyly
  - Clinodactyly (incurving of fifth finger)
  - Contractures
  - Joint hypermobility
  - Syndactyly
  - Polydactyly
  - Broad thumbs and halluces
  - Scoliosis
- Neurologic
  - Muscle tone (hypertonia or hypotonia)
  - Strength
  - Gait
  - Cranial nerve abnormalities (facial palsy, hearing loss, abnormal eye movements)

hospitalizations and surgeries should also be recorded as well as significant illnesses. Information regarding feeding and growth is also important, especially to establish if feeding problems are related to a CP or craniofacial anomaly or perhaps caused by underlying neurologic or other structural anomalies, such as a heart defect. Many genetic disorders, especially chromosomal conditions, are associated with poor growth.

Developmental history also gives important clues to diagnosis and management. Major parameters of development include speech and language development, gross motor skills, fine motor skills and personal–social development. For patients with craniofacial disorders, speech and language delays may indicate hearing deficits, whether from middle ear effusions with recurrent otitis media or possibly other structural neurologic problems causing conductive and/or sensorineural deafness. See **Box 1** for essential components of the genetics medical history.

Family History

A family history is an essential component of a genetics evaluation. Information from family history can provide information regarding hereditary disorders and birth defects. A pedigree is constructed, which is a pictorial representation of the family history. Usually information for at least 3 generations is obtained (**Fig. 3**). Family history should include information about

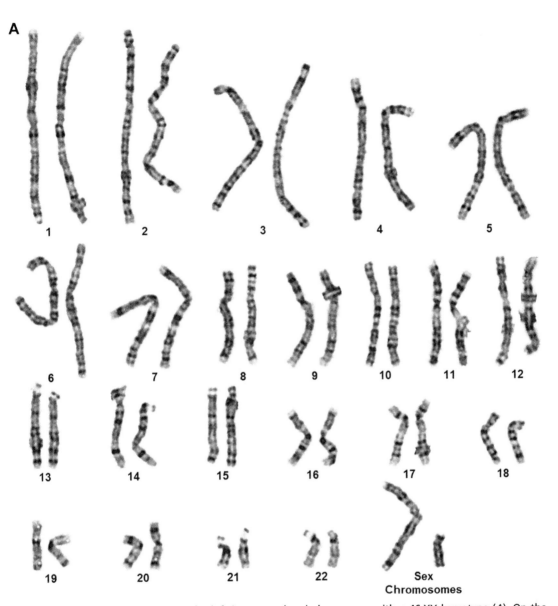

Fig. 4. Chromosome karyograms. On the left is a normal male karyogram with a 46,XY karyotype (*A*). On the right is an abnormal male karyogram with 47 chromosomes and trisomy 21 consistent with a diagnosis of Down syndrome (*B*).

- Birth defects
- Consanguinity
- Pregnancy loss (miscarriages and stillbirths)
- Developmental delay and intellectual disability
- Early or unexpected deaths and causes (if known)
- Mental illness and psychiatric disorders
- Early or unusual cancers
- Blindness
- Deafness
- Chromosome disorders

Physical Examination

A physical examination is an important component of any medical evaluation. The medical genetics physical examination differs from the typical physical examination because in addition to looking for typical findings, the genetics evaluation focuses on looking for atypical or dysmorphic physical features, which may give clues to a genetic or other syndromic disorder or possible etiology. **Box 2** outlines many of the features that may be seen. Any physical examination should include growth

B

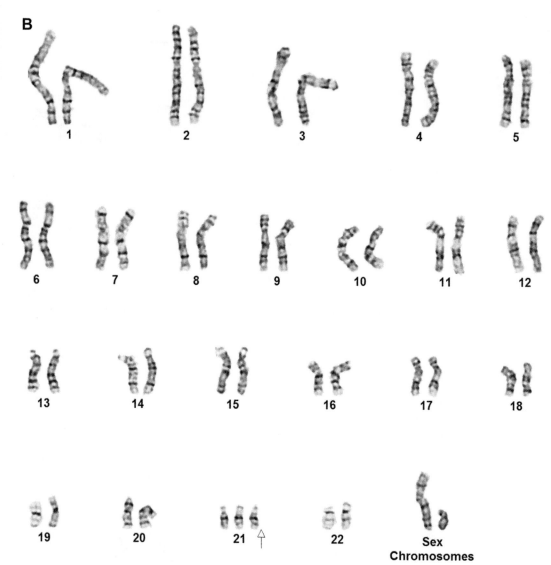

Fig. 4. (*continued*)

parameters, height, weight, and head circumference and should be accompanied by growth percentiles and z scores. These data are essential for diagnosis of short stature, microcephaly, and failure to thrive, all of which may give critical clues to causes of craniofacial disorders and diagnoses.

Laboratory Analysis

There are more than 1000 different disorders that can cause craniofacial anomalies, CLP, and CP. The prenatal, medical, and family histories and the physical examination often give clues as to the specific diagnosis; it then becomes important to confirm the diagnosis if a genetic etiology is suspected. In an analysis of children born with CLP or CP at Cincinnati Children's Hospital Medical Center, chromosomal anomalies were among the most common group of genetic conditions associated with orofacial clefts (**Fig. 4**). There was no clustering of specific chromosome disorders, but several chromosome conditions are associated with CLP and CP, including trisomy 13, trisomy 18, and Wolf-Hirschhorn syndrome (deletion of the short arm of chromosome 4). Velocardiofacial syndrome, or deletion 22q11.2 syndrome, is caused by a microdeletion of the long arm of chromosome 22 and can be diagnosed with a specific fluorescent-tagged DNA sequence, which hybridizes to the specific sequence of chromosome 22 by a test, FISH. In 22q11.2 deletion syndrome, 1 of the 2 chromosome 22 homologues has a deletion of this critical region (**Fig. 5**). Standard chromosome analysis is helpful for many conditions with additional or missing chromosomes or for identifying large chromosomal rearrangements. Chromosomal microarray is a more recently developed test that not only can identify large chromosomal rearrangements but also is able to identify small submicroscopic rearrangements.[23,24] Microarray has many advantages over routine chromosome analysis, including the ability to identify rare chromosomal rearrangements and increase yield of diagnoses.[24]

Many genetic disorders are caused by mutations in single genes. Some common craniofacial disorders and syndromes are single-gene disorders, such as Stickler syndrome and many of the craniosynostosis syndromes. More than 7000 single-gene disorders have been identified (https://globalgenes.org/rare-diseases-facts-statistics/).[25] Genetic testing is available for many of these disorders using gene sequencing. This testing, often called Sanger sequencing, uses polymerase chain reaction to sequence single genes. When ordering gene sequencing for specific genetic disorders, there must be a degree of suspicion of a diagnosis to determine which genetic test or tests to perform.

Many children have rare or even unique genetic disorders for which clinical genetic testing may not be available. These types of cases can now be evaluated using next-generation sequencing. This technology allows for massive parallel sequencing of the human genome. Because the approximately 20,000 human genes comprise only 1% to 2% of the entire human genome, however, only the coding portions of the genome (exons) are sequenced and analyzed and this test is called whole-exome sequencing.[26] Whole-exome sequencing has significantly increased the ability to diagnose genetic disorders, leading to a 25% to 40% increase in diagnostic yield.[27,28] Since the advent of whole-exome sequencing, hundreds of new genetic disorders have been identified.

Additional Evaluations

In addition to these studies, further clinical evaluation is often helpful, including additional medical evaluations, radiographs and other imaging studies, and audiology evaluation. Imaging studies are helpful to identify additional structural anomalies. Ophthalmology evaluation can identify myopia, a clue to Stickler syndrome or Marshall syndrome. Iris and retinal colobomas may be clues to multiple anomaly syndromes, such as CHARGE syndrome (colobomas, heart defects, atresia choanae, retarded growth and/or development, ear anomalies and/or deafness). Children with craniofacial macrosomia may have epibulbar dermoids. An otolaryngology evaluation is important for assessing ear anomalies and laryngotracheal anomalies that may be syndromic. Microtia and absent external auditory canals are seen in the mandibulofacial dysostoses, including Treacher Collins syndrome. Many cases of glottic webs are associated with 22q11.2 deletion syndrome.[29] Cardiology evaluation is essential for diagnosis and management of many syndromes associated with heart defects. The evaluation includes an echocardiogram. Approximately 75% of children with deletion 22q11.2 syndrome have a

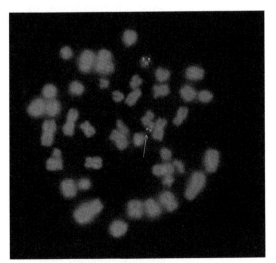

Fig. 5. FISH showing interstitial deletion of chromosome 22q11.2. The arrow points to the chromosome with the deletion; note the absence of the hybridization to the red fluorescence-tagged cDNA, which would hybridize to this region if not deleted.

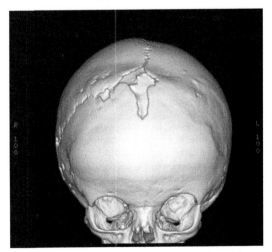

Fig. 6. CT scan with 3-D reconstruction demonstrating fusion of the left coronal suture.

congenital heart defect. Children with chromosome anomalies frequently have heart defects. Congenital heart defects are cardinal findings of CHARGE syndrome.

Imaging studies that can be helpful include radiographs, CT scans, and MRI scans. The radiographs are most helpful when looking for specific skeletal anomalies, including complete skeletal surveys looking for skeletal dysplasia syndromes. Vertebral anomalies are often seen with craniofacial macrosomia, Klippel-Feil syndrome, and diabetic embryopathy. Children with a large

Table 1
Syndromes associated with cleft lip with or without cleft palate

Disorder	Etiology	Gene	Inheritance	Clinical Features
Craniofacial microsomia (see **Fig. 8**)	Sporadic, possibly vascular disruption		Sporadic, Rarely AD	Facial asymmetry, microtia, vertebral anomalies, renal anomalies, heart defect
Amniotic bands (see **Fig. 9**)	Sporadic		Sporadic	CLP, digit or limb amputation, encephalocele
Van der Woude syndrome (**Fig. 7**)	Single-gene mutation	*IRF6*	AD	Lower lip fistulae (pits), CLP, CP, SMCP
Opitz syndrome (G syndrome; hypertelorism-hypospadias syndrome)	Single-gene mutation	*MID1* *SPECCIL*	XLR AD	Hypertelorism, hypospadias, CLP, congenital heart defects
Oral-facial-digital syndrome type I	Single-gene mutation	*OFD1*	XLD	CLP (midline), hyperplastic oral frenulae; tongue lobulations with hamartomas, digital anomalies, syndactyly
CHARGE association	Single-gene mutation	*CHD7*	AD, most cases de novo mutations	Heart defects, deafness, colobomas, genitourinary anomalies, choanal atresia, developmental disabilities
Smith-Lemli-Opitz syndrome	Single-gene mutation	*SLOS*	AR	Growth retardation, microcephaly, CLP, CP, heart defects, genital, syndactyly of toes 2 and 3, anomalies, developmental disabilities
Fetal alcohol syndrome	Teratogenic		Sporadic	Growth retardation, CLP, CP, heart defects, facial dysmorphism, developmental disabilities
Diabetic embryopathy	Teratogenic		Maternal diabetes	Heart defects, CLP, CP, vertebral anomalies, renal anomalies, brain anomalies
Deletion 1p36 syndrome	Chromosomal deletion		Sporadic	CL, CP, facial dysmorphism, speech apraxia, developmental disability
Wolf-Hirschhorn syndrome (4p- syndrome)	Chromosomal deletion		Sporadic	CLP, facial dysmorphism, hypotonia
Trisomy 13	Chromosomal, 3 copies of chromosome 13 (meiotic nondisjunction)		Sporadic (may be familial if there is a translocation)	CLP, CP, brain anomalies including holoprosencephaly, cutis aplasia of scalp, microphthalmia, heart defects, neural tube defects

Abbreviations: AD, autosomal dominant; AR, autosomal recessive; XLD, X-linked dominant; XLR, X-linked recessive.

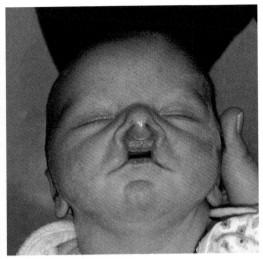

Fig. 7. Infant with Van der Woude syndrome and bilateral cleft lip with CP. Note lip pits of lower lip.

number of genetic disorders may have renal anomalies, including dysplastic kidneys, hydronephrosis, and congenitally absent kidneys. Renal anomalies are common in craniofacial macrosomia, diabetic embryopathy, Klippel-Feil syndrome, and 22q11.2 deletion syndrome. Brain MRI is

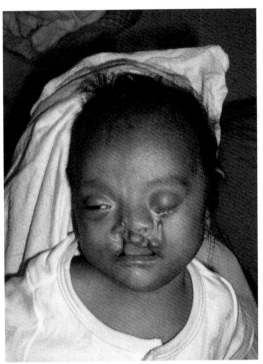

Fig. 9. Infant with cleft lip and CP secondary to amniotic band sequence. Note the remnant of the band below the left eye and lower lid coloboma caused by the band.

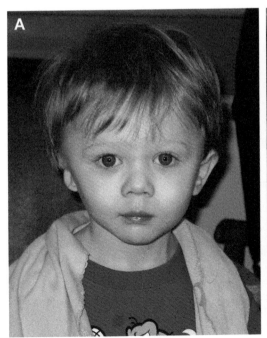

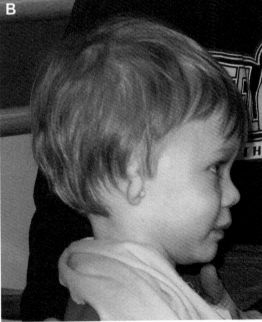

Fig. 8. Young boy with right craniofacial microsomia. Photo on right shows facial asymmetry (*A*) and photo on left shows microtia of right ear (*B*).

useful for identifying structural brain anomalies. It can be a useful test for diagnosis of neurofibromatosis type 1, in which optic pathway gliomas are commonly seen.[30] CT scans are helpful for looking at calcified tissues. This is an important test for evaluation of cranial structures, especially with 3-D reconstruction, and is the test of choice for diagnosing craniosynostosis (**Fig. 6**).

Genetic Counseling

Once all data are gathered and a diagnosis is made (and in many instances no diagnosis is made), it is important to discuss this information with the family. This becomes a time of educating the family regarding genetics and inheritance. Many genetic conditions have a low recurrence risks, either because these are de novo chromosomal anomalies, such as trisomy 13, or are de novo gene mutations for autosomal dominant disorders, such as CHARGE syndrome. Some disorders are inherited. Although 22q11.2 deletion syndrome is de novo in 90% of patients, in 10% of cases 1 of the parents also has a deletion of 22q11.2. Recurrence risk is 50% with each pregnancy.

Many genetic disorders have variable expressivity. For example, if an infant has Stickler syndrome with CP, the affected parent may have myopia as the sole manifestation of Stickler syndrome. Therefore, once a diagnosis is made, it is important to examine the parents and other family members and consider genetic testing of individuals at risk. Recurrence risk analysis should also include information regarding prenatal testing and reproductive options. Prenatal testing, with amniocentesis or

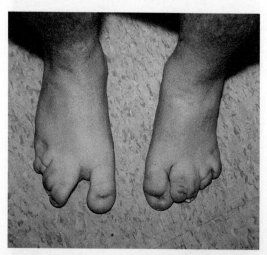

Fig. 10. Feet of a man with popliteal pterygium syndrome. There is triangular tissue over the left great toe and syndactyly.

chorionic villus sampling, is available for most chromosomal and single-gene disorders. Preimplantation testing using assisted reproductive technology can be an option for some conditions.

It is important to discuss the natural history of a genetic disorder or syndrome with the patient and family. Because most genetic disorders involve more than one organ system and frequently are associated with developmental and learning issues, medical and developmental interventions should be discussed. Because most craniofacial disorders are chronic conditions, long-term follow-up by a geneticist can be helpful for anticipatory management and to help address any additional medical issues that may arise.

CRANIOFACIAL DISORDERS
Cleft Lip with or Without Cleft Palate

CLP is among the most common birth defects. In the United States, between the years 2004 and 2006, 4437 infants were born with CLP with an incidence of 1 in 940 live births.[31] The prevalence of CLP depends on race, gender, and socioeconomic factors. Native Americans have the highest prevalence, with 3.6 cases of CLP per 1000 births, compared with Asians, with 1.7 to 2.1 cases per 1000 births, with Africans and African Americans having approximately 1 in 2500 births.[32,33] Boys are more likely to be affected than girls by a 2:1 ratio.[34]

Approximately 30% of cases of CLP are associated with an underlying syndrome or multiple anomalies disorders.[35] The remaining 70% of cases are nonsyndromic. Inheritance is multifactorial, meaning that the condition is caused by both genetic and nongenetic factors. Nongenetic factors may include maternal environment, fetal environment, teratogenic exposures, placental factors, maternal nutritional factors, and as yet several undefined factors.[36] The importance of genetic factors in isolated multifactorial CLP is supported by racial differences in prevalence. In addition, recurrence risk for first-degree relatives of individuals with CLP is elevated to approximately 3% to 5%.[37] This recurrence risk is further elevated as the number of affected individuals in the family increases. In families with 2 affected first-degree relatives, recurrence risk is increased to 5% to 10%. There have been several genes that have been implicated as predisposing to isolated nonsyndromic CLP. In 1 review, 17 genes are listed, including *TGF-A*, *TGF-B3*, *MSX1*, and *IFR6*.[38] Perhaps one of the better studied genes has been *IRF6*, which causes Van der Woude syndrome and popliteal pterygium syndrome. A recent study has demonstrated that 0.24% to

Table 2
Syndromes associated with cleft palate

Disorder	Etiology	Gene	Inheritance	Clinical Features
Craniofacial microsomia (see Fig. 8)	Sporadic, possibly vascular disruption		Sporadic, rarely AD	Facial asymmetry, microtia, vertebral anomalies
Fetal alcohol syndrome	Teratogenic		Environmental	Growth retardation, CLP, CP, heart defects, facial dysmorphism, developmental disabilities
Fetal valproate syndrome (see Fig. 2)	Teratogenic		Environmental	CP, metopic craniosynostosis, microcephaly, spina bifida, developmental disabilities, facial dysmorphism
Van der Woude syndrome	Single-gene mutation	IRF6	AD	Lower lip fistulae (pits), CLP, CP, SMCP
Stickler syndrome (Fig. 11)	Single-gene mutation (genetic heterogeneity)	COL2A1 COL11A1 COL11A2	AD AD AD	Micrognathia, CP, SMCP, myopia, vitreoretinal degeneration (COL2A1 and COL11A1), sensorineural hearing loss, early adult osteoarthritis, facial dysmorphism
Treacher Collins syndrome (Fig. 12)	Single-gene mutation (genetic heterogeneity)	TCOF1 POLR1D POLR1C	AD AD AR	Micrognathia, hypoplastic zygomas, CP, conductive hearing loss, lower eyelid colobomas
22q11.2 Deletion syndrome (Fig. 13)	Chromosomal deletion		AD	Facial dysmorphism, CP, CLP, SMCP, heart defects, developmental disabilities, renal anomalies, psychiatric disorders, hypocalcemia, immunodeficiency
Smith-Lemli-Opitz syndrome	Single-gene mutation	SLOS	AR	Growth retardation, microcephaly, CLP, CP, heart defects, genital, syndactyly of toes 2 and 3, anomalies, developmental disabilities
Diabetic embryopathy	Teratogenic		Maternal diabetes	Heart defects, CLP, CP, vertebral anomalies, renal anomalies, brain anomalies
Deletion 1p36 syndrome	Chromosomal deletion		Sporadic	CL, CP, facial dysmorphism, speech apraxia, developmental disability
Branchio-oto-renal syndrome	Single-gene mutation (genetic heterogeneity)	EYA1 SIX1 SIX5	AD AD AD	Branchial cleft cysts, preauricular fistulae (pits), dysplastic ears, conductive hearing loss, sensorineural hearing loss, CP, SMCP, renal dysplasia, renal cysts, small kidneys
Cornelia de Lange syndrome	Single-gene mutation (genetic heterogeneity)	NIPBL SMC1A HDAC8 RAD21 SMC3	AD XLD XLD AD AD	Growth restriction, microcephaly, CP, facial dysmorphism, micrognathia, synophrys, small mouth, limb and digital anomalies, clinodactyly, brachydactyly, oligodactyly, developmental disabilities
Nager syndrome (Fig. 14)	Single-gene mutation	SF3B4	AD	Growth restriction, micrognathia, CP, conductive hearing loss, hypoplastic zygoma, microtia, thumb aplasia
Loeys-Dietz syndrome (Fig. 15)	Single-gene mutation	TGFBR1 TGFBR2	AD AD	Aortic root dilation, scoliosis, joint hypermobility, pectus deformity, narrow arched palate, SMCP, bifid uvula craniosynostosis, mitral valve prolapse

Abbreviations: AD, autosomal dominant; AR, autosomal recessive; XLD, X-linked.

418

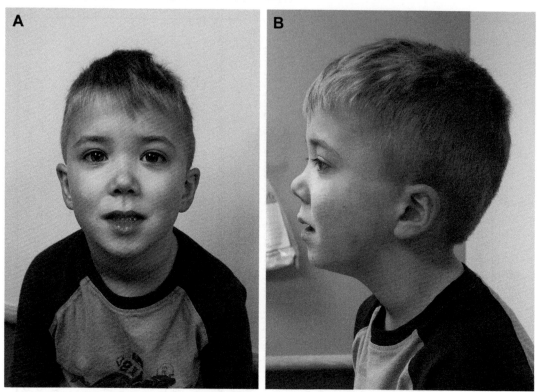

Fig. 11. Young boy with Stickler syndrome. He has a short upturned nose, flat nasal bridge (*A*), and a flat facial profile (*B*).

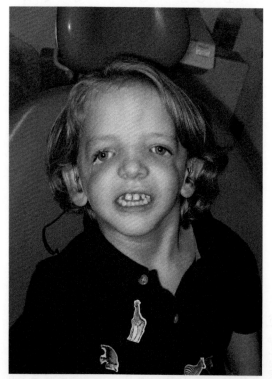

Fig. 12. Young boy with Treacher Collins syndrome caused by a mutation of *TCOF1*. He has micrognathia, down-slanting palpebral fissures, ectropion of lateral lower lids, and low-set ears with conductive hearing loss.

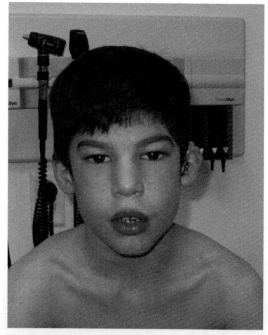

Fig. 13. The 22q11.2 deletion syndrome in a boy. He has an oval-shaped face with prominent nasal tip, prominent nasal pyramid, dysplastic ears, and up-slanting palpebral fissures.

0.44% of isolated multifactorial CLPs are associated with *IRF6* mutations.[39]

Many syndromes have been identified as being associated with CLP. The Online Mendelian Inheritance in Man (OMIM), a catalog of genetic disorders, lists 389 single-gene disorders with CP and 295 disorders with CLP.[40] At Cincinnati Children's Hospital Medical Center, the most common group of disorders associated with CLP is chromosome disorders followed by Opitz syndrome, craniofacial microsomia, diabetic embryopathy, fetal alcohol syndrome and less common disorders such as amniotic band syndrome (**Table 1, Figs. 8** and **9**).

Among the most common syndromes associated with both CLP and CP is Van der Woude syndrome, which is the most common single-gene cause of CLP, responsible for 2% of all CLP cases.[41,42] The classic clinical feature of Van der Woude syndrome is the presence of congenital, bilateral, and paramedian lower lip fistulae (pits) (see **Fig. 7**). Other clinical findings may include elevated mounds of the lower lip with a sinus tract leading from a mucous gland of the lip, CLP, CP, or submucous CP (SMCP).[42] Van der Woude syndrome is one of the few genetic disorders in which affected individuals can have

CLP or CP. The penetrance of lip pits in Van der Woude syndrome is 86%.[42]

Popliteal pterygium syndrome is a genetic disorder also caused by IRF6 mutations.[42,43] In addition to having lip pits with CLP or CP, individuals with popliteal pterygium syndrome have popliteal pterygia, syndactyly, abnormal external genitalia, intraoral adhesions, and pyramidal skin on the hallux (**Fig. 10**).[42]

Cleft Palate

In the United States, between the years 2004 and 2006, the annual incidence of CP was 1 in 1574 live births.[31] Unlike CLP, there is no racial or ethnic predisposition for CP. CP is more likely to be associated with syndromes and multiple anomaly disorders than CLP. Approximately 50% of individuals with CP have an underlying syndrome or multiple anomaly disorder.[34,35] Although some conditions with CP are common, diagnosis of an underlying syndrome with CP can often be challenging because many of these disorders are rare. SMCP is a microform of CP. In SMCP, there is incomplete fusion of the muscular layers of the

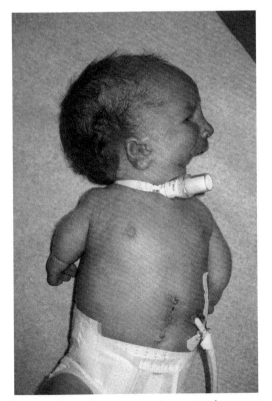

Fig. 14. Infant with Nager syndrome. He has severe micrognathia with PRS and absence of the radii and thumbs.

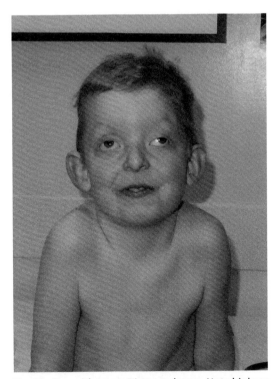

Fig. 15. Boy with Loeys-Dietz syndrome. Note his long oval-shaped face. Individuals with Loeys-Dietz syndrome are at risk for SMCP and craniosynostosis (usually sagittal).

velum (soft palate) with fusion of the overlying mucosa. Presenting features vary ranging from infants with feeding disorders to children with velopharyngeal dysfunction and hypernasal speech. At Cincinnati Children's Hospital Medical Center, the most common disorders associated with CP are Stickler syndrome, 22q11.2 deletion syndrome, fetal alcohol syndrome, and chromosome disorders. See **Table 2** for a list of common CP syndromes (see **Figs. 11** and **13**).

The syndrome most commonly associated with CP is Stickler syndrome. This disorder is genetically heterogeneous, with 6 genes implicated, 3 with autosomal dominant inheritance and 3 with autosomal recessive inheritance.[44] Most cases are autosomal dominantly inherited and associated with mutations in genes for type 2 collagen, *COL2A1*, *COL11A1*, or *COL11A2*. Types I and II Stickler syndrome are caused by mutations in *COL2A1* and *COL11A1*, respectively, and have a similar presentation. The classic features of types I and II Stickler syndrome are micrognathia, RPS, CP, myopia, vitreoretinal degeneration, elevated risk for retinal detachment, early onset of osteoarthritis, and sensorineural hearing loss. Facial features are characterized by micrognathia in infancy with growth of the mandible as the child gets older, flat midface, shallow orbits, flat nasal bridge, and short upturned nose (see **Fig. 11**). Stickler syndrome type III is caused by mutations in *COL11A2* and has similar clinical presentation as types I and II Stickler syndrome with the exception of ocular involvement.[44]

The 22q11.2 deletion syndrome is a common genetic disorder also called velocardiofacial syndrome and DiGeorge syndrome. This disorder is caused by an interstitial deletion of the long arm of chromosome 22.[45] The incidence is approximately 1 in 4000 live births.[46] CP and SMCP are common, seen in approximately 27% of patients. Velopharyngeal dysfunction is also common, even in the absence of CP or SMCP.[47] This condition is also associated with multiple additional anomalies. Congenital heart defects are common, seen in more than 70% of affected individuals. Other significant anomalies are immunodeficiency related to thymus hypoplasia, hypercalcemia secondary to hypoparathyroidism, psychosis and schizophrenia, and developmental disabilities.[48,49] Many patients have typical facial features of narrow face, prominent nasal tip, small mouth, and dysplastic ears (see **Fig. 13**).

Pierre Robin Sequence

PRS is defined by the classic triad of micrognathia, glossoptosis, and obstructive apnea PRS. Patients with PRS frequently have a CP as well (**Fig. 16**). Previous studies have shown that PRS is associated with an underlying syndrome or

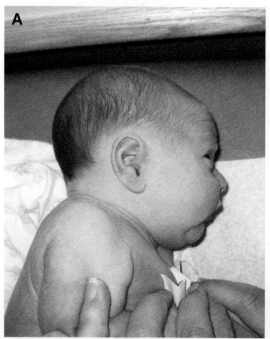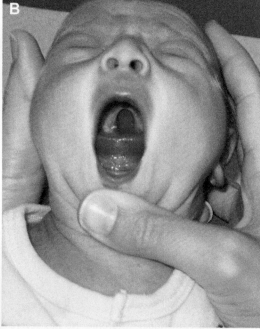

Fig. 16. Infant with PRS. Lateral view shows micrognathia (*A*) and there is a U-shaped cleft of the secondary palate (*B*).

Table 3
Craniosynostosis syndromes

Syndrome	Inheritance	Gene(s)	Chromosome Location	Clinical Features
Antley-Bixler syndrome	AR	POR	7q11.23	Coronal and lambdoid synostosis, radiohumeral synostosis, genital anomalies, developmental disabilities
Apert syndrome (Fig. 17)	AD	FGFR2	10q26.13	Craniosynostosis, syndactyly of hands and feet, midface hypoplasia, developmental disabilities
Baller-Gerold syndrome	AR	RECQLR	8q24.3	Craniosynostosis, radial aplasia
Carpenter syndrome	AR	RAB23	6p22.1-p11.2	Acrocephaly, craniosynostosis, brachydactyly, syndactyly, preaxial polydactyly, developmental disabilities
Craniofrontonasal dysplasia	XLD	EFNB1	Xq13.1	Female: craniofrontonasal dysplasia, craniofacial asymmetry, bifid nasal tip. Male: hypertelorism
Craniosynostosis FGFR3 mutation (Muenke syndrome)	AD	FGFR3	4p16.3	Coronal craniosynostosis
Crouzon syndrome (Fig. 18)	AD	FGFR2	10q26.13	Coronal synostosis, maxillary hypoplasia, mandibular prognathism, exophthalmos
Crouzon syndrome with acanthosis nigricans	AD	FGFR3	4p16.3	Coronal synostosis, maxillary hypoplasia, mandibular prognathism, exophthalmos, acanthosis nigricans
Fetal methotrexate syndrome	Environmental Teratogenic	NA	NA	Craniosynostosis, cleft lip, CP, limb anomalies, syndactyly, brain anomalies, developmental disabilities
Fetal valproate syndrome (see Fig. 2)	Environmental Teratogenic	NA	NA	Metopic suture synostosis, spina bifida, microcephaly, CP, developmental disability
Hyperthyroidism	Environmental Teratogenic	NA	NA	Craniosynostosis. May be neonatal (maternal hyperthyroidism or Graves disease) or acquired hyperthyroidism
Hypophosphatasia, perinatal and infantile	AR	ALPL	1p36.12	Poorly mineralized bone, coronal synostosis, sagittal synostosis, metopic synostosis, limb deformities, narrow thorax, respiratory distress
Jackson-Weiss syndrome	AD	FGFR2	10q26.13	Craniosynostosis, flat midface, hypertelorism, exophthalmos, broad deviated great toe
Loeys-Dietz syndrome (see Fig. 15)	AD	TGFBR1 TGFBR2	9q22.33 3p24.1	Aortic root dilation, scoliosis, joint hypermobility, pectus deformity, narrow arched palate, SMCP, bifid uvula craniosynostosis, mitral valve prolapse

(continued on next page)

Table 3 (continued)				
Syndrome	Inheritance	Gene(s)	Chromosome Location	Clinical Features
Pfeiffer syndrome	AD	FGFR1 FGFR2	8p11.23 1026.13	Type 1: craniosynostosis (coronal), broad thumbs and great toes, maxillary hypoplasia. Type 2: cloverleaf skull, broad thumbs and great toes. Type 3: craniosynostosis (coronal), ankyloses of elbows, tracheobronchial anomalies.
Saethre-Chotzen syndrome (**Fig. 19**)	AD	TWIST	7p21.1	Craniosynostosis, ptosis, folded ear pinna, broad great toes
Shprintzen-Goldberg syndrome	AD	SKI	1p36.33-p36.32	Craniosynostosis, marfanoid body habitus, aortic root dilation, scoliosis, pectus deformity, developmental disabilities

Abbreviations: AD, autosomal dominant; AR, autosomal recessive; NA, not applicable; XLD, X-linked dominant.

multiple anomaly disorder in more than 50% of cases.[50,51] A recent study has shown that in patients with PRS both with and without CP, 54% had syndromes.[52] The most common syndrome was Stickler syndrome, followed by Treacher Collins syndrome (see **Fig. 12**), arthrogryposis multiplex congenita, and chromosome disorders.

nonsyndromic. The etiologies of nonsyndromic craniosynostoses are complex and these seem to be heterogeneous.[55] Multiple genetic and teratogenic causes of craniosynostosis, however, have been identified. The OMIM recognizes 183 single-gene disorders associated with craniosynostosis.[56] Teratogenic causes include valproate

Craniosynostosis

Craniosynostosis is the premature fusion of 1 or more of the cranial sutures.[53] The incidence is between 1 in 2000 to 2500.[54,55] Craniosynostosis can be syndromic or nonsyndromic. Approximately 85% of all cases of craniosynostosis are

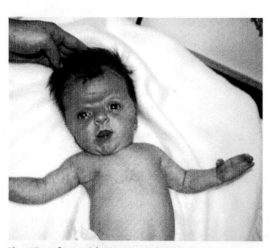

Fig. 17. Infant with Apert syndrome. She has bicoronal craniosynostosis with high forehead, depressed nasal bridge, and beaked nose. She also has the typical syndactyly with deviated thumb.

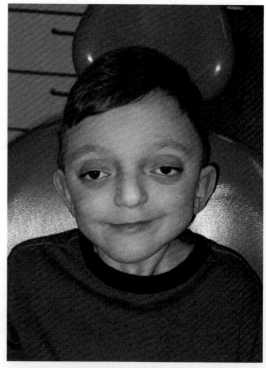

Fig. 18. Boy with Crouzon syndrome. He has shallow orbits and exophthalmos.

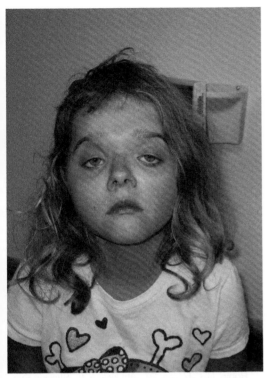

Fig. 19. Girl with Saethre-Chotzen syndrome who was born with bicoronal craniosynostosis. Note the down-slanting palpebral fissures, posteriorly rotated ears, and upturned nose.

embryopathy,[57] which causes metopic suture synostosis, and hyperthyroidism, both neonatal and acquired. Because there is variable expression among the different craniosynostosis syndromes, genetic testing is often required to confirm diagnosis and to give accurate recurrence risks. See **Table 3** for a list of the common craniosynostosis syndromes (see **Figs. 17–19**).

REFERENCES

1. Leppig KA, Werler MM, Cann CI, et al. Predictive value of minor anomalies. I. Association with major malformations. J Pediatr 1987;110(4):531–7.
2. American Cleft Palate –Craniofacial Association. Standards for Cleft Palate and Craniofacial Teams. 2016. Available at: http://www.acpa-cpf.org/team_care/standards.
3. Liu S, Rouleau J, Leon JA, et al. Impact of prepregnancy diabetes mellitus on congenital anomalies, Canada, 2002-2012. Health Promot Chronic Dis Prev Can 2015;35(5):79–84.
4. Kesby G. Repeated adverse fetal outcome in pregnancy complicated by uncontrolled maternal phenylketonuria. J Paediatr Child Health 1999;35(5):499–502.
5. Zimmerman D. Fetal and neonatal hyperthyroidism. Thyroid 1999;9(7):727–33.
6. Wayne C, Cook K, Sairam S, et al. Sensitivity and accuracy of routine antenatal ultrasound screening for isolated facial clefts. Br J Radiol 2002;75(895):584–9.
7. Maarse W, Berge SJ, Pistorius L, et al. Diagnostic accuracy of transabdominal ultrasound in detecting prenatal cleft lip and palate: a systematic review. Ultrasound Obstet Gynecol 2010;35(4):495–502.
8. Lind K, Aubry MC, Belarbi N, et al. Prenatal diagnosis of Pierre Robin Sequence: accuracy and ability to predict phenotype and functional severity. Prenat Diagn 2015;35(9):853–8.
9. Saleem SN. Fetal MRI: An approach to practice: a review. J Adv Res 2014;5(5):507–23.
10. Dorrie N, Focker M, Freunscht I, et al. Fetal alcohol spectrum disorders. Eur Child Adolesc Psychiatry 2014;23(10):863–75.
11. Manning MA, Eugene Hoyme H. Fetal alcohol spectrum disorders: a practical clinical approach to diagnosis. Neurosci Biobehav Rev 2007;31(2):230–8.
12. Munger RG, Romitti PA, Daack-Hirsch S, et al. Maternal alcohol use and risk of orofacial cleft birth defects. Teratology 1996;54(1):27–33.
13. Lammer EJ, Chen DT, Hoar RM, et al. Retinoic acid embryopathy. N Engl J Med 1985;313(14):837–41.
14. Schorry EK, Oppenheimer SG, Saal HM. Valproate embryopathy: clinical and cognitive profile in 5 siblings. Am J Med Genet Part A 2005;133A(2):202–6.
15. Jentink J, Dolk H, Loane MA, et al. Intrauterine exposure to carbamazepine and specific congenital malformations: systematic review and case-control study. BMJ 2010;341:c6581.
16. Hanson JW, Smith DW. The fetal hydantoin syndrome. J Pediatr 1975;87(2):285–90.
17. Hyoun SC, Obican SG, Scialli AR. Teratogen update: methotrexate. Birth Defects Res A Clin Mol Teratol 2012;94(4):187–207.
18. Lam PK, Torfs CP. Interaction between maternal smoking and malnutrition in infant risk of gastroschisis. Birth Defects Res A Clin Mol Teratol 2006;76(3):182–6.
19. Honein MA, Paulozzi LJ, Watkins ML. Maternal smoking and birth defects: validity of birth certificate data for effect estimation. Public Health Rep 2001;116(4):327–35.
20. Honein MA, Rasmussen SA, Reefhuis J, et al. Maternal smoking and environmental tobacco smoke exposure and the risk of orofacial clefts. Epidemiology 2007;18(2):226–33.
21. Carmichael SL, Ma C, Rasmussen SA, et al. Craniosynostosis and maternal smoking. Birth Defects Res A Clin Mol Teratol 2008;82(2):78–85.
22. Beaty TH, Taub MA, Scott AF, et al. Confirming genes influencing risk to cleft lip with/without cleft palate in a case-parent trio study. Hum Genet 2013;132(7):771–81.

23. Manning M, Hudgins L. Array-based technology and recommendations for utilization in medical genetics practice for detection of chromosomal abnormalities. Genet Med 2010;12(11):742–5.

24. Hayeems RZ, Hoang N, Chenier S, et al. Capturing the clinical utility of genomic testing: medical recommendations following pediatric microarray. Eur J Hum Genet 2015;23(9):1135–41.

25. Genes G. 2015. Available at: https://globalgenes.org/rare-diseases-facts-statistics/. Accessed February 1, 2016.

26. Biesecker LG, Green RC. Diagnostic clinical genome and exome sequencing. N Engl J Med 2014;370(25):2418–25.

27. Sawyer SL, Hartley T, Dyment DA, et al. Utility of whole-exome sequencing for those near the end of the diagnostic odyssey: time to address gaps in care. Clin Genet 2016;89(3):275–84.

28. Yang Y, Muzny DM, Reid JG, et al. Clinical whole-exome sequencing for the diagnosis of mendelian disorders. N Engl J Med 2013; 369(16):1502–11.

29. Miyamoto RC, Cotton RT, Rope AF, et al. Association of anterior glottic webs with velocardiofacial syndrome (chromosome 22q11.2 deletion). Otolaryngol Head Neck Surg 2004;130(4):415–7.

30. Prada CE, Hufnagel RB, Hummel TR, et al. The use of magnetic resonance imaging screening for optic pathway gliomas in children with neurofibromatosis type 1. J Pediatr 2015;167(4):851–6.e1.

31. Parker SE, Mai CT, Canfield MA, et al. Updated National Birth Prevalence estimates for selected birth defects in the United States, 2004-2006. Birth Defects Res A Clin Mol Teratol 2010;88(12): 1008–16.

32. Croen LA, Shaw GM, Wasserman CR, et al. Racial and ethnic variations in the prevalence of orofacial clefts in California, 1983-1992. Am J Med Genet 1998;79(1):42–7.

33. Suleiman AM, Hamzah ST, Abusalab MA, et al. Prevalence of cleft lip and palate in a hospital-based population in the Sudan. Int J Paediatr Dent 2005; 15(3):185–9.

34. Tolarova MM, Cervenka J. Classification and birth prevalence of orofacial clefts. Am J Med Genet 1998;75(2):126–37.

35. Jugessur A, Farlie PG, Kilpatrick N. The genetics of isolated orofacial clefts: from genotypes to subphenotypes. Oral Dis 2009;15(7):437–53.

36. Stanier P, Moore GE. Genetics of cleft lip and palate: syndromic genes contribute to the incidence of non-syndromic clefts. Hum Mol Genet 2004;13(Spec No 1):R73–81.

37. Sivertsen A, Wilcox AJ, Skjaerven R, et al. Familial risk of oral clefts by morphological type and severity: population based cohort study of first degree relatives. BMJ 2008;336(7641):432–4.

38. Rahimov F, Jugessur A, Murray JC. Genetics of non-syndromic orofacial clefts. Cleft Palate Craniofac J 2012;49(1):73–91.

39. Leslie EJ, Koboldt DC, Kang CJ, et al. IRF6 mutation screening in non-syndromic orofacial clefting: analysis of 1521 families. Clin Genet 2015;90(1):28–34.

40. Online Mendelian Inheritance in Man, OMIM®. McKusick-Nathans Institute of Genetic Medicine, Johns Hopkins University (Baltimore, MD), January 5, 2016. Available at: http://omim.org/.

41. Murray JC, Daack-Hirsch S, Buetow KH, et al. Clinical and epidemiologic studies of cleft lip and palate in the Philippines. Cleft Palate Craniofac J 1997; 34(1):7–10.

42. Schutte BC, Saal HM, Goudy S, et al. IRF6-Related Disorders. 2003 Oct 30 [Updated 2014 Jul 3]. In: Pagon RA, Adam MP, Ardinger HH, et al, editors. GeneReviews® [Internet]. Seattle (WA): University of Washington, Seattle; 1993–2016. Available from: http://www.ncbi.nlm.nih.gov/books/NBK1407/.

43. Lees MM, Winter RM, Malcolm S, et al. Popliteal pterygium syndrome: a clinical study of three families and report of linkage to the Van der Woude syndrome locus on 1q32. J Med Genet 1999;36(12): 888–92.

44. Robin NH, Moran RT, Ala-Kokko L. Stickler Syndrome. 2000 Jun 9 [Updated 2014 Nov 26]. In: Pagon RA, Adam MP, Ardinger HH, et al, editors. GeneReviews® [Internet]. Seattle (WA): University of Washington, Seattle; 1993–2016. Available from: http://www.ncbi.nlm.nih.gov/books/NBK1302/.

45. Goldmuntz E, Driscoll D, Budarf ML, et al. Microdeletions of chromosomal region 22q11 in patients with congenital conotruncal cardiac defects. J Med Genet 1993;30(10):807–12.

46. Goodship J, Cross I, LiLing J, et al. A population study of chromosome 22q11 deletions in infancy. Arch Dis Child 1998;79(4):348–51.

47. McDonald-McGinn DM, Kirschner R, Goldmuntz E, et al. The Philadelphia story: the 22q11.2 deletion: report on 250 patients. Genet Couns 1999;10(1): 11–24.

48. Bassett AS, McDonald-McGinn DM, Devriendt K, et al. Practical guidelines for managing patients with 22q11.2 deletion syndrome. J Pediatr 2011; 159(2):332–9.e1.

49. Hacihamdioglu B, Hacihamdioglu D, Delil K. 22q11 deletion syndrome: current perspective. Appl Clin Genet 2015;8:123–32.

50. Tomaski SM, Zalzal GH, Saal HM. Airway obstruction in the Pierre Robin sequence. Laryngoscope 1995; 105(2):111–4.

51. Izumi K1 KL, Mitchell AL, Jones MC. Underlying genetic diagnosis of Pierre Robin sequence: retrospective chart review at two children's hospitals and a systematic literature review. J Pediatr 2012; 160(4):645–50.

52. Weaver KN, Zhang X, Bender PL, et al. Diagnosis, treatment and outcomes of Robin sequence at Cincinniati Children's. American Cleft Palate-Craniofacial Association Annual Meeting. Scottsdale, AZ, April 24, 2015.

53. Cohen MM, MacLEan RE. Craniosynostosis: diagnosis, evaluation, and management. 2nd edition. New York: Oxford University Press; 2000.

54. Boulet SL, Rasmussen SA, Honein MA. A population-based study of craniosynostosis in metropolitan Atlanta, 1989-2003. Am J Med Genet Part A 2008;146A(8):984–91.

55. Heuze Y, Holmes G, Peter I, et al. Closing the gap: genetic and genomic continuum from syndromic to nonsyndromic craniosynostoses. Curr Genet Med Rep 2014;2(3):135–45.

56. Online Mendelian Inheritance in Man, OMIM®. Baltimore, MD: McKusick-Nathans Institute of Genetic Medicine; Johns Hopkins University; 2016. Available at: http://omim.org/.

57. Jentink J, Loane MA, Dolk H, et al. Valproic acid monotherapy in pregnancy and major congenital malformations. N Engl J Med 2010;362(23):2185–93.

Early Airway Intervention for Craniofacial Anomalies

Lauren A. Bohm, MD[a,b,c],*, James D. Sidman, MD[a,b], Brianne Roby, MD[a,b]

KEYWORDS

- Craniofacial anomalies • Airway obstruction • Airway intervention • Distraction osteogenesis
- Tracheostomy

KEY POINTS

- The area of craniofacial skeleton involved in different syndromes is predictive of the airway problems typically encountered in affected patients.
- Most episodes of upper airway obstruction in children with craniofacial anomalies present in the immediate neonatal period.
- A majority of infants with Pierre Robin sequence (PRS) are able to be managed nonsurgically.
- The need for early endotracheal intubation is associated with an increased rate of subsequent surgical airway intervention.
- Tracheostomy rates are highest among children with combined midface and mandible hypoplasia.

INTRODUCTION

The medical management of children with craniofacial anomalies is complex. Therefore, their care is best addressed by a multidisciplinary team consisting of a geneticist, pediatrician, otolaryngologist, craniofacial surgeon, neurosurgeon, dentist, orthodontist, oral maxillofacial surgeon, audiologist, speech-language pathologist, and social services provider. The otolaryngologist plays a critical role in the evaluation and management of the airway in these children.

This patient population is uniquely predisposed to upper airway obstruction. Children with craniofacial anomalies often present with varying degrees of respiratory insufficiency during the neonatal period, requiring acute intervention. The airway management of these patients should be

tailored to the degree and anatomic site of obstruction. Possible interventions range from positioning maneuvers to surgical airway establishment. This article presents a classification system of craniofacial anomalies by the site of airway obstruction, along with algorithms to guide the initial management of these patients.

DIAGNOSTIC EVALUATION
Bedside Clinical Assessment

All patients with suspected craniofacial anomalies should undergo a complete head and neck physical examination, along with flexible fiberoptic laryngoscopy. The physical assessment should focus on the cranial vault shape and suture patency, maxillomandibular relation, palatal clefting, tongue position, presence of stertor,

---

Conflict of Interest and Financial Disclosures: None.
[a] Children's ENT and Facial Plastic Surgery, Children's Hospitals and Clinics of Minnesota, 2530 Chicago Avenue South, Suite 450, Minneapolis, MN 55404, USA; [b] Department of Otolaryngology, University of Minnesota, 420 Delaware Street Southeast, MMC 396, Minneapolis, MN 55455, USA; [c] Division of Pediatric Otolaryngology, University of Michigan CW5702, 1540 E. Hospital Drive, Ann Arbor, MI 48109, USA
* Corresponding author. Division of Pediatric Otolaryngology, University of Michigan CW5702, 1540 E. Hospital Drive, Ann Arbor, MI 48109.
E-mail address: lbohm@med.umich.edu

presence of stridor, and overall work of breathing.

An endoscopic examination is most useful to determine the anatomic location of the obstruction. Nasal endoscopy should always be performed bilaterally to ensure patency of both nasal passages. Difficulty passing the endoscope through the nasal vestibule is diagnostic of pyriform aperture stenosis, whereas the inability to pass it more posteriorly suggests choanal atresia. In children with micrognathia, endoscopy can be used to confirm the presence of tongue-base obstruction.

Laboratory Studies

In select cases, laboratory studies may be helpful to diagnose subclinical respiratory insufficiency. Blood gas analysis can demonstrate elevated carbon dioxide levels, which is indicative of inadequate gas exchange and may predict impending hypercarbic respiratory failure.

Polysomnography

Prior studies have demonstrated a strong correlation between obstructive sleep apnea (OSA) and craniofacial anomalies.[1] The overall incidence of positive OSA screening in children with craniofacial anomalies is 28.2%, but can affect at least 50% of children with particular craniosynostosis syndromes and facial clefts.[2,3]

In the authors' experience, however, polysomnography usually does not provide additional information that would alter management in the acute setting. The necessity of early airway intervention is most often a clinical decision based on a patient's degree of respiratory compromise and feeding ability, and is unrelated to sleep.

CRANIOFACIAL SYNDROME CLASSIFICATION

Major craniofacial anomalies may be categorized into those with midface hypoplasia, mandible hypoplasia, combined midface and mandible hypoplasia, and midline deformities. This approach provides an anatomic classification of the most common craniofacial anomalies (Table 1).

MIDFACE HYPOPLASIA
Pathophysiology

Many craniosynostosis syndromes involve premature fusion of the cranial sutures with concomitant midface hypoplasia. The midfacial growth tends to occur more slowly and arrests prior to 10 years of age, resulting in a short anterior cranial base, acute cranial base angle, and class III occlusion.[4] Additionally, the maxilla is constricted and highly

Table 1 Craniofacial classification	
Site	**Syndrome**
Midface	Apert Carpenter Crouzon Down Pfeiffer Saethre-Chotzen
Mandible	PRS Nager Stickler
Combined	Bilateral hemifacial microsomia Treacher Collins syndrome
Midline	Choanal atresia Midline cleft Pyriform aperture stenosis

arched, which may impinge on the vertical dimension of the nasal cavity.

These anatomic abnormalities, along with the normal development of lymphatic tissue within the Waldeyer ring, leads to nasopharyngeal and oropharyngeal obstruction. The degree of obstruction can be so severe that it mimics bilateral choanal atresia during presentation.[5] In addition to a routine physical examination, all children with suspected craniosynostosis syndromes should undergo a nasopharyngeal evaluation with passage of a 5/6 French suction catheter or fiberoptic endoscope.

CT is the initial imaging modality of choice to evaluate the bony anatomy of the midface. Three-dimensional reconstructions can also be obtained to plan for future craniofacial surgery (Fig. 1). Finally, MRI is indicated to rule out associated central nervous system abnormalities, such as hydrocephalus or Chiari malformation.

Airway Management Techniques

A previous study demonstrated that approximately half of patients with midface hypoplasia require some form of airway intervention.[6] Medical therapy with topical vasoconstrictors represents a minimally invasive intervention that can relieve mild nasal obstruction, particularly during periods of concurrent infection.

Nasopharyngeal airways, also known as nasal trumpets, offer another potential method to relieve midface obstruction. In the authors' experience, however, placement of a nasopharyngeal airway is not always possible nor beneficial in these patients. Nasopharyngeal airways themselves are space occupying and, therefore, compromise the

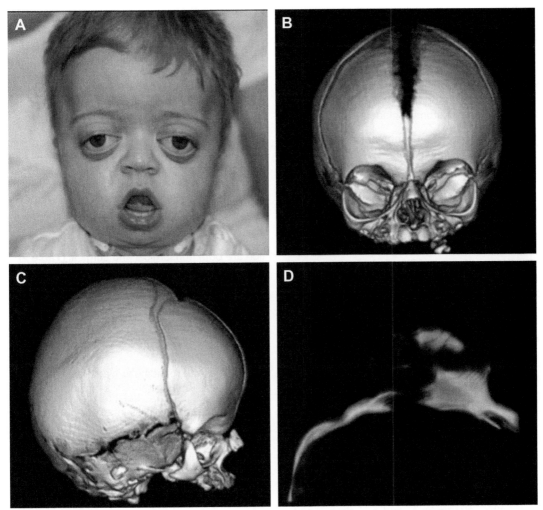

Fig. 1. (*A*) Infant with characteristic craniofacial features of Pfeiffer syndrome. (*B*) Coronal and (*C*) sagittal 3-D CT reconstructions demonstrating the craniofacial anatomy of Pfeiffer syndrome. (*D*) Sagittal bone-subtraction CT reconstruction showing the nasal and nasopharyngeal airway narrowing in midface hypoplasia.

cross-sectional area of the nasal passage. They are also prone to crust formation and may incite further mucosal inflammation. If a nasopharyngeal airway is implemented, frequent saline irrigation with gentle suctioning should be performed to maintain its patency.

Noninvasive positive pressure ventilation may serve as a short-term method of ventilation in patients with respiratory compromise not requiring emergent intubation. The presence of midface hypoplasia and exorbitism can interfere, however, with the fit of a face mask. Should bag-valve mask ventilation be necessary, it is recommended that the mouth be held in an open position while firmly applying pressure on the face mask to form a seal.[7]

Acute airway obstruction not responsive to noninvasive measures should be managed with orotracheal intubation. Orotracheal intubation usually does not pose a unique challenge in this patient population, unless there are other sites of airway obstruction or vertebral abnormalities limiting neck extension. Conversely, nasotracheal intubation may be difficult and require the use of a smaller endotracheal tube. The need for initial endotracheal intubation is predictive of an increased rate of subsequent airway intervention.

The final step of the management algorithm for upper airway obstruction is tracheostomy. The overall incidence of tracheostomy among children with craniofacial anomalies is approximately 20%.[6,8] In a recent retrospective cohort study, craniofacial anomalies were cited as the second most common reason for infant tracheostomy.[9]

Children with midface hypoplasia and resultant nasal and/or nasopharyngeal obstruction commonly require tracheostomy.[6] Infants who undergo tracheostomy placement secondary to craniofacial anomalies generally have a long period of cannulation with a mean length of 6.7 years.[8] There is evidence, however, that long-term pediatric tracheostomy is associated with morbidity and mortality.[10,11] Potential complications of a tracheostomy include

- Pneumothorax or pneumomediastinum
- Accidental decannulation
- Cannula obstruction
- Hemorrhage
- Infection
- Stoma maintenance issues
- Tracheal stenosis
- Speech and swallowing impairment

Finally, caregivers of children with tracheostomy tubes experience a significant burden with respect to the child's illness severity and associated costs.[12]

MANDIBLE HYPOPLASIA
Pathophysiology

Mandible development begins during the fourth week of gestation with neural crest cell migration to the head and neck region. Mandible hypoplasia is thought to be the result of inadequate neural crest cell incorporation into the first branchial arch.[13] Congenital hypoplasia usually occurs bilaterally. More than 60 syndromes with mandible hypoplasia have been identified to date.[14]

Pierre Robin sequence refers to the triad of micrognathia, glossoptosis, and a U-shaped cleft palate (**Fig. 2**). It is considered a sequence because multiple anomalies are caused by a series of in utero events initiated by a single anomaly. The initial

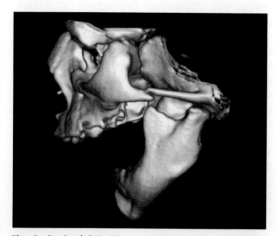

Fig. 2. Sagittal 3-D CT reconstruction of mandibular hypoplasia in an infant with PRS.

event, mandible hypoplasia, positions the tongue posterosuperiorly in the oral cavity between the palatal shelves. This abnormal tongue position then causes a mechanical disruption in palatal closure with resultant cleft formation. Approximately 20% to 40% of PRS cases are isolated and the remainder occur as part of a syndrome, such as Stickler syndrome.

Airway Management Techniques

Airway interventions for children with mandibular hypoplasia aim to reposition the tongue anteriorly and alleviate pharyngeal obstruction. Approximately three-fourths of these patients require an airway intervention.[6] Options for the management of upper airway obstruction in this patient population are both nonsurgical and surgical (**Table 2**).

The most conservative treatment of mandibular hypoplasia involves prone or decubitus positioning. Previous studies have shown high success rates with positioning maneuvers alone for the management of PRS.[15–17] The long-term efficacy of such positioning techniques, however, has not been demonstrated.[18]

If a child with mandibular hypoplasia continues to experience mild obstructive episodes despite prone positioning, nasopharyngeal airway placement should be performed. A nasopharyngeal airway maintains a lumen between the tongue base and posterior pharyngeal wall during periods of collapse. Published success rates of nasopharyngeal airway placement range from 48% to 100%.[17,19,20] Most children require continuation of the nasopharyngeal airway for several weeks to months, but its use has been described up to 27 months without complication.[20] Often, a nasopharyngeal airway is used in the short term until a more definitive intervention is completed (**Fig. 3**).

Endotracheal intubation is a safe and effective method of airway management in PRS infants when performed by experienced providers. Indications for endotracheal intubation include nonsurgical treatment of severe airway obstruction

Table 2		
Airway interventions for mandible hypoplasia		
	Intervention	
Nonsurgical	Positioning Nasopharyngeal airway Endotracheal intubation	
Surgical	Glossopexy procedures Mandibular distraction osteogenesis Tracheostomy	

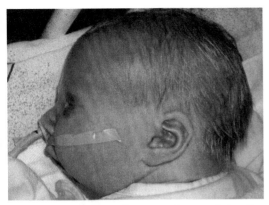

Fig. 3. Management of upper airway obstruction in an infant with PRS by nasopharyngeal airway placement.

and airway management during elective surgical procedures. Prior studies have shown that approximately one-third of infants with PRS are able to be intubated by direct laryngoscopy.[21,22] Intubation over a flexible fiberoptic bronchoscope is a reliable alternative method in those patients, who fail direct laryngoscopy.[22]

Although a majority of infants with PRS are able to be managed nonsurgically, some necessitate operative intervention.[17,23,24] Several glossopexy procedures have previously been reported in the literature, including the tongue-lip adhesion. Since its original description by Douglas in 1946,[25] the tongue-lip adhesion procedure has undergone several modifications, including a genioglossal release and circummandibular suture.[26–28]

The authors no longer practice tongue-lip adhesions for the management of infant micrognathia due to the potential for further feeding impairment. Retrospective reviews have shown that more than half of patients undergoing tongue-lip adhesions require gastrostomy placement.[29,30] A recent survey of the American Cleft Palate-Craniofacial Association (ACPA) members revealed that only 28% of surgeons prefer tongue-lip adhesion for airway management in PRS patients, who failed nonsurgical treatment.[31]

Mandibular distraction osteogenesis has become an increasingly popular method of surgical intervention that offers definitive micrognathia correction. The same ACPA survey indicated that 48% of the society's membership choose to treat PRS infants with mandibular distraction.[31] Bilateral mandibular advancement is accomplished by slow distraction after osteotomy creation via either external or internal hardware.

During the past 15 years, numerous studies have confirmed the efficacy of mandibular distraction in appropriately selected patients. It has proved an effective means of tracheostomy avoidance in isolated PRS or syndromic PRS without neurologic impairment.[32] Potential complications of the procedure include

- Infection
- Scar formation
- Hardware failure
- Inferior alveolar nerve paresthesia
- Facial nerve palsy
- Dental loss or malformation
- Mandibular growth deformity

Tracheostomy is typically reserved as a final means of relieving upper airway obstruction in mandibular hypoplasia (**Fig. 4**). In the authors' experience, syndromic children with neurologic involvement tend to fare best with tracheostomy and gastrostomy placement to effectively manage

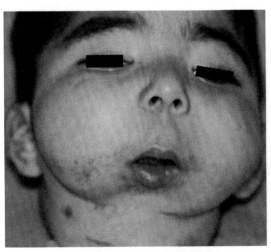

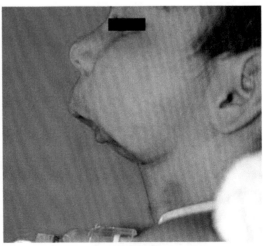

Fig. 4. Frontal and lateral views of a child with Nager syndrome (acrofacial dysostosis), who required neonatal tracheostomy placement due to severe airway obstruction.

their associated hypotonia and poor swallowing coordination.

COMBINED MIDFACE AND MANDIBLE HYPOPLASIA
Pathophysiology

A few syndromes, such as Treacher Collins and bilateral hemifacial microsomia, are characterized by hypoplasia of both the midface and the mandible. Affected children pose a unique challenge to airway management due to their multiple levels of obstruction and frequent involvement of the temporomandibular joint. Approximately three-fourths of patients with combined midface and mandible hypoplasia ultimately require airway intervention.[6] Furthermore, tracheostomy rates are highest among children with this craniofacial morphology.[6]

Treacher Collins syndrome or mandibulofacial dysostosis is an autosomal dominant disorder with incomplete penetrance and variable expressivity.[33] Defining clinical features include bilateral malar hypoplasia, micrognathia, auricular malformation, lower lid colobomas, and lateral downward slanting palpebral fissures.[34] It is associated with PRS in 35% of cases.

Hemifacial microsomia refers to a collection of abnormalities of the first and second branchial arches that manifest as hypoplasia of the orbit, maxilla, mandible, ear, and soft tissue. Although hemifacial microsomia is predominantly a unilateral condition, the incidence of bilateral involvement is estimated to be 10% to 33%.[35–38] The Pruzansky classification system,[39] later modified by Kaban and colleagues,[40] differentiates 3 types of hemifacial microsomia based on the size and function of the temporomandibular joint.

Airway Management Techniques

Prior studies have documented the highest rates of intubation difficulty among this unique patient population.[41,42] High-grade laryngoscopic views have been reported in more than 50% of children with Treacher Collins syndrome, often resulting in multiple intubation attempts and modalities.[41,42] Many techniques for airway management have been suggested, including laryngeal mask airway, direct laryngoscopy with or without a stylet, light wand intubation, retrograde intubation, and flexible fiberoptic intubation.

It is the authors' preference to use flexible fiberoptic nasotracheal intubation for perioperative airway control in this patient population, particularly if there is temporomandibular joint involvement. It has been shown that fiberoptic intubation is a safe and effective method of airway management in children with limited oral opening precluding conventional orotracheal intubation.[43] Advancing age and prior mandibular distraction are not associated with an improved ability to perform direct laryngoscopy in Treacher Collins syndrome patients.[41,44]

MIDLINE DEFORMITIES
Pathophysiology

Children with midline facial deformities often present with a unique set of airway problems and are, therefore, deserving of recognition as a distinct category of craniofacial anomalies (**Figs. 5 and 6**). Facial clefting involves sagittally oriented fissures within the craniofacial skeleton that result from failure of embryonic facial process fusion. Facial clefts confined to the midline are described by the Tessier classification system numbers 0 to 5 and 12 to 14.[45,46]

Pyriform aperture stenosis and choanal atresia are both causes of nasal obstruction that can lead to respiratory distress due to obligate nasal breathing in the neonate. Pyriform aperture stenosis, however, affects the anterior nasal inlet, whereas choanal atresia causes narrowing of the posterior choanae. Pyriform aperture stenosis

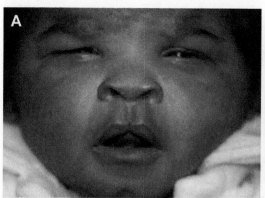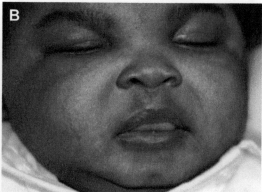

Fig. 5. Infant with a midline microform cleft lip (A) before and (B) 2 months after surgical repair.

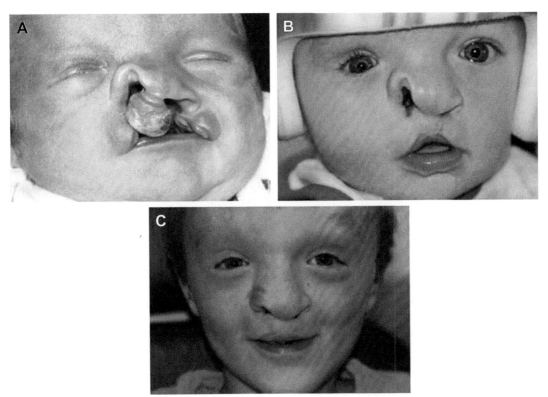

Fig. 6. Infant with a facial cleft (*A*) before and (*B*) 4 months after cleft lip repair. (*C*) A 7-year-old after tip rhinoplasty with composite grafting, local skin flap reconstruction, and hypertelorism repair.

occurs at approximately one-fifth the frequency of choanal atresia.[47] It can occur as an isolated finding or in conjunction with other midline congenital anomalies, such as holoprosencephaly, hypopituitarism, or a single central megaincisor.[48]

Both diagnoses may be confirmed with thin-cut (1.5–3.0 mm) CT imaging. An individual pyriform aperture width less than 3 mm or total pyriform aperture width less than 8 mm in a term infant is diagnostic for pyriform aperture stenosis (**Fig. 7**).[47] Choanal atresia is differentiated by medial bowing and thickening of the lateral nasal wall, enlargement of the vomer, and bony (30%) or mixed bony/membranous (70%) choanal obstruction.[49,50]

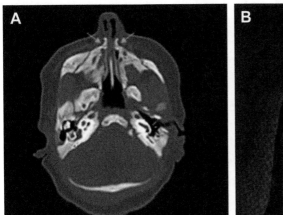
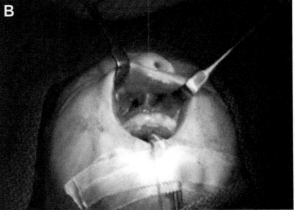

Fig. 7. (*A*) Axial CT image demonstrating narrowing of the nasal processes of the maxilla, resulting in a 4-mm pyriform aperture (*arrows*). (*B*) Intraoperative photograph of a corrected bilateral pyriform aperture stenosis via a sublabial approach.

Airway Management Techniques

Extra perioperative planning must be undertaken before deciding to proceed with repair of a midline facial cleft. The risk of postoperative nasal airway obstruction is significant and may be worsened by subsequent edema and crusting. In select cases, the surgical repair may be delayed or staged to allow for additional facial growth. Alternatively, temporary nasal stents or conformers may be used to maintain patency of the nasal vestibule in the immediate postoperative period. Finally, a short period of intubation may be instituted to allow for healing.

Surgical repair of pyriform aperture stenosis is indicated in cases of severe respiratory insufficiency unresponsive to medical therapy and failure to thrive. A sublabial approach provides exposure to surgically widen the bony aperture with otologic drills and microinstruments.[51] An adjunctive inferior turbinate reduction and/or outfracture may be performed in the same setting.

Since the first blind transnasal puncture was reported by Emmert in 1854,[52] many articles have been published describing various techniques for the surgical repair of choanal atresia. Endoscopic resection has become increasingly popular over the past few decades. After topical decongestion, the atretic plate is perforated under endoscopic visualization. Then, the choanae are gradually enlarged with removal of the posterior nasal septum using sinus surgery instruments, microdébriders, or drills (**Fig. 8**). No definitive evidence exists to support the routine use of topical mitomycin C, nasal stents, or lasers.[53] Children with craniofacial anomalies often have abnormal skull base anatomy; therefore, care must be taken to avoid a potential intracranial injury.

ADDITIONAL CONSIDERATIONS
Bronchoscopic Examination

In addition to the common causes of upper airway obstruction (described previously), children with craniofacial syndromes may also have accompanying anomalies of the laryngotracheal complex. As such, rigid bronchoscopy serves as an invaluable tool in these patients, who may be ineffectively managed with standard airway stabilization techniques.

Although the incidence remains unknown, tracheal stenosis due to complete tracheal rings is more common among children with Down syndrome and Pfeiffer syndrome (**Fig. 9**). Neonatal respiratory difficulty in this population should raise suspicion for underlying tracheal pathology, especially with a history of a difficult intubation or necessity of a smaller-than-expected endotracheal tube.

A tracheal cartilaginous sleeve is a rare malformation in which distinct tracheal rings are replaced by a continuous cartilaginous segment that may extend to the carina or mainstem bronchus. All reported cases to date have been associated with craniosynotosis syndromes, the most common of which include Apert, Crouzon, and Pfeiffer syndromes.[54]

The diagnosis of a tracheal cartilaginous sleeve portends a poor prognosis with a reported 90% mortality by 2 years of age in children with craniosynostosis syndromes.[55] A recently conducted meta-analysis demonstrated, however, a survival

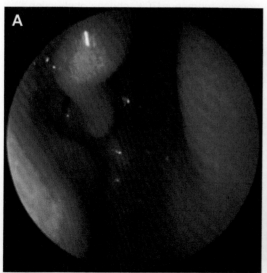
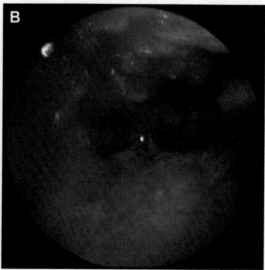

Fig. 8. (*A*) Preoperative and (*B*) postoperative right nasal endoscopy in a patient with bilateral choanal atresia undergoing surgical repair.

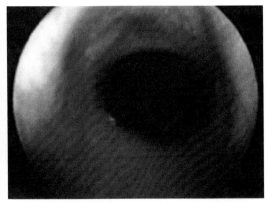

Fig. 9. Distal tracheal stenosis due to the presence of complete tracheal rings.

advantage of tracheostomy performed in this patient population.[56] Finally, short-segment tracheal sleeves may be amenable to surgical resection with primary anastomosis.[57]

REFERENCES

1. Lam DJ, Jensen CC, Mueller BA, et al. Pediatric sleep apnea and craniofacial anomalies: a population-based case-control study. Laryngoscope 2010;120(10):2098–105.

2. Paliga JT, Tahiri Y, Silvestre J, et al. Screening for obstructive sleep apnea in children treated at a major craniofacial center. J Craniofac Surg 2014; 25(5):1762–5.

3. Pijpers M, Poels P, Vaandrager JM, et al. Undiagnosed obstructive sleep apnea syndrome in children with syndromal craniofacial synostosis. J Craniofac Surg 2004;15(4):670–4.

4. Mann DG. Parturient with pre-existing congenital anomalies. In: Suresh M, Segal BS, Preston RL, et al, editors. Shnider and Levinson's anesthesia for obstetrics. 5th edition. Philadelphia: Lippincott Williams & Wilkins; 2013. p. 664–5.

5. Boston M, Rutter MJ. Current airway management in craniofacial anomalies. Curr Opin Otolaryngol Head Neck Surg 2003;11(6):428–32.

6. Perkins JA, Sie KC, Milczuk H, et al. Airway management in children with craniofacial anomalies. Cleft Palate Craniofac J 1997;34(2):135–40.

7. Nargozian C. The airway in patients with craniofacial abnormalities. Paediatr Anaesth 2004;14(1): 53–9.

8. Sculerati N, Gottlieb MD, Zimbler MS, et al. Airway management in children with major craniofacial anomalies. Laryngoscope 1998;108(12):1806–12.

9. Lewis CW, Carron JD, Perkins JA, et al. Tracheostomy in pediatric patients: a national perspective. Arch Otolaryngol Head Neck Surg 2003;129(5): 523–9.

10. Carr MM, Poje CP, Kingston L, et al. Complications in pediatric tracheostomies. Laryngoscope 2001; 111(11 Pt 1):1925–8.

11. Carron JD, Derkay CS, Strope GL, et al. Pediatric tracheotomies: changing indications and outcomes. Laryngoscope 2000;110(7):1099–104.

12. Hartnick CJ, Bissell C, Parsons SK. The impact of pediatric tracheotomy on parental caregiver burden and health status. Arch Otolaryngol Head Neck Surg 2003;129(10):1065–9.

13. Moore KL, Persaud TVN. The pharyngeal (branchial) apparatus. In: Moore KL, Persaud TVN, editors. The developing human: clinically oriented embryology. Philadelphia: WB Saunders; 1998. p. 215–56.

14. Singh DJ, Bartlett SP. Congenital mandibular hypoplasia: analysis and classification. J Craniofac Surg 2005;16(2):291–300.

15. Schaefer RB, Stadler JA 3rd, Gosain AK. To distract or not to distract: an algorithm for airway management in isolated Pierre Robin sequence. Plast Reconstr Surg 2004;113(4):1113–25.

16. Marques IL, de Sousa TV, Carneiro AF, et al. Clinical experience with infants with Robin sequence: a prospective study. Cleft Palate Craniofac J 2001;38(2): 171–8.

17. Meyer AC, Lidsky ME, Sampson DE, et al. Airway interventions in children with Pierre Robin sequence. Otolaryngol Head Neck Surg 2008;138(6):782–7.

18. Sher AE. Mechanisms of airway obstruction in Robin sequence: implications for treatment. Cleft Palate Craniofac J 1992;29(3):224–31.

19. Wagener S, Rayatt SS, Tatman AJ, et al. Management of infants with Pierre Robin sequence. Cleft Palate Craniofac J 2003;40(2):180–5.

20. Abel F, Bajaj Y, Wyatt M, et al. The successful use of the nasopharyngeal airway in Pierre Robin sequence: an 11-year experience. Arch Dis Child 2012;97(4):331–4.

21. Stricker PA, Budac S, Fiadjoe JE, et al. Awake laryngeal mask insertion followed by induction of anesthesia in infants with Pierre Robin sequence. Acta Anaesthesiol Scand 2008;52(9):1307–8.

22. Marston AP, Lander TA, Tibesar RJ, et al. Airway management for intubation in newborns with Pierre Robin sequence. Laryngoscope 2012;122(6):1401–4.

23. Evans AK, Rahbar R, Rogers GF, et al. Robin sequence: a retrospective review of 115 patients. Int J Pediatr Otorhinolaryngol 2006;70(6):973–80.

24. Kirschner RE, Low DW, Randall P, et al. Surgical management in Pierre Robin sequence: is there a role for tongue-lip adhesion? Cleft Palate Craniofac J 2003;40(1):13–8.

25. Douglas B. The treatment of micrognathia associated with obstruction by a plastic procedure. Plast Reconstr Surg 1946;1(3):300–8.

26. Routledge RT. The Pierre Robin syndrome: a surgical emergency in the neonatal period. Br J Plast Surg 1960;13:204–18.

27. Randall P. The Robin anomalad: micrognathia and glossoptosis with airway obstruction. In: Converse JM, editor. Reconstructive plastic surgery. Philadelphia: WB Saunders; 1977. p. 2235–45.

28. Argamaso RV. Glossopexy for upper airway obstruction in Robin sequence. Cleft Palate Craniofac J 1992;29(3):232–8.

29. Denny AD, Amm CA, Schaefer RB. Outcomes of tongue-lip adhesion for neonatal respiratory distress caused by Pierre Robin sequence. J Craniofac Surg 2004;15(5):819–23.

30. Rogers GF, Murthy AS, LaBrie RA, et al. The GILLS score: part I. Patient selection for tongue-lip adhesion in Robin sequence. Plast Reconstr Surg 2011; 128(1):243–51.

31. Collins B, Powitzky R, Robledo C, et al. Airway management in Pierre Robin sequence: patterns of practice. Cleft Palate Craniofac J 2014;51(3):283–9.

32. Scott AR, Tibesar RJ, Lander TA, et al. Mandibular distraction osteogenesis in infants younger than 3 months. Arch Facial Plast Surg 2011;13(3):173–9.

33. Dixon MJ. Treacher Collins syndrome. Hum Mol Genet 1996;5(Spec No):1391–6.

34. Jones KL, Jones MC, del Campo M. Facial defects as major feature. In: Jones KL, Jones MC, del Campo M, editors. Smith's recognizable patterns of human malformation. 7th edition. Philadelphia: Sauders Elsevier; 2013. p. 334–5.

35. Rollnick BR, Kaye CI, Nagatoshi K, et al. Oculoauriculovertebral dysplasia and variants: phenotypic characteristics of 294 patients. Am J Med Genet 1987;26(2):361–75.

36. Grabb WC. The first and second branchial arch syndrome. Plast Reconstr Surg 1965;36(5):485–508.

37. Burck U. Genetic aspects of hemifacial microsomia. Hum Genet 1983;64(3):291–6.

38. Nargozian C, Ririe DG, Bennun RD, et al. Hemifacial microsomia: anatomical prediction of difficult intubation. Paediatr Anaesth 1999;9(5):393–8.

39. Pruzansky S. Not all dwarfed mandibles are alike. Birth Defects 1969;5:120.

40. Kaban LB, Moses MH, Mulliken JB. Surgical correction of hemifacial microsomia in the growing child. Plast Reconstr Surg 1988;82(1):9–19.

41. Frawley G, Espenell A, Howe P, et al. Anesthetic implications of infants with mandibular hypoplasia treated with mandibular distraction osteogenesis. Paediatr Anaesth 2013;23(4):342–8.

42. Sinkueakunkit A, Chowchuen B, Kantanabat C, et al. Outcome of anesthetic management for children with craniofacial deformities. Pediatr Int 2013;55(3):360–5.

43. Meyers JA, Sidman J. Children with limited oral opening can safely be managed without a tracheostomy. Otolaryngol Head Neck Surg 2014;150(1):133–8.

44. Hosking J, Zoanetti D, Carlyle A, et al. Anesthesia for Treacher Collins syndrome: a review of airway management in 240 pediatric cases. Paediatr Anaesth 2012;22(8):752–8.

45. Tessier P. Anatomical classification facial, craniofacial and latero-facial clefts. J Maxillofac Surg 1976;4(2):69–92.

46. David DJ, Moore MH, Cooter RD. Tessier clefts revisited with a third dimension. Cleft Palate J 1989;26(3):163–84.

47. Belden CJ, Mancuso AA, Schmalfuss IM. CT features of congenital nasal piriform aperture stenosis: Initial experience. Radiology 1999;213(2):495–501.

48. Robson CD, Hudgins PA. Pediatric airway disease. In: Head and neck imaging. 4th edition. St. Louis (MO): Mosby; 2003. p. 1521–93.

49. Slovis TL, Renfro B, Watts FB, et al. Choanal atresia: precise CT evaluation. Radiology 1985; 155(2):345–8.

50. Brown OE, Pownell P, Manning SC. Choanal atresia: a new anatomic classification and clinical management applications. Laryngoscope 1996;106(1 Pt 1):97–101.

51. Devambez M, Delattre A, Fayoux P. Congenital nasal pyriform aperture stenosis: diagnosis and management. Cleft Palate Craniofac J 2009;46(3):262–7.

52. Emmert C. Stenochorie und atresie der choannen. Lehrback der Speciellen Chirurgie 1854;2:535–8.

53. Ramsden JD, Campisi P, Forte V. Choanal atresia and choanal stenosis. Otolaryngol Clin North Am 2009;42(2):339–52.

54. Stater BJ, Oomen KP, Modi VK. Tracheal cartilaginous sleeve association with syndromic midface hypoplasia. JAMA Otolaryngol Head Neck Surg 2015; 141(1):73–7.

55. Noorily MR, Farmer DL, Belenky WM, et al. Congenital tracheal anomalies in the craniosynostosis syndromes. J Pediatr Surg 1999;34(6):1036–9.

56. Lertsburapa K, Schroeder JW Jr, Sullivan C. Tracheal cartilaginous sleeve in patients with craniosynostosis syndromes: a meta-analysis. J Pediatr Surg 2010;45(7):1438–44.

57. Nguyen CV, Javia LR. Craniofacial syndromes with airway anomalies: an overview. In: Lioy J, Sobol SE, editors. Disorders of the neonatal airway: fundamentals for practice. New York: Springer; 2015. p. 15–24.

Feeding Management in Infants with Craniofacial Anomalies

Jill M. Merrow, MA, CCC-SLP

KEYWORDS

- Cleft • Craniofacial • Feeding management • Dysphagia • Breastfeeding
- Fiberoptic endoscopic evaluation of swallowing • Modified barium swallow study
- Video swallow study

KEY POINTS

- Feeding and swallowing abilities in infants born with craniofacial anomalies show great variability.
- Difficulties with feeding mechanics in infants with cleft lip and/or palate include limited labial seal and stability of the nipple within the oral cavity, suboptimal intraoral pressure, suction, and milk transfer.
- Feeding difficulties with cleft lip and/or palate can be more complicated in the presence of an associated syndrome or sequence.
- Common feeding goals for infants with craniofacial anomalies include improvement of milk flow to meet caloric intake requirements, prevention of excessive air intake, minimalization of nasal regurgitation, and attainment of physiologic stability accomplished through various management strategies.
- Instrumental assessment via fiberoptic endoscopic evaluation of swallowing and/or modified barium swallow study can be used when appropriate to gain further objective data regarding swallow function and to devise strategies to promote safe feeding and swallowing.

  Video content accompanies this article at http://www.facialplastic.theclinics.com.

INTRODUCTION

Feeding abilities in all children gain prompt attention and demand vigilance from parents immediately after birth. Whether receiving a prenatal diagnosis of a craniofacial anomaly by fetal ultrasound or receiving the diagnosis at birth, the anxiety and worry can be overwhelming. The sooner that caregivers are educated regarding feeding management, the sooner they feel empowered to adequately feed their infant. Referrals to cleft and craniofacial teams for prenatal consultations after identification of a cleft on fetal ultrasound have been found to be both informative and anxiety-reducing to the parents.[1,2] Specifically, Davalbhatka and Hall[3] (2000), reported that antenatal counseling prepared parents for the birth of an infant with a cleft in 85% of respondents; 89% of parents felt they benefitted from knowing the diagnosis ahead of time. Although feeding and swallowing issues persist beyond infancy, this section focuses on typical development of infant feeding and swallowing skills, feeding difficulties and their causes, evaluation, and management.

Disclosure: The author has nothing to disclose.
State University of New York (SUNY) Upstate Medical Center, 750 East Adams Street, Syracuse, NY 13210, USA
E-mail address: merrowj@upstate.edu

Facial Plast Surg Clin N Am 24 (2016) 437–444
http://dx.doi.org/10.1016/j.fsc.2016.06.004
1064-7406/16/© 2016 Elsevier Inc. All rights reserved.

Typical Feeding and Swallowing Development

In a healthy, typically developing newborn, feeding is reflexive. The rooting reflex encourages the newborn to find the nipple and the suck reflex to pull milk from the nipple. Milk is extracted from the nipple by both positive and negative pressure, otherwise known as compression and suction. Milk extraction results from the coordinated movements of the following oral structures.

Jaw
The supportive structure of the jaw moves in a vertical dimension. Its inferior movement assists with creating suction.

Lips
The lips assist with the anterior seal around the nipple and support stabilization of the nipple within the oral cavity.

Tongue
The tongue tip compresses the nipple. The posterior aspect of the tongue seals the oral cavity against the soft palate. When the tongue drops, it enlarges the oral cavity creating suction. The tongue also forms a midline groove for the transfer of the liquid bolus from the mouth to the oropharynx.

Cheeks
The cheeks provide stability. The greater the fat pads, the greater the stability.

Hard palate
The hard palate assists the tongue with nipple compression and stability.

Soft palate
The soft palate assists the tongue in closing off the oral cavity posteriorly. During the swallow, it rises to seal off the nasal cavity, prevent nasal regurgitation and create suction.

Sucking These oral movements coordinate with respiration and swallowing to produce a suck-swallow-breathe sequence ideally in a 1:1 suck-swallow ratio. Suckling is the first phase of the suck to emerge. The tongue moves in an anterior-to-posterior dimension and, according to Arvedson and Brodsky[4] (2002), "liquid is drawn into the mouth through a rhythmic licking action of the tongue, combined with pronounced opening and closing of the jaw. Lips are loosely approximated." This pattern changes by the sixth month of life with onset of differentiation between the jaw, tongue, and lips, including increased lip closure and more vertical excursion of the tongue.

Swallowing Swallowing, or deglutition, is not a synonymous term to pair with feeding. Swallowing is a complex process of both volitional and reflexive behaviors involving the action of coordinated, sequential motor movements from the mouth to the esophagus. Hence, there are 4 stages to swallowing that are generally accepted: the oral preparatory phase, the oral phase, the pharyngeal phase, and the esophageal phase. The oral preparatory phase involves the suckling or sucking, biting, and chewing actions that bring the food into the mouth and form the bolus. The oral phase consists of bolus transit to the oropharynx by the tongue. The pharyngeal phase involves the closure of the nasopharyngeal port, anterior and vertical excursion of the larynx, inverse movement of the epiglottis, vocal fold closure at midline and relaxation of the upper esophageal sphincter (UES), and inverse movement of the epiglottis with coverage of but not a tight seal for the laryngeal vestibule. The pharyngeal muscle constriction triggers pharyngeal peristalsis. As the bolus moves from the hypopharynx through the open UES, the esophageal phase begins. The involuntary peristaltic action of the esophagus propels the bolus through the relaxed lower esophageal sphincter to allow the bolus to enter the stomach.

Progression Reaching oral sensorimotor milestones allows the typically developing infant to progress to solid foods. According to Arvedson and Brodsky[4] (2002), spoon-feeding skills emerge between 4 to 6 months of age. At about 6 months, munching with vertical jaw movements emerges. Infants become ready for thicker textures. Rotary jaw action begins at about 7 months and is refined by 12 months of age. New textures should be gradually introduced in order for the child to gain competence in chewing ability and to prevent choking.

Feeding Difficulties: the Mechanics

Parents of infants with clefts often make the following observations regarding limited feeding ability: "My baby isn't sucking well. My baby doesn't want to feed. He pushes the nipple out of his mouth. My baby is lazy. My baby isn't swallowing correctly. It comes out of his nose. My baby is always hungry. My baby acts hungry but then falls asleep as soon as he starts feeding." These symptoms are often influenced by the mechanical issues that emerge due to the cleft lip and/or palate. In simple terms, the lip latches to the nipple and the palate maintains the latch. Given lip and palatal deficiencies, the latch and its maintenance are adversely affected. The type and severity of the cleft directly influence the intensity of the modifications needed for feeding success. Clefts are classified as unilateral or bilateral and complete versus incomplete. Peterson-Falzone and colleagues[5] (2001) remind us that "clefts vary in three other dimensions: anterior to posterior, width and 'depth.'" These dimensions are important when deciding on the most efficacious nipple placement within the mouth. Infants with cleft lip and palate innately exhibit a sucking reflex similar to typically developing infants; however, they have limited ability to create suction efficiently and consistently.

Cleft lip

Cleft lip causes a limited labial seal around the nipple of the breast or bottle that may decrease negative pressure to a minor degree and contribute to limited stability of the nipple within the oral cavity. These issues are usually very mild with cleft lip only. The nipple of the breast or bottle will often fill the space of the cleft to create a seal and stability of the nipple. Nutritive breastfeeding is typically preserved in this population.

Cleft lip and alveolus

With significant involvement of the alveolus, it becomes more difficult for the infant to anchor the nipple between supporting structures to achieve a good latch and seal of the oral cavity (ie, lips, tongue, primary palate) and may limit negative pressure generation. The infant has less ability to compress the nipple in a vertical plane (ie, tongue and primary palate). Infants often show a greater extent of vertical jaw excursion to improve compression contributing to fatigue. Nutritive breastfeeding is typically achieved given assistance with milk delivery.

Cleft palate

With compromise of the hard palate comes decreased stability of the nipple within the oral cavity and decreased compression of the nipple. These infants are more reliant on suction for milk extraction. With compromise of the soft palate comes decreased intraoral pressure, decreased suction, and limited milk transfer. This results in decreased sucking efficiency and lengthy feeding times with limited intake. Excessive air intake occurs due to the poor seal between the oral and nasal cavities. As the tongue drops in preparation for the swallow, air is pulled into the oropharynx and hypopharynx from the nasal cavity. This can lead to aerophagia, a false sense of satiation, excessive spit up, and emesis. This also provides a conduit for milk to propel from the mouth into the nasopharyngeal region, otherwise known as nasal regurgitation, before or during the swallow. This leads to nasal congestion and trouble breathing while feeding given that infants are obligate nasal breathers. With a small cleft of the soft palate, the tongue often occludes the cleft for at least part of the transition from suck to swallow, thereby reducing effect on negative pressure generation. With a submucous cleft palate, there may be mild reduction in negative pressure due to the dysfunction of the velopharyngeal valve. Nutritive breastfeeding is most likely possible with a small cleft of the soft palate or submucous cleft palate; however, nutritive breastfeeding is rarely successful in an infant with a large cleft palate.

Cleft lip and palate

The combination of cleft lip and palate will result in the aforementioned feeding issues but likely to a greater degree. Nutritive breastfeeding is rarely successful in an infant with complete cleft lip and palate.

Poor longitudinal feeding outcomes may include general fatigue with limited alertness and interaction, refusal behaviors, limited urinary and fecal output, and limited weight gain. These unfortunate circumstances may negatively affect infant and caregiver interaction over time. Masarei and colleagues[6] (2007) compared feeding skills in infants with unrepaired clefts to healthy infants without clefts. All comparisons were statistically significant in demonstrating the decreased sucking efficiency in infants with unrepaired isolated cleft palate and unilateral cleft lip and palate. The infants with unrepaired clefts demonstrated shorter lengths of individual sucks and shorter lengths of sucking bursts (number of suck-swallow sequences) while rate of sucking, suck-swallow ratio, and positive pressure generation were greater (**Table 1**).

Reid and colleagues[7] (2007) examined the suction capabilities of 40 2-week-old infants with clefts. All 8 infants with cleft lip demonstrated suction. One out of 10 infants with cleft lip and palate demonstrated suction. Thirteen out of 22 infants with cleft palate demonstrated suction. Of the 13 infants, 10 had clefts of the soft palate only and only 3 maintained regular pressure changes over time. The investigators found significant between-group differences, concluding that infants with cleft lip or minor clefts of the soft palate were more likely to generate normal levels of suction and compression than infants with larger clefts.

Special Populations

Pierre Robin sequence

Sucking in infants with Pierre Robin sequence is negatively affected by the limitations in positive pressure generation given the maxillary-mandibular discrepancy of the micrognathia, the

Table 1
Sucking differences in infants with clefts

	Infants with Unilateral Cleft Lip and Palate or Isolated Cleft Palate	Infants without Clefts
Length of sucking bursts	8.97 s	13.28 s
Rate of sucking	109.26 sucks/min	75.07 sucks/min
Length of individual sucks	0.57 s	0.87 s
Positive pressure generation	71.68%	25.71%
Suck-swallow ratio	2.97:1	1.20:1

Data from Masarei AG, Sell D, Habel A, et al. The nature of feeding in infants with unrepaired cleft lip and/or palate compared with healthy noncleft infants. Cleft Palate Craniofac J 2007;44:321–8.

misaligned forces of compression by the dental arches, and the lack of contact to the superior surface of the nipple secondary to the typically wide U-shaped cleft palate. The tongue often sits retracted in the mouth (glossoptosis) with minimal ability to produce an anterior tongue carriage to compress the nipple effectively. If the infant is able to produce an anterior tongue carriage to secure the nipple, airway patency typically improves. Suction ability depends on the size of the cleft palate. There is variability in the phenotypic expression of Pierre Robin sequence and there may be absence of a cleft palate in some cases. With less pharyngeal space for airway patency and swallowing mechanics due to micrognathia and glossoptosis, these infants may experience significant chest retractions, nasal flaring, snorting, stertor, and stridor at baseline and while feeding. These infants tend to pause more frequently and tolerate only short sucking bursts. Longer sucking bursts often tax efforts at coordination and lead to extended swallow apneas, gasping, gagging, and possibly aspiration. Furthermore, airway issues may also mask underlying neuromotor dysfunction.

Hemifacial microsomia

This broad group of first and second branchial arch malformations results in mandibular hypoplasia and facial weakness of varying degrees.[4]

According to Peterson-Falzone and colleagues[5] (2001), both sides of the face may be involved but typically one side is more affected than the other. Feeding and swallowing difficulties may result from structural anomalies of the jaw, tongue, face, and pharynx, or from neurologic dysfunction and/or congenital heart defects.

22q deletion syndrome

These infants may experience feeding and swallowing problems of multiple causes given the great variability in phenotypic expression. Airway anomalies and cardiac defects can negatively affect the suck-swallow-breathe cycle, induce significant fatigue, and lead to aspiration from an antegrade process. Cardiac defects can cause extrinsic compression of the trachea or of the esophagus, and obstruct the passing of food and liquid. Gastrointestinal tract dysfunction can occur due to hypotonia with reflux, slowed motility, and structural anomalies. These issues can lead to limited caloric intake, feeding refusal, poor weight gain, and failure to thrive. It is important to keep in mind the linear growth trajectory predicted for these infants and the tendency to exhibit slower growth than their same-age peers in early childhood.

Treacher Collins syndrome

These infants often experience poor airway patency and respiratory difficulties. Tracheotomies are frequently required.[5] Surgical repair of a cleft palate may lead to greater risk of airway compromise. Conservative oral feeding measures may be needed with supplemental or alternate enteral feedings to meet nutritional needs but, certainly, variability is present.

SOCIAL–EMOTIONAL INTERACTIONS

The technical aspects of feeding infants with clefts and other craniofacial anomalies are of utmost importance to ensure adequate growth; however, attention should also be paid to the feeding interaction between parent and child. Speltz and colleagues[8] (1994) assessed 3-month-old infants with clefts and their mothers. The infants were divided into 3 groups: cleft lip and palate; cleft palate only; and healthy, typical infants. Infants' temperament and mothers' emotional and attitudinal factors were critiqued. Infants in the typical group rated higher than both cleft groups on the clarity of cues scale. Infants with cleft lip and palate were less likely to signal readiness to eat and less likely to display changes in tension at the onset of the feeding and shortly thereafter. Both cleft groups were less likely than the typical infants to smile or laugh during feeding. Of interest, the mothers of infants in the cleft groups showed no significant difference from the mothers of typical infants in their responsiveness to their infants who smiled less; however, the mothers of the infants with cleft lip and palate showed decreased sensitivity to their infants' cues. The investigators suggest that the lowered maternal sensitivity in this group was likely due to the additional problems of the cleft lip. In feeder-assisted interactions, infants exhibited less control of feeding pace and length of feeding. There is valuable suggestion that training of feeding technique should be combined with attention to the quality of social interaction. The prenatal consultation can help parents feel more comfortable in learning the technical aspects of feeding, thereby more expeditiously shifting the focus from feeding technique to social interactions and enjoyment of their infant sooner after birth.

Outcomes and Goals

Outcome measures help compare the effectiveness of feeding skills of the infant born with a craniofacial anomaly to typically developing infants while considering other variables in the feeding process, such as infant–caregiver interaction and milk supply to the infant. Outcomes within the feeding session may include the quantity of intake during the feeding, as well as change in physiologic stability from baseline, endurance, and tolerance of the food and liquid offered. Generally, an infant should complete his or her full feeding within 20 to 30 minutes; otherwise, she or he tends to burn more calories than consumed. The hospital-based neonatologist, community-based pediatrician, or cleft and craniofacial team may guide the feeding plan with a daily intake goal. The daily intake for an infant with a cleft, daily output, and weight gain over time (due to significant day-to-day variability) are quantifiable factors by which to assess the adequacy of the infant's intake. If the infant is reaching feeding goals safely, further evaluation may not be necessary. If an infant has other diagnosed congenital anomalies (eg, micrognathia, cardiac defect, short stature as a phenotypic characteristic of a diagnosed syndrome), goals and expectations for intake may be altered. The World Health Organization growth charts are recommended by the Center for Disease Control and Prevention (CDC) and are supported by the American Academy of Pediatrics for use from birth to 2 years of age. The CDC growth charts are recommended by the CDC for use with children from 2 years of age and older.[9]

FEEDING EVALUATION

To best manage these feeding issues, thorough assessment is necessary, including a detailed history, physical examination with baseline physiologic assessment, feeding observation, and stimulability trials. In some instances, further evaluation of the swallowing mechanism is necessary via instrumental testing. This may include a fiberoptic endoscopic evaluation of swallowing (FEES) or modified barium swallow study (MBSS). Disorders of swallowing can be classified as oral and/or pharyngeal dysphagia, and as described by Darrow and Harley[10] (1998): mechanical, neurologic, or developmental dysphagia.

History

Detailed history and discussion of current feeding practices provide valuable insight into the nature of the feeding problem. The outline below is helpful to address the major variables in the feeding process:

- History of the problem: caregiver description of the feeding difficulties, signs and symptoms of intolerance, medical restrictions.
- Environment: place of feeding, caregivers involved with feeding, distractions.
- Nutrition: breastmilk, formula (type, calories per ounce, supplements trialed), other liquids or foods offered, intake goals
- Feeding method: breast (discuss milk supply, use of manual expression, pumping), bottle (type, nipple, flow rate), enteral feedings (type, formula, rate).
- Feeding efficiency: optimal state for feeding, duration of feedings, frequency of feedings, sleep and feeding schedule, changes in feeding from beginning to end of session, changes in feeding from first feedings until present, physiologic stability.
- Other pertinent details: positioning, work of breathing, burping, presence of nasal regurgitation and/or emesis, output.

Observation at rest

Observe the infant's behavior and ability to communicate his needs, as well as the caregiver's responses to these requests, to gain insight regarding potential issues with child–caregiver interaction. Physiologic observations at rest include posture and positioning, airway patency and respiratory effort (audible and visual observation-stridor, stertor, halted breathing or apnea, chest retractions, nasal flaring), neuromotor function, airway protection, including frequency of spontaneous swallows, presence of drooling (anterior and posterior), coughing, phonation (vocal quality, pitch, intensity), vital sign monitoring (oxygen saturation, heart rate and respiratory rate), color, oral examination, and anthropometric measurements.

Feeding observation

The amount of change in physiologic parameters with onset of the feeding session and the infant's tolerance thereof will determine whether the work of feeding is functional or excessive, requiring modifications. Observations of the typical feeding (simulated as best as possible given a likely change from home to a clinical setting) should include state, motor control, tactile reflexes and behavioral responses, oral motor movements, suck-swallow-breathe coordination, and outcomes of the feeding (eg, quantity consumed, length of feeding).[11] Oral, pharyngeal and esophageal phases of swallowing should be monitored as well.

Stimulability testing

Stimulability testing assesses effectiveness of modifications to promote successful feeding outcomes. This is performed during the feeding evaluation, if possible, following observation of the infant with his or her caregiver, in attempt to immediately alleviate feeding issues for the family. This involves making milk flow easily to meet caloric requirements, preventing excessive air intake, minimizing nasal regurgitation, and maintaining physiologic stability through changes in positioning, feeding modality, flow rate, liquid viscosity, assistance with milk delivery, and other strategies (eg, pacing techniques).

Instrumental evaluation

Despite thorough historical investigation and complete clinical feeding and swallowing evaluation, an instrumental evaluation may be necessary to further examine unanswered clinical questions. FEES and MBSS are common instrumental procedures used for objective evaluation of swallowing. Both tools provide a baseline anatomic and physiologic assessment of the swallowing mechanism, gauge swallowing function for trialed foods and liquids, and host therapeutic trials with use of positional strategies, changes in food texture and liquid viscosities, as well as changes in modalities used for presentations (eg, bottle, cup, spoon). There are conflicting reports regarding diagnostic agreement between FEES and MBSS in children.[12,13] There are inherent advantages and disadvantages to both procedures. Each can be used solely or in combination to obtain qualitative information from multiple views.

Fiberoptic Endoscopic Evaluation of Swallowing

A FEES provides the most direct view of the laryngeal structures and observation of laryngeal function. Real-time video in color makes examination of the integrity of the mucosa and the abundance of secretions easily visible (Video 1). FEES should be considered initially instead of the MBSS if it will provide the quality of information desired to avoid radiation exposure during MBSS. Furthermore, if transportation to the radiology suite or positioning within the videofluoroscopic space is not possible, FEES should be considered. Willging and colleagues[14] (2001) reported indications for pediatric FEES to include assessment of readiness for oral feedings, to determine if a structural abnormality is present, and to determine if there is need to further assess airway protection and devise strategies to improve safe swallowing. FEES with the component of sensory testing has been proven a useful tool in the diagnosis and management of laryngopharyngeal sensation in children.[15] Recent studies examining the effects of topical nasal anesthetic on swallowing have shown differing results. Kamarunas and colleagues[16] (2013) found no change in comfort, ease of examination, or quality of view between conditions of viscous lidocaine hydrochloride versus gel Surgilube during FEES. Fife and colleagues[17] (2015) found no statistical significance for impairment of swallowing ability in patients with dysphagia given use of aerosolized lidocaine during FEES; however, "topical nasal anesthesia significantly reduces subjective pain and discomfort and improved tolerance during FEES." O'Dea and colleagues[18] (2015) reported significant lower pain ratings during scope insertion without significant change in swallow function or residue between anesthetized and nonanesthetized conditions when using a dose of 0.2 mL of 4% atomized lidocaine during FEES. The investigators suggest that the quantity of anesthetic used during the evaluation and the length of the evaluation may be variables affecting pain tolerance.

Modified Barium Swallow Study

The MBSS provides the most comprehensive view of the oropharyngeal swallowing mechanism for examination of the oral, pharyngeal, and esophageal stages of swallowing (Video 2). This examination allows for observations not visible with endoscopy (eg, tongue base contact with the posterior pharyngeal wall that is seen as a whiteout during FEES, deep laryngeal penetration during the swallow). Consecutive swallows, often seen with infants feeding from a bottle or a neurologically impaired child who has difficulty with self-pacing, are better evaluated by MBSS; otherwise, the view from the endoscope is obstructed by the repetitive peristaltic movement of the bolus through the hypopharynx. Globus complaints, possible cricopharyngeal dysfunction, and nonspecific complaints are better evaluated by MBSS.[19] If a patient would have poor tolerance of endoscopy or refusal thereof, an MBSS would be indicated. A prospective study by Weir and colleagues[20] (2011) supported the use of MBSS to identify silent aspiration in children, including those with aspiration lung disease and neurologic impairment. MBSS is also a helpful assessment tool when diagnosing functional effects of asymmetric movement given the lateral, anteroposterior, and Towne views available.

FEEDING MANAGEMENT

If an infant is showing feeding difficulty, modifications should be trialed during the evaluative session, including the following:

Positioning of the feeder: Supported position to maintain stability throughout the feeding.

Positioning of the infant: Upright or elevated side lying to minimize the effects of nasal regurgitation and glossoptosis (if applicable).

Occlusion of the cleft lip and alveolus: With the breast or a wide nipple. Stabilize the jaw and cheeks for better oral closure, being mindful that the infant may rely on oral versus nasal breathing if airway patency issues are present.

Occlusion of the cleft palate: Obturators are not necessary and used infrequently.

Nipple modifications: Wide base and shaft for better occlusion of the cleft, length depends on size of the mouth and cleft, softness for easier compression, and variable hole size to adjust the flow rate of milk.

Infant-directed, assisted milk flow by bottle (**Fig. 1**): Use a soft-sided bottle and pliable nipple or a one-way flow valve.

Feeder-directed, assisted milk flow by bottle: Use a soft-sided bottle and pliable nipple, angle the nipple to contact a portion of bone for better positive pressure generation, squeeze the bottle when the infant sucks to synchronize positive pressure application with the infant's suck-swallow-breathe pattern (see **Fig. 1**).

Other: Burp frequently, irrigate the nose only if needed.

Breastfeeding (if applicable depending on the type and severity of the cleft): Nurse through let down, use manual expression, use assisted milk flow at the breast (eg, a supplemental nursing system), and close monitoring of growth.

Breastfeeding (if the infant is not a good candidate for nutritive feeding at the breast): Put the infant to breast briefly either at the onset of the feeding or after nutritive feeding from the bottle, encourage infant to breast for skin-to-skin contact and stimulation of milk production, elicit assistance from a lactation consultant for milk production strategies.

Compensatory strategies for poor feeding: Add supplement to the breastmilk, increase caloric

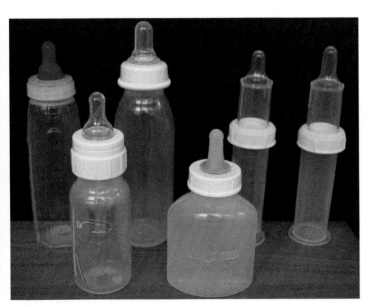

Fig. 1. Bottles commonly used to assist with milk delivery during feeding. From left to right: Ross bottle with Similac Premature Nipple & Ring, Dr. Brown's Specialty Feeding System, Respironics Pigeon feeder, Mead Johnson Cleft Lip/Palate Nurser, Medela's Special-Needs feeder with Mini teat, Medela's SpecialNeeds Feeder. The second, third, fifth, and sixth systems include a one-way valve to promote more controlled, infant-directed feeding.

concentration of the formula, provide temporary enteral feedings if necessary.

Monitoring: Weight checks with the pediatrician, follow-up with clinician, referral to other specialists as needed, hospital admission for failure to thrive or if physiologic stability is significantly compromised.

Postoperative Feeding: Recommendations based on surgeon's preferences, practice preoperatively.

SUMMARY

Feeding and swallowing abilities in infants born with craniofacial anomalies show great variability. Those infants with the same medical diagnosis or craniofacial anomaly may present very differently in their intrinsic management of food and liquid consumption. The instinctual drive to gain nourishment can become complicated by structural differences, physiologic instability, and environmental influences. These factors assessed individually and in combination will assist in producing the most favorable feeding outcomes possible with overall goals of providing adequate nutrition and hydration for brain development and growth, and facilitating the most positive feeding experience for both infant and caregiver.

SUPPLEMENTARY DATA

Supplementary data related to this article can be found at http://dx.doi.org/10.1016/j.fsc.2016.06.004.

REFERENCES

1. Berggman H, Hansson E, Uvemark A, et al. Prenatal compared with postnatal cleft diagnosis: what do the parents think? J Plast Surg Hand Surg 2012; 46:235–41.

2. Jones MC. Prenatal diagnosis of cleft lip and palate: detection rates, accuracy of ultrasonography, associated anomalies, and strategies for counseling. Cleft Palate Craniofac J 2002;39(2):169–73.

3. Davalbhatka A, Hall PN. The impact of antenatal diagnosis on the effectiveness and timing of counselling for cleft lip and palate. Br J Plast Surg 2000;53:298–301.

4. Arvedson J, Brodsky L. Pediatric swallowing and feeding: assessment and management. 2nd edition. New York: Singular; 2002.

5. Peterson-Falzone SJ, Hardin-Jones MA, Karnell MP. Cleft palate speech. St Louis (MO): Mosby; 2001.

6. Masarei AG, Sell D, Habel A, et al. The nature of feeding in infants with unrepaired cleft lip and/or palate compared with healthy noncleft infants. Cleft Palate Craniofac J 2007;44:321–8.

7. Reid J, Reilly S, Kilpatrick N. Sucking performance of babies with cleft conditions. Cleft Palate Craniofac J 2007;44(3):312–20.

8. Speltz M, Goodell EW, Endriga MC, et al. Feeding interactions of infants with unrepaired cleft lip and/or palate. Infant Behav Dev 1994;17:131–40.

9. Growth charts. Center for Disease Control and Prevention Web site. Page reviewed September 9, 2010. Available at: http://www.cdc.gov/growth-charts/index.htm. Accessed February 1, 2016.

10. Darrow DH, Harley CM. Evaluation of swallowing disorders in children. Otolaryngol Clin North Am 1998;31(3):405–18.

11. Wolf LS, Glass RP. Feeding and swallowing disorders in infancy: assessment and management. San Antonio (TX): Therapy Skill Builders; 1992.

12. Leder SB, Karas DE. Fiberoptic endoscopic evaluation of swallowing in the pediatric population. Laryngoscope 2000;110(7):1132–6.

13. DaSilva AP, Lubianco Neto J, Santoro PP. Comparison between videofluoroscopy and endoscopic evaluation of swallowing for the diagnosis of dysphagia in children. Otolaryngol Head Neck Surg 2010;143:204–9.

14. Willging JP, Miller CK, Thompson Link D, et al. Use of FEES to assess and manage pediatric patients. In: Langmore SE, editor. Endoscopic evaluation and treatment of swallowing disorders. New York: Thieme; 2001. p. 213–34.

15. Link DT, Willging JP, Miller CK, et al. Pediatric laryngopharyngeal sensory testing during flexible endoscopic evaluation of swallowing: feasible and correlative. Ann Otol Rhinol Laryngol 2000;109:899–905.

16. Kamarunas EE, McCullough GH, Guidry TJ, et al. Effects of topical nasal anesthetic on fiberoptic endoscopic examination of swallowing with sensory testing (FEESST). Dysphagia 2014;29:33–43.

17. Fife TA, Butler SG, Langmore SE, et al. Use of topical nasal anesthesia during flexible endoscopic evaluation of swallowing in dysphagic patients. Ann Otol Rhinol Laryngol 2015;124(3):206–11.

18. O'Dea MB, Langmore SE, Krisciunas GP, et al. Effect of lidocaine on swallowing during FEES in patients with dysphagia. Ann Otol Rhinol Laryngol 2015; 124(7):537–44.

19. Langmore SE, Aviv JE. Endoscopic procedures to evaluate oropharyngeal swallowing. In: Langmore SE, editor. Endoscopic evaluation and treatment of swallowing disorders. New York: Thieme; 2001. p. 213–34.

20. Weir KA, McMahon S, Taylor S, et al. Oropharyngeal aspiration and silent aspiration in children. Chest 2011;140(3):589–97.

Evaluation of Speech and Resonance for Children with Craniofacial Anomalies

CrossMark

Ann W. Kummer, PhD, CCC-SLP, ASHA-F

KEYWORDS

- Cleft palate • Velopharyngeal insufficiency • Velopharyngeal dysfunction • Hypernasality
- Resonance • Speech evaluation

KEY POINTS

- Speech and resonance disorders are common in patients with craniofacial anomalies, particularly those with clefts.
- Dental and occlusal anomalies can affect lingual-alveolar and bilabial sounds, whereas velopharyngeal insufficiency can cause hypernasality and/or nasal emission on pressure-sensitive sounds.
- In addition to an assessment of speech sound placement, manner of production, and voicing, the speech evaluation should also include an assessment of the presence of obligatory distortions or compensatory errors when there are oropharyngeal anomalies. The presence, audibility, and consistency of nasal emission on speech sounds are also important to note.
- The speech evaluation should always include an assessment of the type of resonance (normal, hypernasal, hyponasal, or cul-de-sac resonance). Severity ratings typically are not useful in determining appropriate management.
- Instrumental measures (whether high-tech or low-tech) can augment the perceptual evaluation and provide useful information for surgical management and measurement of outcomes.

 Video content accompanies this article at http://www.facialplastic.theclinics.com.

INTRODUCTION

Children with craniofacial anomalies often demonstrate disorders of speech and/or resonance due to structural anomalies of the jaws, oral cavity, and velopharyngeal (VP) valve. These anomalies are most commonly caused by clefts of the primary palate and secondary palate.

Clefts of the primary palate (particularly complete clefts that go through the alveolus) often result in dental anomalies and/or malocclusion. Dental anomalies, such as misplaced or supernumerary teeth, can interfere with tongue tip movement, and affect lingual and even bilabial placement during speech. Because the tongue tip needs to be positioned under the alveolar ridge and the lips need to come together easily for production of many speech sounds, malocclusion of the jaws is an even bigger problem for speech. With a class III malocclusion (and often with just an anterior crossbite), the tongue tip is positioned anterior to the alveolar ridge, which can affect the production of lingual-alveolar sounds (t, d, n, l, s, z) and even bilabial sounds (p, b, m). With a severe class II maloclussion secondary to micrognathia,

Disclosure Statement: The author receives royalties from Cengage Learning for a text book entitled: *Cleft Palate and Craniofacial Anomalies: The Effects on Speech and Resonance*, 3rd edition. The author also receives royalties for a clinical device called the Oral & Nasal Listener (Super Duper Publications, Greenville, SC).
Division of Speech-Language Pathology, Cincinnati Children's Hospital Medical Center, 3333 Burnet Avenue, MLC 4011, Cincinnati, OH 45229-3039, USA
E-mail address: Ann.Kummer@cchmc.org

the tongue tip may be positioned behind the alveolar ridge and under the palatal vault, making lingual-alveolar and bilabials sounds virtually impossible to produce normally.

Clefts of the secondary palate often result in VP insufficiency (VPI), which is defined as abnormal structure of the VP valve. It is estimated that, despite palatoplasty, 20% to 30% of children with repaired cleft palate will demonstrate some degree of VPI, resulting in abnormal speech.[1,2] Depending on the size of the opening, VPI can cause hypernasality (an abnormality of resonance) and/or nasal air emission (an abnormality of airflow).

PERCEPTUAL ASSESSMENT OF SPEECH AND RESONANCE

Children with clefts and other craniofacial anomalies should receive yearly speech evaluations by a speech-language pathologist (SLP) (preferably one associated with a craniofacial team) during the preschool years until speech is age-appropriate. These children should continue to receive at least screening evaluations through puberty.[3]

What to Evaluate

As part of a typical examination of a child with craniofacial anomalies, the SLP will assess speech sound production, the presence of nasal emission on pressure-sensitive phonemes (speech sounds), and resonance.[3-10] The examiner will also attempt to determine the cause of abnormalities in speech and/or resonance that are found.

Speech sound production

After listening to an inventory of all speech sounds in the child's language, the SLP will note errors of placement, errors of manner (eg, nasal, plosive, fricative, affricate), and errors of voicing (eg, use of voiced for voiceless phonemes or vice versa). The examiner will determine if multiple errors are related phonologically, which is important for therapeutic intervention. The examiner will also determine if the errors are consistent (eg, the error occurs in all conditions and all word positions) or are not consistent. Developmental errors (those that are normal for the child's age) are also noted. Finally, when there are structural anomalies, including dental anomalies, occlusal anomalies, and VPI, the examiner will determine if there are obligatory distortions and/or compensatory errors.

Obligatory distortions occur when the child's articulation placement is normal but the abnormal structure causes distortion of the sounds. These distortions will self-correct with correction of the structure and, therefore, are not appropriate for speech therapy. Compensatory errors occur with the child alters his or her articulation to compensate for the structural abnormality. Common compensatory errors for anterior crowding of the tongue tip or for class III malocclussion are palatal-dorsal substitutions. Common compensatory errors for VPI include glottal stops and pharyngeal fricatives. These errors require speech therapy, ideally after the structure is corrected or at least improved.[5,6]

Nasal emission

Nasal emission is a release of air flow through the nasal cavity during the production of oral sounds. Nasal emission is most audible on voiceless plosives (p, t, k), voiceless fricatives (f, s, sh), and the voiceless affricate (ch). Therefore, these sounds are typically used for assessment. The examiner will determine if there is audible nasal emission, the loud and distracting nasal rustle (AKA nasal turbulence), or if the nasal emission is inaudible. **Box 1** describes the diagnostic characteristics of nasal emission.[10]

Inaudible nasal emission occurs with a very large VP opening where the airflow travels through the valve with relatively low impedance to the flow. The sound of this nasal emission is very low in volume and is masked by the hypernasality. Inaudible nasal emission will significantly reduce airflow in the oral cavity causing certain

---

Box 1
Nasal emission

Nasal emission affects oral airflow and the ability to build up air pressure during speech. Nasal emission:

- Is characterized by abnormal escape of the air stream through the nasal cavity during production of pressure-sensitive consonants (plosives, fricatives, and affricates).

- Is typically caused by VPI but can also be caused by an anterior oronasal fistula or even by abnormal articulation placement in the pharynx.

- Affects voiceless pressure-sensitive phonemes the most (ie, p, t, k, f, s, sh, ch).

- May be audible or inaudible. If inaudible (due to a large VP opening), it will also cause consonants to be very weak in intensity and pressure, short utterance length (due to the need to take more breaths during speech), and may cause a nasal grimace during speech.

other characteristics, including weak or omitted consonants. In addition, the patient will take frequent breaths while speaking to replace the airflow that has leaked through the valve. A nasal grimace (contraction near the nasal bridge and/or around the nostrils) may also occur as an overflow muscle reaction to excessive effort in achieving VP closure. Finally, with a large VP opening, the nasal emission will typically be accompanied by hypernasality.

When the VP opening is very small, there is more impedance to the airflow, resulting in increased audibility of the airflow as it goes through the opening. In addition, the air passes with increased pressure so that as it is released it causes bubbling of secretions on the nasal surface of the VP valve.[10–12] The sound associated with bubbling, a nasal rustle (nasal turbulence) is very audible and distracting.[5,6,10–12] Video 1 demonstrates the sound of a nasal rustle. Because a nasal rustle is due to a small opening, it does not occur with inadequate intraoral air pressure needed for consonant production.

In addition to the quality of nasal emission, the examiner will judge its consistency. If nasal emission occurs inconsistently but on all pressure-sensitive phonemes, the cause is typically VPI. On the other hand, if it occurs consistently but only on specific phonemes, it is considered phoneme-specific nasal emission (PSNE). PSNE is caused by the use of pharyngeal or nasal fricative substitutions for some or all of the sibilant sounds (s, z, sh, zh, ch, j) and is only due to abnormal articulatory placement. Because this is a functional disorder, this can be corrected with speech therapy, rather than surgery.

Resonance

Determining the type of resonance (normal, hypernasal, hyponasal, cul-de-sac, or mixed) is very important because it gives clues as to the cause of the resonance disorder and the type of management required for correction. **Box 2** describes the diagnostic characteristics of these resonance disorders.[10] Video 2 shows an example of hypernasality and Video 3 is an example of hyponasality. Severity ratings of abnormal resonance are now being used for comparison of outcomes, although adequate interjudge reliability requires training.[13,14] From a clinical standpoint, if the parents want the abnormal resonance due to VPI or obstruction corrected, the severity rating is not relevant because it does not determine the type of physical management (usually surgery) that is required. Hypernasality due to VPI, which is a structural anomaly, will require surgical

---

Box 2
Resonance disorders

A resonance disorder affects the phonated sounds (all vowels and voiced consonants) during speech. It is characterized by an abnormal balance of sound energy in the cavities of the vocal tract (pharyngeal cavity, oral cavity, and nasal cavity) during speech.

Hypernasality

- Is characterized by too much sound resonating in the nasal cavity during the production of oral sounds.
- Is particularly perceptible on vowels and is also manifested as nasalization of voiced consonants (eg, m/b, n/d).
- Is typically caused by VPI or a large oronasal fistula.

Hyponasality

- Occurs when there is not enough nasal resonance during speech production.
- Is noted on the nasal consonants (m, n, ng).
- Is associated with chronic mouth breathing, snoring, and obstructive sleep apnea.
- Is caused by sources of upper airway obstruction, including maxillary retrusion.

Cul-de-sac resonance

- Is characterized by a muffled quality and reduced volume.
- Occurs when there is obstruction at the exit of one of the cavities of the vocal tract (pharyngeal, oral or nasal cavity).
  - Oral cul-de-sac resonance can be caused by microstomia (a small mouth opening).
  - Pharyngeal cul-de-sac resonance can be caused by very large tonsils.
  - Nasal cul-de-sac resonance can be caused by a combination of VPI and anterior nasal obstruction (eg, stenotic naris), and is seen in many patients with a cleft lip and palate.

Mixed nasality

- Occurs when there is some degree of hypernasality on oral consonants and vowels, and also hyponasality on nasal consonants.
- Can occur when there is VPI and co-occurring nasopharyngeal obstruction (ie, enlarged adenoids).

---

intervention, whereas hyponasality may benefit from pharmacologic management (eg, nasal sprays) or surgical treatment to decrease nasopharyngeal obstruction. Structural anomalies always require surgical management for correction. Speech therapy is not appropriate unless the abnormal resonance is phoneme-specific and due to misarticulation.

Based on the speech characteristics (and the laws of physics), the examiner can predict the approximate size of the VP opening (**Fig. 1**).[5,6,11,12]

Speech Samples

When assessing speech sound production (articulation), resonance, and VP function, it is important to select an appropriate speech sample to obtain the information that is needed for a definitive diagnosis.[5,6] There are many factors to consider when obtaining a speech sample, including the child's age, developmental status, articulation and language skills, language spoken, type and severity of the speech problem, and previously noted speech sound errors. For a child age 3 years or older, the examiner should attempt to elicit a variety of speech contexts, which may include single words, syllables, sentences, and spontaneous speech.

Single words

There are a variety of formal single word articulation tests that allow the examiner to evaluate each speech phoneme in all word positions (initial, medial, and final). These tests are expensive, time-consuming, and do not reveal problems that occur in connected (running) speech.

Syllable repetition

To isolate individual phonemes and eliminate the effects of other speech sounds, the examiner may ask the patient to produce consonants (particularly plosives, fricatives, and affricates) in a repetitive manner (eg, "pah, pah, pah"; "pee, pee, pee"; "tah, tah, tah"; "tee, tee, tee").[6,12,13] Each of the phonemes should be tested with both a low vowel (eg, "ah" as in "father") and then with a high vowel (eg, "ee" as in "heat").[5,6]

Sentence repetition

Perhaps the best way to test speech sound production and VP function for speech is to use a battery of sentences that the patient is asked to repeat.[6] It is preferable to use sentences that contain multiple productions of the same phoneme placement (eg, "Buy baby a bib," "Do it for Daddy," and "Take Teddy to town."). This method allows the examiner to quickly and easily assess articulation placement, the presence of nasal emission, and determine the type of resonance in a connected speech environment.

INTRAORAL EXAMINATION

An evaluation of the oral cavity is an important part of a speech and resonance evaluation.[15] The examiner typically evaluates bilabial competence, dental occlusion, and the position of the tongue tip relative to the alveolar ridge. The examiner must rule out the presence of a fistula (if the child

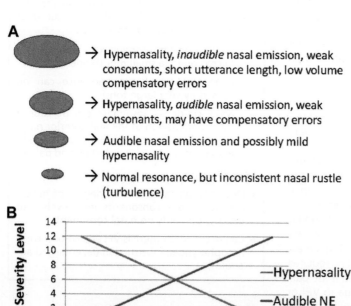

A

→ Hypernasality, *inaudible* nasal emission, weak consonants, short utterance length, low volume compensatory errors

→ Hypernasality, *audible* nasal emission, weak consonants, may have compensatory errors

→ Audible nasal emission and possibly mild hypernasality

→ Normal resonance, but inconsistent nasal rustle (turbulence)

B

Severity Level / Velopharyngeal Gap Size (Large, Medium, Small)
—Hypernasality
—Audible NE

Fig. 1. Prediction of velopharyngeal gap size based on perceptual features of speech and resonance. (*A*) Large gaps typically cause hypernasality with inaudible nasal emission, whereas small gaps cause audible nasal emission with no hypernasality. (*B*) The relationship between gap size and perceptual features of hypernasality and nasal emission.

had a cleft), rule out a submucous cleft (if the child did not have a cleft), and examine the tonsils. During phonation, it is important to assess the position of the velar dimple, where the levator muscles interdigitate.[16] The examiner also looks for signs of upper airway obstruction, which can cause hyponasality or cul-de-sac resonance.

To obtain the best view of the posterior oral cavity and pharynx (often without a tongue blade), the examiner asks the child to say the vowel /æ/ as in "hat" rather than /a/ as in "father."[15] This will bring the back of the tongue down. The patient can also be instructed to stick the tongue out and down as far as it will go during production of this vowel, which will further open the back of the oral cavity for the best view (**Fig. 2**).

INTRUMENTAL ASSESSMENT OF SPEECH AND RESONANCE AND VELOPHARYNGEAL FUNCTION

VPI, as the cause of hypernasality and/or nasal emission, can be diagnosed by an experienced SLP based on the characteristics of the speech. However, instrumental assessment can provide important additional information.[17]

Nasometry

Nasometry is an objective method of measuring the acoustic correlates of VP function (eg, resonance and audible nasal emission).[18] The Nasometer II (PENTAX Medical, Montvale, NJ, USA) is a computer-based system that includes a sound separator plate that has 2 directional microphones on either side. The sound separator plate is placed between the child's upper lip and nose (**Fig. 3**).

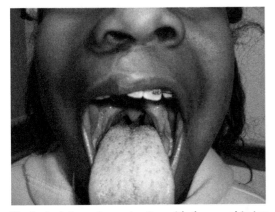

Fig. 2. An intraoral examination with the vowel /æ/ as in "hat." (*From* Kummer AW. Cleft palate and craniofacial anomalies: the effects on speech and resonance. 3rd edition. Clifton Park (NY): Cengage Learning; 2014; with permission.)

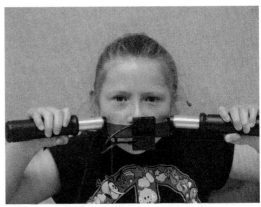

Fig. 3. Use of the nasometer for objective measurement of nasal acoustic energy during speech. (*From* Kummer AW. Cleft palate and craniofacial anomalies: the effects on speech and resonance. 3rd edition. Clifton Park (NY): Cengage Learning; 2014; with permission.)

Standardized speech samples are used, such as the passages in the Simplified Nasometric Assessment Procedures-Revised (SNAP-R).[19] The nasometer computes an objective nasalance score (ratio of oral/total [oral + nasal] energy) for the passage. See Video 1 and Video 3 for examples of the nasograms, which are visual representations of the percentage of nasal acoustic energy (from either hypernasality and/or audible nasal emission) during speech. When an individual's score is compared with normative data for each passage, a judgment can be made regarding the normalcy of VP function. High scores, in comparison with normative data, suggest hypernasality and/or audible nasal emission. Low scores, in comparison with normative data, suggest hyponasality or cul-de-sac resonance and upper airway obstruction. Nasometry can provide objective information regarding changes resulting from surgery or therapeutic intervention.

Nasopharyngoscopy

Nasopharyngoscopy is a minimally invasive nasopharyngeal endoscopic procedure that allows direct visual observation and analysis of the VP mechanism during speech.[20,21] See Video 2, which shows a nasopharyngoscopy examination of a patient with a large coronal VP opening. Nasopharyngoscopy has some specific advantages compared with videofluoroscopy, in that it allows the examiner to better:

- View the nasal surface of the velum to rule out an occult submucous cleft (**Fig. 4**)
- Identify small VP gaps

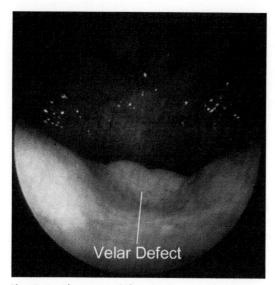

Fig. 4. A submucous cleft palate as viewed through nasopharyngoscopy. (*From* Kummer AW. Cleft palate and craniofacial anomalies: the effects on speech and resonance. 3rd edition. Clifton Park (NY): Cengage Learning; 2014; with permission.)

- Determine the location of the openings, which helps in surgical planning
- Closely examine the position of a pharyngeal flap or sphincter and the function of the ports.

In addition, nasopharyngoscopy does not involve radiation and the parent can hold and calm the child during the procedure.[20,21]

Nasopharyngoscopy can provide important information about the size, location, and usually the cause of the VP opening. This information is helpful in determining the best surgical procedure for the patient.

Low-Tech Instruments

Low-tech instruments, such as a stethoscope, a piece of tubing, or even a straw, can be used to determine if there is hypernasality, nasal emission, or even hyponasality. Just like a stethoscope, a piece of tubing or a bending straw will amplify sound.[5,6] The examiner places one end of the tube in the child's nostril and the other end next to the examiner's ear (**Fig. 5**). The child is first asked to repeat only oral sounds. Hypernasality or nasal emission will be heard loudly through the tube. Next, the child is asked to repeat syllables with nasal phonemes (m, n) or prolong one of these sounds (preferably m). If there is not much sound heard through the tube, this indicates hyponasality due to obstruction.

SUMMARY

Speech and resonance disorders are common in patients with craniofacial anomalies, particularly those with clefts of the primary and/or secondary palate. An evaluation of speech, resonance and VP function should be done for all at-risk patients soon after age 3. A knowledgeable and experienced SLP will be able to determine the type of disorder and the probable cause. If there is VPI, the speech characteristics will give a clue as to the size of the VP gap. Nasopharyngoscopy can help to identify the location of a VP opening, which can be useful in surgical planning. Nasometry can provide objective data regarding changes after

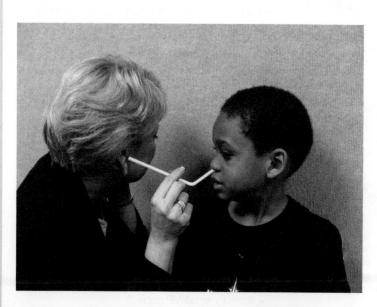

Fig. 5. Use of a straw to amplify sound from the nasal cavity during speech. (*From* Kummer AW. Cleft palate and craniofacial anomalies: the effects on speech and resonance. 3rd edition. Clifton Park (NY): Cengage Learning; 2014; with permission.)

surgical management. Finally, children with clefts or other craniofacial anomalies should be managed by a craniofacial team for coordinated care and the best overall outcomes.

SUPPLEMENTARY DATA

Supplementary data related to this article can be found at http://dx.doi.org/10.1016/j.fsc.2016.06.003.

REFERENCES

1. Witt PD, Wahlen JC, Marsh JL, et al. The effect of surgeon experience on velopharyngeal functional outcome following palatoplasty: is there a learning curve? Plast Reconstr Surg 1998;102(5):1375–84.
2. Rintala AE, Haapanen ML. The correlation between training and skill of the surgeon and reoperation rate for persistent cleft palate speech. Br J Oral Maxillofac Surg 1995;33(5):295–371 [discussion: 297–8].
3. American Cleft Palate-Craniofacial Association (ACPA). Parameters for evaluation and treatment of patients with cleft lip/palate or other craniofacial anomalies. Cleft Palate Craniofac J 2009; 30(Suppl):1–16.
4. Kuehn DP, Henne LJ. Speech evaluation and treatment of patients with cleft palate. Am J Speech Lang Pathol 2003;12:103–9.
5. Kummer AW. Perceptual assessment of resonance and velopharyngeal function. Semin Speech Lang 2011;32(2):159–67.
6. Kummer AW. Speech and resonance assessment. In: Kummer AW, editor. Cleft palate and craniofacial anomalies: the effects on speech and resonance. Clifton Park (NY): Cengage Learning; 2014. p. 324–51.
7. Marsh JL. The evaluation and management of velopharyngeal dysfunction. Clin Plast Surg 2004;31(2): 261–9.
8. Smith B, Guyette TW. Evaluation of cleft palate speech. Clin Plast Surg 2004;31(2):251–60.
9. Smith BE, Kuehn DP. Speech evaluation of velopharyngeal dysfunction. J Craniofac Surg 2007;18(2): 251–60.
10. Kummer AW. Disorders of resonance and airflow secondary to cleft palate and/or velopharyngeal dysfunction. Semin Speech Lang 2011;32(2):141–9.
11. Kummer AW, Briggs M, Lee L. The relationship between the characteristics of speech and velopharyngeal gap size. Cleft Palate Craniofac J 2003; 4(6):590–6.
12. Kummer AW, Curtis C, Wiggs M, et al. Comparison of velopharyngeal gap size in patients with hypernasality, hypernasality and nasal emission, or nasal turbulence (rustle) as the primary speech characteristic. Cleft Palate Craniofac J 1992;29(2):152–6.
13. Sell D, Harding A, Grunwell P. GOS.SP.ASS/98: an assessment for speech disorders associated with cleft palate and/or velopharyngeal dysfunction (revised). Int J Lang Commun Disord 1999;34(1): 17–33.
14. Chapman KL, Baylis A, Trost-Cardamone J, et al. The Americleft speech project: a training and reliability study. Cleft Palate Craniofac J 2016;53(1): 93–108.
15. Kummer AW. Orofacial examination. In: Kummer AW, editor. Cleft palate and craniofacial anomalies: the effects on speech and resonance. Clifton Park (NY): Cengage Learning; 2014. p. 352–86.
16. Boorman JG, Sommerland BC. Levator veli palati and palatal dimples: their anatomy, relationship, and clinical significance. Br J Plast Surg 1995;38: 326–32.
17. Pannbacker M, Middleton G. Integrating perceptual and instrumental procedures in assessment of velopharyngeal insufficiency. Ear Nose Throat J 1990; 69(3):161–75.
18. Kummer AW. Nasometry. In: Kummer AW, editor. Cleft palate and craniofacial anomalies: the effects on speech and resonance. Clifton Park (NY): Cengage Learning; 2014. p. 400–34.
19. Kummer AW. Simplified nasometric assessment procedures- revised (SNAP-R). In PENTAX Medical Instruction Manual Nasometer Model 6450. 2005.
20. Kummer AW. Nasopharyngoscopy. In: Kummer AW, editor. Cleft palate and craniofacial anomalies: the effects on speech and resonance. Clifton Park (NY): Cengage Learning; 2014. p. 488–528.
21. Lam DJ, Starr JR, Perkins JA, et al. A comparison of nasendoscopy and multiview videofluoroscopy in assessing velopharyngeal insufficiency. Otolaryngol Head Neck Surg 2006;134(3):394–402.

Cleft Lip Repair, Nasoalveolar Molding, and Primary Cleft Rhinoplasty

Aditi A. Bhuskute, MD[a], Travis T. Tollefson, MD, MPH[b],*

KEYWORDS

- Cleft lip • Cleft palate • Subunit cleft repair • Nasoalveolar molding • Cleft rhinoplasty

KEY POINTS

- The cleft lip design should be measured carefully and executed to reduce variability.
- Primary rhinoplasty at the time of the lip repair repositions the ala improves the stigmata of the cleft lip nasal deformity.
- Specialized orthodontists can be very effective using nasoalveolar molding to simplify the lip repair and ultimate outcome.
- Specialized orthodontia is a labor-intensive therapy that requires parental compliance and motivation.

 Video content accompanies this article at http://www.facialplastic.theclinics.com.

INTRODUCTION

Orofacial clefts occur in a spectrum that include cleft lip–cleft palate and are the most common craniofacial birth defect. Cleft lip repair is just the beginning of sequential, interdisciplinary care that this patient population requires. Presurgical care can be optimized by partnering with specialized orthodontists and the use of nasoalveolar molding (NAM) with presurgical infant orthopedics (PSIO). This therapy can enhance the surgical repair. The cleft lip and its corresponding nasal deformity should be considered a complex dentofacial problem in most cases. Often, the residual cleft nasal deformity results in permanent cleft stigmata. An interdisciplinary cleft team can effectively identify and guide treatment in dentition, speech, swallowing, hearing, and psychosocial issues. The objectives of this manuscript are to describe an evidenced-based review of presurgical care (eg, lip taping and NAM), as well as preferred techniques for lip repair and primary rhinoplasty.

EPIDEMIOLOGY

Orofacial clefting is the fourth most common birth defect after congenital heart deformities, spina bifida, and limb deformities. The incidence of cleft lip–cleft palate in the United States is between 1 in 600 and 1 in 750 live births, with some ethnic variability.[1] A higher incidence in Native American and Asian populations is noted, and the lowest incidence is in African Americans and Africans.[2] Isolated cleft palate is considered separate from a cleft lip occurring with or without cleft palate. Approximately two-thirds of orofacial clefts are cleft lip with or without cleft palate, whereas

[a] Department of Otolaryngology-Head and Neck Surgery, UC Davis Medical Center, 2521 Stockton Boulevard, Suite 7200, Sacramento, CA 95817, USA; [b] Facial Plastic and Reconstructive Surgery, Department of Otolaryngology-Head and Neck Surgery, UC Davis Medical Center, 2521 Stockton Boulevard, Suite 7200, Sacramento, CA 95817, USA
* Corresponding author.
E-mail address: tttollefson@ucdavis.edu

Facial Plast Surg Clin N Am 24 (2016) 453–466
http://dx.doi.org/10.1016/j.fsc.2016.06.015
1064-7406/16/© 2016 Elsevier Inc. All rights reserved.

one-third are isolated cleft palate. The majority of cleft lip with or without cleft palate cases are unilateral and are more commonly left sided. Isolated cleft palate is more common in females, whereas cleft lip with or without cleft palate is more common in males.[3]

The classification of an orofacial cleft based on laterality of the cleft lip (unilateral or bilateral), severity, and involvement of lip, alveolus, and/or palate. A complete cleft lip extends through the lip and nasal sill, whereas an incomplete cleft involves diastasis of the orbicularis oris and skin, but remains intact for at least three-quarters of the lip length. The microform, and less described nanoform, cleft is characterized by a philtral skin groove, minor nasal alar hooding and alar base asymmetry, furrowing of the orbicularis oris muscle, and a notch at the vermilion–cutaneous junction. A microform cleft lip, also called a form fruste, does not extend to more than one-quarter of the labial height, measured from the normal peak of Cupid's bow to the nasal sill. The cleft alveolus can be complete or notched. Independent of the cleft lip type, a cleft palate can be unilateral (1 palatal shelf is attached to the nasal septum) or bilateral, and include the primary palate, portions of the hard and soft palate, or soft palate only.[4]

TIMING OF INTERVENTIONS

Interdisciplinary cleft team management of a child with a cleft lip–cleft palate follows a typical timeline. The cleft lip is typically repaired at 3 to 5 months of age, but may be later if NAM is chosen. Those with cleft palate have a higher incidence of Eustachian tube dysfunction, which is managed with bilateral tympanostomy tube placement based on tympanogram and otomicroscopy. We use a selective tube placement and obtain a behavioral audiogram around 8 months of age. Routine speech assessment and therapy begins in the first 2 years with routine 6-month follow-up. This leads to velopharyngeal dysfunction assessment and potential secondary speech

surgery. Alveolar bone grafting usually needs orthodontic preparation at around 7 to 10 years old, with definitive orthognathic surgery reserved for those with dentofacial malocclusion after full skeletal growth. This may be followed by a cleft septorhinoplasty.

BILATERAL CLEFT LIP

The bilateral cleft lip presents a more involved defect of both sides of the premaxilla/prolabium, but obtaining the general symmetry is inherently easier than in the grossly asymmetric unilateral cleft lip deformity. The greatest challenges of the bilateral cleft lip repair are dealing with the short columella and upper lip, protruding premaxilla, and persistent nasal deformities, including hooding of nostrils and lack of tip projection and definition. Some surgeons choose a 2-stage repair with primary lip repair in infancy and a secondary columellar lengthening between 1 to 5 years of age. More commonly, a 1-stage Mulliken or Millard approach is performed with PSIO and/or NAM used for the more complex, wide cases.

Bilateral cleft lip
- Premaxilla is not attached to the lateral palatal shelves.
- Forward projected premaxilla.
- Absent or small anterior nasal spine.
- Posteriorly displaced lateral piriform apertures.
- Widely splayed lower lateral cartilages.

A wide bilateral cleft lip (**Fig. 1**) may have a protruding premaxilla and excessive tension on the lip segments with the pinch test to allow a primary 1-staged repair. In these situations, we prefer to partner with our cleft team orthodontist team using NAM (see NAM section) to set the premaxilla back, establish the maxillary arch and increase columellar length with nasal prongs (**Fig. 2**). In cases where NAM is not possible, the repair is delayed and lip taping is applied (**Fig. 3**).

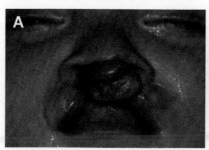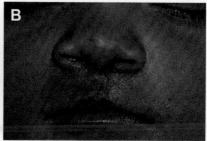

Fig. 1. Infant with a complete bilateral cleft lip and palate (*A*) preoperatively and (*B*) postoperatively.

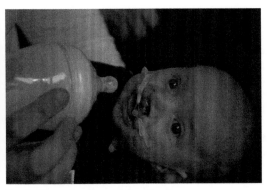

Fig. 2. Nasoalveolar molding feeding.

A staged cleft lip repair (lip adhesion) in a child with any of the following: (1) too old to start NAM (owing to rigidity of maxillary segments), (2) grossly asymmetric cleft, or (3) diminutive prolabium (<6 mm in height) A delayed definitive cleft lip repair is completed months later. In rare cases, premaxillary repositioning with vomer osteotomy is an option. Caution is advised owing to the risks of premaxilla devascularization and potential growth inhibition.[5]

Surgical Technique: Bilateral Cleft Lip Repair with Primary Rhinoplasty

No matter what technique is chosen, precise planning and markings are of utmost importance. When one can see the landmarks well enough to create the correct markings, the lip repair becomes a calculated method with less trial and error. Cupid's peak, the vermillion–cutaneous junction, and the junction of the columella and lip are examples of landmarks that should not be distorted by local anesthesia injections.

Measurements begin with design of a lozenge-shaped philtrum from the prolabial skin and soft tissues (there is no muscle in the prolabium in a complete bilateral cleft lip). Keys to this repair, based on Mulliken's techniques, are to use back cuts on the lateral lip vermilion, which create flaps

that will be sewn under the prolabium.[6,7] Infraorbital nerve block and vasoconstriction of the superior labial arteries, buccal sulcus, and nose (columella and ala) is completed with gentle injection of bupivacaine 0.25% with 1:200,000 epinephrine injections.

Design of Prolabial Flaps

Initial the markings are made with a temporary tattoo of methylene blue using a 27- or 30-gauge needle and include the following (**Fig. 4**):

- *Subnasale*—midline prolabium at the junction of the lip and columella;
- *Alare*—lateral-most aspects of bilateral nasal ala;
- *Cupid's bow peaks* (4–5 mm apart) at the vermilion–cutaneous junction; and
- The columella–nasal sill junction.

Next the philtral heights (6–8 mm) and distance from subnasale to alare are measured. The philtrum is designed to be in the shape of a lozenge or standard necktie. Perpendicular lines from the columella–nasal sill junction extend below the nasal sill (these will receive the lateral lip flaps). The neophiltral flap is incised centrally and the lateral prolabial flaps are deepithelialized.

Design of the Lateral Lip Segments

Markings in the lateral lip include the following (see **Fig. 4**):

- *Noordhoff's point*—vermilion–cutaneous junction where the cutaneous roll and vermillion (dry lip) fade as you trace superiomedially.
- *Noordhoff's red line*—the (wet–dry) vermillion–mucosal junction.
- High point of flaps are chosen to include dermal hairs but not vibrissae of nose.
- Vermillion flap back cut marks approximately 3 to 4 mm inferior lip flap mark (dry vermillion).

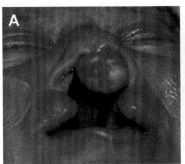
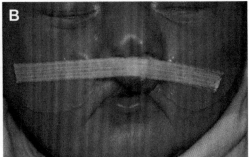

Fig. 3. (*A*) Infant before lip taping. (*B*) Infant after taping.

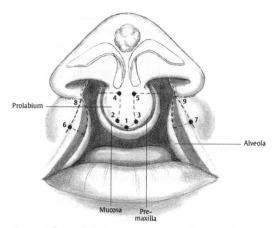

Fig. 4. Bilateral design (choose from 2 options).

The vertical philtral lip height was measured on the prolabium and is juxtaposed to advancement flap height (~8 mm). Similar markings are made on the opposite side.

Flap Mobilization and Muscle Dissection

A 15-C blade or ophthalmologic cornea knife is used for the cutaneous incisions, which are made with a tourniquet squeeze of the lip using thumb and index fingers. The vermillion flaps are incised about 3 mm proximal to most inferior advancement flap point. Mucosal incisions using a cut setting on cautery are followed by blunt dissection of the lateral lip from the supraperiosteal plane of the maxilla. In wider clefts, cautery dissection is continued down to the insertion of the inferior turbinate to facilitate digital release of the alar base from the piriform aperture. This is repeated on the contralateral lip. The lateral lip segments are retracted medially to test the tension.

The prolabial incisions are made second to avoid dependent bleeding onto the lateral lip markings. The philtral columns are incised just through the dermis to maximize blood supply. The lateral circular prolabial incisions are made down to but not including the sulcus mucosa, which is preserved to cover the anterior face of the premaxilla (to prevent adherence to the reconstructed orbicularis oris muscle). Bilateral septal mucoperichondrial flaps are raised with a Freer elevator for nasal floor closure.

The orbicularis oris muscle layer is dissected free from the "sandwich" of overlying dermis and underlying mucosa just deep to the minor salivary glands. Adequate muscle release is when muscle approximation is tension free. Countertraction with a small double prong retractor and forceps facilitates muscle release.

Primary Rhinoplasty

Bilateral partial marginal incisions are created to expose the nasal tip fat pad, which is freed and passed superiorly. The lower lateral cartilages are sewn together in the midline in a lateral crural steal maneuver. The cephalic borders of the lower lateral cartilages are secured cephalad onto the upper lateral cartilages, similar to Skoog. When there is excessive hooding, an elliptical excision of the soft tissue triangle hooding is completed (Tajima's reverse U).

Closure

The prolabium mucosa is laid superiorly and sewn to the premaxillary periosteum to create the gingivobuccal sulcus, which the orbicularis oris muscle will glide across. The nasal floor is closed with 5-0 chromic. An alar base cinching suture is placed using a "key" suture of 4-0 Vicryl or polydiaxone. The alare–alare distance is typically set as narrow as possible (~25 mm in infants).

The intraoral lip mucosa is joined in the midline with 4-0 absorbable sutures. Simple and vertical mattress sutures (3-0 or 4-0 monocryl or polydiaxone) are used to join the lateral lip muscle flaps. The superior-most orbicularis oris is sewn to the periosteum of the nasal spine to accentuate the nasolabial angle.

A discrepancy in prolabium height to the lateral lip height is addressed with a standing cone repair at the alar base (minimal alotomy). A dermal suture from the philtrum to the deep muscle can create a philtral dimple. Deep 6-0 monocryl subcuticular sutures approximate the vermillion and philtrum. Lip closure creates tension on the columella and nasal tip flattening. The 2 dry vermilion flaps are sewn together, and the dart of the philtral column is inset. Cyanoacrylate surgical glue (Dermabond) in thin layers is used for final skin closure, and the lip is completed with 5-0 chromic. Nasal conformers are secured to the caudal septum. These stent open the collapsed nostrils, supporting the primary rhinoplasty maneuvers for up to 6 weeks (**Fig. 5**).

UNILATERAL CLEFT LIP

Cleft lip repair can be as simple as approximating the medial and lateral lip elements with preservation of natural lip landmarks. More severe clefts can involve the lip, alveolus, nasal sill, and extend back to the palate. Presurgical treatment for wider clefts can decrease wound tension and untoward results. Each surgeon will have a slightly different opinion about their favorite technique,

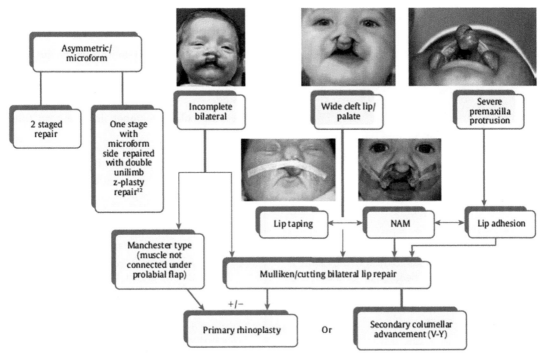

Fig. 5. Bilateral algorithm. NAM, nasoalveolar molding. (*From* Goudy S, Tollefson TT, editors. Complete cleft care. New York: Thieme; 2015; with permission.)

but the general principles will align a concentric orbicularis oris muscle to establish symmetry and proportionality of the perioral and nasal landmarks.

Unilateral cleft lip
- Septal displacement out of the vomerine groove to the noncleft nostril.
- Shortened columella on the cleft side.
- Hypoplastic and malformed alar cartilage with short medial crus and elongated lateral crus.
- Inferior and posterior displacement of the lateral crus.
- Widened and asymmetric nasal tip owing to medial crus deformity and columella.
- Nostril asymmetry with widened nostril on the cleft side.

The design of the unilateral cleft lip repair can be categorized into 3 general schools: (1) straight-line closure, (2) geometric, and (3) rotation–advancement techniques. The rotation–advancement technique is the most common in the United States, which included the original Millard, and the Noordhoff, and the Mohler modifications (**Fig. 6**).[8] The Fisher subunit approach is a geometric approach that is increasingly more popular.[9] The senior author uses a hybrid of this technique and describes it in detail.

Surgical Technique: A Hybrid Subunit Approach

This is a simplified version of Fisher's description that focuses on basic landmarks instead of the 25 lip and nasal points in his original description (**Fig. 7**).[9] The natural anatomy landmarks

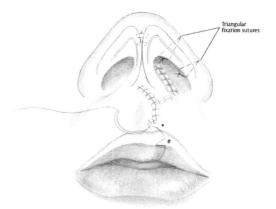

Fig. 6. Mohler rotation–advancement design with primary rhinoplasty demonstrated the triangular fixation sutures used to suspend the left alar cartilages. * represents the skin closure just about the cutaneous (white) roll. # represents the Noordhoff red line (ie, the wet-dry vermillion-mucosal lip junction). (*From* Goudy S, Tollefson TT, editors. Complete cleft care. New York: Thieme; 2015; with permission.)

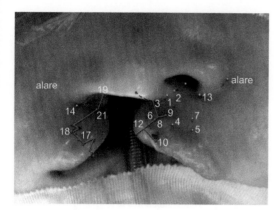

Fig. 7. Subunit design.

are similar to those used from a rotation-advancement cleft lip repair. Similar to the bilateral lip repair technique, this description of the hybrid subunit cleft lip repair will include design and lip markings, flap mobilization and muscle dissection, rhinoplasty, and closure.

Design and Lip Markings

The design of the cleft lip repair is marked with temporary skin tattoos (methylene blue) using a 30-G needle. Markings are shown in **Box 1** and also noted in **Fig. 7**. The principles of the repair are to create the essential symmetric lip height and alar bases between the noncleft and cleft sides, while maintaining proportionality to the lip fullness and nostril shapes. Measurements are recorded as follows:

1. The cleft side height is subtracted from the normal (noncleft side) lip height to determine the difference. This difference (eg, 7 – 5 mm = 2 mm) is then used as the size of the lateral lip triangle flap, which is placed at the inferior limb of the lateral lip design. This noncleft side measurement is simply from just above the cutaneous roll at the peak of Cupids' bow on the noncleft side (point 7) to the lateral columella/lip crease (point 2). The cleft side is from points 8 to 3.
2. The difference in nostril size is measured at the alar base from subnasale to alare bilaterally, and the difference used to determine nasal base width.
3. The normal philtral height from step one is (points 2–7) is transferred with a caliper to the lateral lip starting at Noordhoff's point, which was marked point 18. The caliper extends superiorly (eg, 7 mm) and the superior site (point 21) is marked. Adjustments are needed to prevent nasal vibrissae from being in the lip

closure. An angled line is drawn up to point 19, which mimics the opposing columellar flap. In incomplete cleft lips, the excision of nasal sill skin must be conservative to prevent nostril stenosis.

4. The inferior limb triangle of the lateral lip is set with a caliper to be 1 mm less than the difference in lip heights measured in step one, owing to the Rose Thompson effect.[9] This is extended superiorly from point 18 (just above the cutaneous roll at Noordhoff's point). Triangles larger than 3 mm are to be avoided. When the lateral lip height is deficient, the triangle can be opened up in a method similar to Tennison's description (**Fig. 8**).[10]
5. Similar to Noordhoff's vermillion triangle flap, the dry lip triangle from the lateral lip is marked and a recipient back cut (line from points 10–12) on the cleft side is marked.[11]
6. A back cut (from point 8–9) is made on the cleft side lip height just above the cutaneous roll, which will be the recipient of the isosceles triangle flap form the lateral lip. This back cut

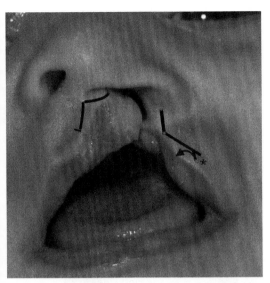

Fig. 8. Subunit design showing lateral lip marking with a Tennison-like opening triangle to increase the height of the lateral lip.

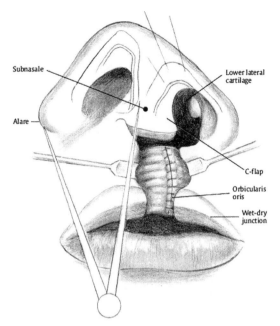

Fig. 9. Primary cleft rhinoplasty showing lower lateral cartilage malposition. Caliper is illustrating the need to create alar base symmetry. (*From* Goudy S, Tollefson TT, editors. Complete cleft care. New York: Thieme; 2015; with permission.)

is made perpendicular to the line from points 3 to 8.

7. The alar base widths (alare-sn) measured in step 2 can be only different by 2 to 3 mm in an incomplete cleft lip, but conservative removal of the alar sill in a wedge resection is advised, so as not to create nostril stenosis. The difference in alar base widths can be greater than 10 mm in complete clefts and are used as a guideline for the alar base tightening suture.

Flap Mobilization and Muscle Dissection

The incisions and muscle dissection are described for the bilateral cleft lip repair and are not repeated. The release of the lip soft tissues from the maxilla is completed in a supraperiosteal plane and is expanded for more severe clefts to release tension for closure. Orbicularis oris dissection on the philtral side is minimized to preserve the philtral dimple.

Primary Rhinoplasty

The lower lateral cartilages are dissected bluntly from the skin soft tissue envelope through the columellar lip incision (**Fig. 9**). Transcutaneous plication is achieved with a resorbable 5-0 monocryl suture passed while forceps push the cleft side lower lateral cartilage in a cephalad and medial position. The needle is passed from inside the nostril through the alar crease, and then back in the needle hole before tying inside the nose (see **Fig. 6**). In severe nostril hooding cases, a

Tajima reverse U rim incision is created on the cleft side. Interdomal sutures (5–0 polydiaxone suture) are placed through this incision.

Closure

The closure is not repeated, because it is similar to the bilateral technique. Narrow nasal bases can be created using the subunit approach if the surgeon fails to respect the need for conservation of nasal sill skin. Gingivobuccal sulcus mucosa is closed. The orbicularis oris margins are closed with 4-0 monocryl sutures. The needle path is slightly more cephalic on the medial (cleft side) muscle, which increases the cleft side lip height. The vermilion–cutaneous and cutaneous–roll junctions are approximated using subcuticular sutures with 6-0 monocryl, and the triangular flap from the lateral lip is placed into the back cut at points 8 to 9. The vermillion, vermillion triangle flap, and mucosa are trimmed and inset with 7-0 vicryl and 5-0 chromic suture. Surgical glue is applied to the cutaneous lip. The nostrils are stented with silicone for 6 weeks (**Fig. 10**).

NASOALVEOLAR MOLDING

PSIO includes a gamut of palatal appliances that are fabricated for the neonate with both unilateral and bilateral cleft lip.[12] The senior author reserves

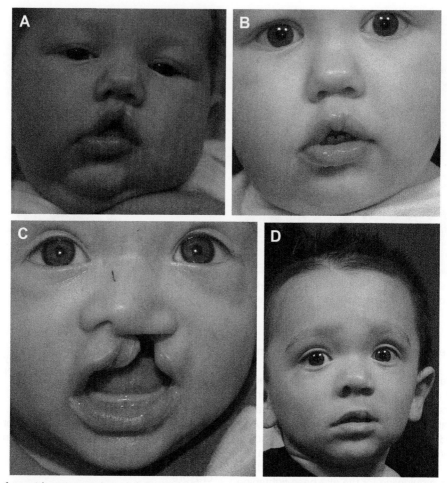

Fig. 10. Infant with an incomplete cleft lip (*A*) before and (*B*) after hybrid subunit cleft lip repair. A 3-month-old infant with a complete cleft lip and palate (*C*) before and (*D*) after hybrid subunit cleft lip repair. Note the slight excess of the mucosal fullness at the site of the vermillion triangle flap, which will be addressed with a revision at the time of another procedure.

the use of these appliances for the wide, complete cleft lip–cleft palate cases. The major goal is to reduce the overall wound tension at the time of the lip repair and to position the maxillary segments and nasal structures into a more anatomic position (**Fig. 11**).

With the advent of NAM therapy, Grayson and Cutting suggested improved nasal appearance, reduced need for secondary nasal surgeries, and a decreased need for alveolar bone grafting.[13,14] The oral appliance is adapted to the cleft alveolus and can function as a static palatal plate (eg, Hotz appliance or Zurich plates).

Physiologically, the nasal cartilages are amenable to molding owing to elevated serum maternal estrogens. These estrogens stimulate the release of proteoglycans and hyaluronic acid, making the cartilage more pliable. This pliability of the cartilage is present in newborns as a

mechanism to relax ligaments, cartilage, and connective tissue as it passes through the birth canal.[15] Matsuo and Hirose[16] recognized the unique qualities of newborn cartilage as a means to mold it to a newly desired state.

Historical Perspective

Manipulation of the protruding premaxilla in cleft lip–palate has been reported as early as the 16th century.[13] As the years progressed, cleft lip preparation for surgery has included lip taping, elastics, orthodontics, and acrylic appliances. This then progressed to maxillary arch devices that were screwed into the lateral arch segments attached to pins connected in the premaxilla.[17,18] Other devices include the Latham device, which also acts to deproject the premaxilla and reposition the lateral alveolar segments.[19,20]

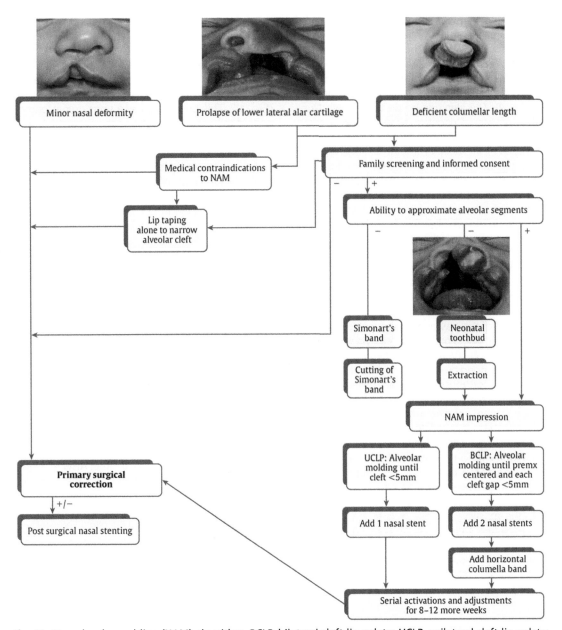

Fig. 11. Nasoalveolar molding (NAM) algorithm. BCLP, bilateral cleft lip palate; UCLP, unilateral cleft lip palate.

Grayson and colleagues[21] introduced the modern NAM appliance. This device combines the orthodontic device on the premaxilla and lateral alveolar segments with nasal stents. This appliance is secured with taping after fitting of the device to the maxilla with molding.

Objectives of Nasoalveolar Molding

The principle objectives of NAM therapy are reduction in the severity of the cleft deformity, which decreases the lip repair tension and potentially improves the nasal outcome.[14] When the

NAM therapy has brought the maxillary segments together, the nasal prongs can improve symmetry of the lower lateral alar cartilages, tissue expand the nasal mucosal lining, and bring the lip segments together. In the bilateral cleft, the columella is elongated, with the premaxilla centered retracted back to near the maxillary segments.[22]

Presurgical Nasoalveolar Molding Consultation

Parents are educated about weight gain goals, feeding, surgical timing, and the practical aspects of NAM. NAM requires time commitment, regular travel to a clinic, adjustment of tape, and awareness of problems. Parental compliance is a major factor in determining whether an infant will complete a NAM therapy protocol. The lip edges can be taped using Steri-strips after the first meeting (see **Fig. 2**). The skin can be protected with Duoderm (Convatee, Princeton, New Jersey).

If the parents and orthodontist agree to PSIO, the maxillary impression (mold) is taken so that the appliance can be fabricated. The infant is cradled in an inverted position to keep the tongue forward. We prefer for a nurse, orthodontist, and surgeon to be present in case the molding material becomes an airway obstruction. Using an acrylic resin impression tray, the appropriately sized tray is fit to the child's mouth to cover the maxillary arch but also remain inside the mouth. Polyvinyl siloxane is mixed and applied to the arch. During this entire process, the child's airway is monitored closely, watching for airway obstruction and need for removal of the tray and material.[12,23]

Once the impression is obtained, it is poured in a hard dental stone (Velmix, Kerr, Orange, CA). This design, developed by Grayson and Cutting is fabricated using orthodontic acrylic (Procryl; GAC, Bohemia, New York), which prevents pressure on the vomer and reduces irritation (**Fig. 12**).[14] The device is then secured to bilateral cheeks with surgical tape applied to elastic bands. The elastic bands loop over a retention button over the anterior portion of the plate (**Fig. 13**). Steps for NAM application can be seen in **Box 2**.

Appliance adjustments by the orthodontist will guide the maxillary segments until the cleft segments are less than or equal to 5 mm apart. At this point, the nasal prongs are added to the appliance. The stent is lined with soft silicone, which contacts the dome and extends the columella (**Fig. 14**).

In infants with bilateral clefts, the protruded premaxilla must be moved posteriorly and medially in addition to moving the lateral alveolar clefts medially. Once this is achieved, the nasal stents are added to the retention arms with a soft denture material added as a bridge between the 2 sides (**Fig. 15**). This bridge acts as a nonsurgical lengthener of the columella, defining the nasolabial junction. Gentle pressure applied to this area also works to lengthen the prolabium. This lengthening is thought to reduce the need for secondary columellar lengthening (V-Y of the upper lip into the columella).[22] A video of the placement of a NAM device is available in the supplemental materials (Video 1).

Gingivoperiosteoplasty and Nasoalveolar Molding

Skoog[24] has described gingivoperiosteoplasty (GPP) at the time of cleft lip repair in the literature in 1967 and later by Millard and Latham. The gingiva of the premaxillary and maxillary segments are sewn together, which may stimulate alveolar cleft bone continuity. NAM may bring these segments close enough together for closure, but critics suggest that maxillary growth may be inhibited by GPP. The decreased need for secondary alveolar bone grafting is a secondary benefit of NAM plus GPP.[25,26] With respect to cost effectiveness, the cost of the NAM plus the surgical time added for GPP was less costly than ABG at a later age. Also, NAM plus GPP reduced the need for ABG as the child grew 60% of the time.[27]

Evidence-Based Approach to Nasoalveolar Molding

There are vigorous arguments for and against PSIO at international cleft meetings. The long-term results of NAM therapy before primary

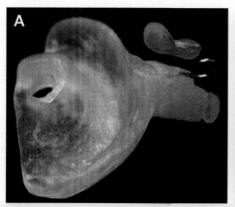
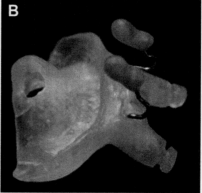

Fig. 12. Nasoalveolar molding appliance for (*A*) unilateral and (*B*) bilateral cleft lip. (*From* Goudy S, Tollefson TT, editors. Complete cleft care. New York: Thieme; 2015; with permission.)

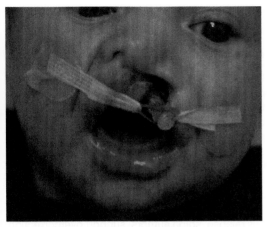

Fig. 13. Infant with maxillary appliance taped to cheeks (before nasal prongs being added).

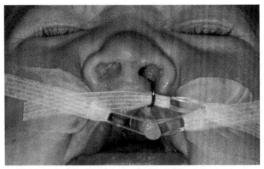

Fig. 14. Nasoalveolar molding appliance for an incomplete right cleft lip and complete unilateral cleft lip, which taped with nasal prong applying cephalad soft tissue expansion of the columella and nasal ala. (*From* Goudy S, Tollefson TT, editors. Complete cleft care. New York: Thieme; 2015; with permission.)

surgical repair remains controversial. In short, opponents to NAM suggest that (1) moving the maxillary segments may inhibit midface growth

---

Box 2
Nasoalveolar molding appliance therapy

- Retention of the oral appliance can be assisted by
  1. Denture adhesive,
  2. Increased angle of the Steri-strip tapes on to the cheek, and
  3. Orthodontic adjustment of the appliance buttons.
- Cleaning the appliance is best with mild soap and water without sterilization.
- The appliance should be adjusted to protect the maxillary frenum.
- Skin irritation is best managed by:
  1. Cheek protective tape (Duoderm sheets [ConvaTec, Princeton NJ]; position changed at least weekly after thorough drying);
  2. Moisturize the exposed cheek with Aquaphor–type product; and
  3. Consider a tape holiday and apply denture adhesive to appliance for retention.
- Appliance lengthening can prevent the infant from protruding the appliance with the tongue.
- Excess posterior appliance length may cause gagging.

Modified from Garfinkle JS, Kapadia H. Presurgical treatment. In: Goudy S, Tollefson TT, editors. Complete cleft care. New York: Thieme; 2015; with permission.

---

and dental arch shape and (2) that the nasal improvements have significant relapse. A 10% to 20% relapse rate is noted after NAM and unilateral cleft lip repair, specifically in nostril width and height in the first year.[28] Overcorrection of the cleft side nostril my counter this relapse.[16,29]

Some factors that influence this disagreement include the lack of clear objective outcome assessments, inconsistency of technique between cleft centers, and a moving threshold for what is considered successful.[12] Systematic reviews have been unable to identify negative impacts of PSIO (excluding NAM itself). However, the potential benefits were also unable to be supported owing to insufficient evidence, such as benefits on ultimate facial growth, maxillary form, dental occlusion, or speech. Potential secondary benefits of parental satisfaction or improvement in feeding were also not substantiated (level II evidence).[30,31]

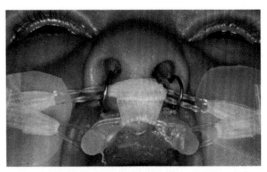

Fig. 15. Nasoalveolar molding appliance for an infant with bilateral cleft lip with a diminutive prolabium. Taping assists in redirecting forces on the columella and philtrum. (*From* Goudy S, Tollefson TT, editors. Complete cleft care. New York: Thieme; 2015; with permission.)

Abbott and Meara[32] presented a review in support of NAM's effectiveness on the nasal form in the unilateral cleft lip (level III evidence). They reviewed the evidence (levels II–V) and concluded that negative effects were not likely, whereas benefits for the bilateral cleft deformity were not demonstrated clearly. This is partially attributable to the paucity of well-designed, controlled outcomes assessments. Confounding variables in the existing studies are difficult to control, and include variable techniques of NAM and lip repair, cleft severity, and long duration of necessary follow-up needed. Future studies should include interdisciplinary, multiple sites, rigid inclusion criteria, and rigorous controls. The senior author currently uses NAM in both unilateral and bilateral cleft cases, while considering the social and economic effects on parents (eg, long distance from cleft center), parental compliance, and severity of cleft.[33,34]

PRIMARY CLEFT RHINOPLASTY

Primary rhinoplasty at the time of cleft lip repair is now a common practice among cleft surgeons since the 1970s. Although definitive rhinoplasty does not occur until nasal growth is achieved, primary rhinoplasty can minimize the severity of the deformity as well as reduce the number of revisions needed in adulthood.[35] Opponents rightly suggest that inappropriate rhinoplasty dissection can lead to disastrous scarring and stenosis, and should be avoided. The goals of the unilateral cleft lip primary rhinoplasty are to restore nasal tip symmetry and correct the nasal ala hooding. The bilateral cleft nasal deformity goals are to reduce alar flare, reconstruct the nasal sill, restore columellar length, correct the malposition of the lower lateral cartilages, and restore projection of the nasal tip.[11,36–39]

The senior author's primary rhinoplasty technique for unilateral or bilateral clefts have been described elsewhere in this article; general guidelines are to use existing lip incisions or a Tajima reverse U alar rim incisions. A conservative septoplasty may be performed. After repositioning of the nasal cartilages, nasal stents should be sized to the nostrils and not cause blanching of the nasal tip.[40]

The creation of a natural nasolabial relationship has been an area of controversy for some time in cleft lip repair. The senior author is in agreement with others who propose that the skin and soft tissue from the nostril can be rotated with NAM, primary rhinoplasty, and nostril stenting to create columellar height. In rare cases, columellar lengthening procedures that borrow tissue from the lip to lengthen the nose can be used (eg, forked flaps, or V-Y columellar advancement).

Outcomes

Ultimately, the proponents of primary cleft rhinoplasty site the improved cartilaginous and soft tissue changes, whereas opponents are swayed by the potential adverse effects on nasal growth, potential for nostril stenosis, loss of vascularity, and gradual relapse of surgical changes.[41] Studies investigating this relapse have demonstrated an increase in nostril width with maintenance of height, which gives the impression of tip collapse and relapse of cleft nasal deformity. To counter this relapse, some authors' support overcorrection of the nasal base width and nostril height deformities.[28] The senior author agrees that the nasal hooding should be slightly overcorrected, and the nasal base is best set at near proportional dimensions. An overly narrow alar base may cause nasal obstruction and is difficult to correct.[42]

SUMMARY

The surgeon who is fortunate enough to treat children with cleft lip–cleft palate greatly benefits from an interdisciplinary team approach. Presurgical preparation can make the surgical procedure more effective. Feeding and nursing support, lip taping, orthodontic care using NAM, and possible primary rhinoplasty at the time of lip repair are all implemented into the algorithms of major cleft centers. The key to understanding the most effective care is in comparative outcomes research, which should be supported.

ACKNOWLEDGMENTS

Video 1 was provided by Dr Richard Gere, DDS, UC Davis Cleft Team Orthodontist.

SUPPLEMENTARY DATA

Supplementary data related to this article can be found online at http://dx.doi.org/10.1016/j.fsc.2016.06.015.

REFERENCES

1. Wyszynski DF, Beaty TH, Maestri NE. Genetics of nonsyndromic oral clefts revisited. Cleft Palate Craniofac J 1996;33(5):406–17.
2. Tollefson TT, Shaye D, Durbin-Johnson B, et al. Cleft lip-cleft palate in Zimbabwe: estimating the distribution of the surgical burden of disease using geographic information systems. Laryngoscope 2015;125(Suppl 1):S1–14.

3. Tollefson TT, Sykes JM. Differences in brain structure related to laterality of cleft lip. Arch Facial Plast Surg 2010;12(6):431–2.

4. Tollefson TT, Humphrey CD, Larrabee WF Jr, et al. The spectrum of isolated congenital nasal deformities resembling the cleft lip nasal morphology. Arch Facial Plast Surg 2011;13(3):152–60.

5. Aburezq H, Daskalogiannakis J, Forrest C. Management of the prominent premaxilla in bilateral cleft lip and palate. Cleft Palate Craniofac J 2006;43(1):92–5.

6. Mulliken JB, Wu JK, Padwa BL. Repair of bilateral cleft lip: review, revisions, and reflections. J Craniofac Surg 2003;14(5):609–20.

7. Mulliken JB. Bilateral complete cleft lip and nasal deformity: an anthropometric analysis of staged to synchronous repair. Plast Reconstr Surg 1995;96(1):9–23 [discussion: 24–6].

8. Sitzman TJ, Girotto JA, Marcus JR. Current surgical practices in cleft care: unilateral cleft lip repair. Plast Reconstr Surg 2008;121(5):261e–70e.

9. Fisher DM. Unilateral cleft lip repair: an anatomical subunit approximation technique. Plast Reconstr Surg 2005;116:61–71.

10. Randall P. A triangular flap operation for the primary repair of unilateral clefts of the lip. Plast Reconstr Surg Transplant Bull 1959;23:331–47.

11. Chen PKT, Noordhoff MS. Bilateral cleft lip and nose repair. In: Losee JE, Kirschner RE, editors. Comprehensive cleft care. New York: McGraw-Hill; 2009. p. 331–42.

12. Garfinkle JS, Kapadia H. Presurgical treatment. In: Goudy S, Tollefson TT, editors. Complete cleft care. New York: Thieme; 2015. p. 10–20.

13. McNeil C. Orthodontic procedures in the treatment of congenital cleft palate. Dent Rec (London) 1950;72:126–32.

14. Grayson B, Cutting C. Presurgical nasoalveolar orthopedic molding in primary correction of the nose, lip, and alveolus of infants born with unilateral and bilateral clefts. Cleft Palate Craniofac J 2001;35:193–8.

15. Singh G, Moxham B, Langley M, et al. Changes in the composition of glycosaminoglycans during normal palatogenesis in the rat. Arch Oral Biol 1994;39:401–7.

16. Matsuo K, Hirose T. Preoperative nonsurgical overcorrection of cleft lip nasal deformity. Br J Plast Surg 1991;44:5–11.

17. Georgiade N, Latham R. Maxillary arch alignment in bilateral cleft lip and palate infant, using the pinned coaxial screw appliance. Plast Reconstr Surg 1975;56:52–60.

18. Georgiade N, Mladick R, Thorne F. Positioning of the premaxilla in bilateral cleft lips by oral pinning and traction. Plast Reconstr Surg 1968;41:240–3.

19. Millard D, Latham R. Improved primary surgical and dental treatment of clefts. Plast Reconstr Surg 1990;86:856–71.

20. Latham R. Orthodontic advancement of the cleft maxillary segment: a preliminary report. Cleft Palate J 1980;17:227–33.

21. Grayson B, Cutting C, Wood R. Preoperative columella lengthening in bilateral cleft lip and palate. Plast Reconstr Surg 1993;92:1422–3.

22. Grayson B, Maull D. Nasoalveolar molding for infants born with clefts of the lip, alveolus, and palate. Clin Plast Surg 2004;31:149–58.

23. Spengler A, Chavarria C, Teichgraeber J, et al. Presurgical nasoalveolar molding therapy for the treatment of bilateral cleft lip and palate: a preliminary study. Cleft Palate Craniofac J 2006;43:321–8.

24. Skoog T. The use of periosteum and Surgicel for bone restoration in congenital clefts of the maxilla. Scand J Plast Reconstr Surg 1967;1:113–30.

25. Santiago P, Grayson B, Cutting C, et al. Reduced need for alveolar bonegrafting by presurgical orthopedics and primary gingi-voperiosteoplasty. Cleft Palate Craniofac J 1998;35:77–80.

26. Wood R, Grayson B, Cutting C. Gingivoperiosteoplastyand midfacial growth. Cleft Palate Craniofac J 1997;34:17–20.

27. Pfeifer T, Grayson B, Cutting C. Nasoalveolar molding and gingivoperiosteoplasty versus alveolar bone graft: an outcome analysis of costs in the treatment of unilateral cleft alveolus. Cleft Palate Craniofac J 2002;39:26–9.

28. Liou E, Subramanian M, Chen P, et al. The progressive changes of nasal symmetry and growth after nasoalveolar molding: a three-year follow-up study. Plast Reconstr Surg 2004;114:858–64.

29. Pai B, Ko E, Huang C, et al. Symmetry of the nose after presurgical nasoalveolar molding in infants with unilateral cleft lip and palate: a preliminary study. Cleft Palate Craniofac J 2005;42:658–63.

30. de Ladeira PR, Alonso N. Protocols in cleft lip and palate treatment: systematic review. Plast Surg Int 2012;2012:562892.

31. Uzel A, Alparslan ZN. Long-term effects of presurgical infant orthopedics in patients with cleft lip and palate: a systematic review. Cleft Palate Craniofac J 2011;48(5):587–95.

32. Abbott MM, Meara JG. Nasoalveolar molding in cleft care: is it efficacious? Plast Reconstr Surg 2012;130(3):659–66.

33. Tollefson TT, Senders CW, Sykes JM. Changing perspectives in cleft lip and palate: from acrylic to allele. Arch Facial Plast Surg 2008;10(6):395–400.

34. Aminpour S, Tollefson TT. Recent advances in presurgical molding in cleft lip and palate. Curr Opin Otolaryngol Head Neck Surg 2008;16(4):339–46.

35. Bennum R, Perandones C, Sepliarsky V, et al. Nonsurgical correction of nasal deformity in

unilateral complete cleft lip: a 6-year follow-up. Plast Reconstr Surg 1999;104:616–30.

36. Mulliken JB. Mulliken repair of bilateral cleft lip and nasal deformity. In: Losee JE, Kirschner RE, editors. Comprehensive cleft care. New York: McGraw-Hill; 2009. p. 343–60.

37. Mulliken JB. Repair of bilateral cleft lip and its variants. Indian J Plast Surg 2009;42(Suppl): S79–90.

38. Mulliken JB. Primary repair of bilateral cleft lip and nasal deformity. Plast Reconstr Surg 2001;108: 181–94 [examination: 195].

39. Mulliken JB. Repair of bilateral complete cleft lip and nasal deformity: state of the art. Cleft Palate Craniofac J 2000;37:342–7.

40. Yeow VK, Chen PK, Chen YR, et al. The use of nasal splints in the primary management of unilateral cleft nasal deformity. Plast Reconstr Surg 1999;103: 1347–54.

41. Tollefson TT, Senders CW. Bilateral cleft lip. In: Goudy S, Tollefson TT, editors. Complete cleft care. New York: Thieme; 2015. p. 63–85.

42. Tollefson TT, Sykes JM. Unilateral cleft Lip. In: Goudy S, Tollefson TT, editors. Complete cleft care. New York: Thieme; 2015. p. 37–62.

Cleft Palate Repair, Gingivoperiosteoplasty, and Alveolar Bone Grafting

Ashley M. Dao, MD[a], Steven L. Goudy, MD[b],*

KEYWORDS

- Cleft palate • Cleft palate repair • Furlow palatoplasty • Gingivoperiosteoplasty
- Alveolar bone grafting

KEY POINTS

- A multidisciplinary approach is essential in providing the best care for patients with a cleft palate.
- The type and width of the cleft palate determine the appropriate surgical palatoplasty technique to adequately achieve a tension-free and multilayered closure with repositioning of the velar muscle sling.
- Intravelar veloplasty is a critical step during palatoplasty to ensure that children have proper velopharyngeal closure.
- Use of adjunctive surgical techniques and biologic materials can decrease the occurrence of fistula formation.

INTRODUCTION

The primary goal of cleft care is to optimize function and appearance while minimizing surgical interventions and complications. Although cleft palate usually is an isolated finding, greater than 30% may have additional comorbidities or an associated syndrome, which must be considered and may affect surgical candidacy, overall prognosis, and surgical outcomes. There are numerous surgical techniques that may be chosen based on cleft classification, cleft width, and surgeon experience and preference. Management and repair of the alveolar cleft is also an important aspect of care and secondary bone grafting is often required to treat alveolar defects. Primary gingivoperiosteoplasty (GPP) closes the alveolar cleft at the time of cleft lip repair, decreasing the likelihood for alveolar bone graft, although it has produced inconsistent results and is controversial. It is essential to recognize and address the emotional and psychological needs of the family, at birth and before surgical care. Overall, assessment and treatment of those with cleft lip and/or palate requires a multidisciplinary team approach.

Genetics and Prenatal Diagnosis

Cleft lip and/or palate is the most common congenital malformation of the head and neck and occurs in the setting of multiple genetic and environmental factors.[1] The condition is linked to more than 400 genes, occurs in an autosomal-dominant or autosomal-recessive or nonmendelian inheritance pattern, and most (70%) patients present without an associated syndrome.[2]

As genetic advances continue it is necessary to counsel expecting families on advanced

The authors have nothing to disclose.

[a] Department of Otolaryngology, Emory University School of Medicine, 550 Peachtree Street NE, 9th Floor MOT, Atlanta, GA 30308, USA; [b] Division of Pediatric Otolaryngology, Emory University School of Medicine, Children's Healthcare of Atlanta, 2015 Uppergate Drive, Atlanta, GA 30322, USA

* Corresponding author.

E-mail address: Steven.goudy@emory.edu

facialplastic.theclinics.com

diagnostic options available for future children. Ultrasound screening is routinely done in the first trimester to document viability, although the fetal face is typically not imaged adequately at this time. Three-dimensional ultrasound images of the face were first obtained in 1986 and became widely used in the mid-1990s, prenatally identifying many more cleft lip and palate patients. In 2000 this technology was used for multiplanar volume rendering[3] and the 2007 American Institute of Ultrasound in Medicine Guidelines for Prenatal Ultrasound Screening require the fetal face to be imaged in the second trimester. Addition of four-dimensional ultrasounds has improved accuracy, although diagnosing an isolated cleft palate remains difficult[4] and false-positives may occur because of shadowing.[5]

Classification

Multiple classification schemes have been created for orofacial clefts.[6] These models are usually based on several features of the cleft including laterality, completeness, severity (wide vs narrow), and presence of any abnormal tissue. Diminutive orofacial clefts may also be described as microform, occult, or minor.[7] Laterality is described as being either unilateral or bilateral. A complete cleft lip extends through the lip and the nasal sill and an incomplete cleft lip extends only through the lower part of the lip with some intact lip tissue above the cleft. The cleft alveolus can be considered complete or only notched. Weblike tissue may extend from the lip's cleft side to the noncleft side at the nasal sill, which is termed a Simonart band and is not equivalent to an incomplete cleft. A cleft palate is unilateral if one palatal shelf attaches to the nasal septum, or bilateral. The four group classification scheme introduced by Veau[8] is the most frequently used system:

- Group I: defect of the soft palate only.
- Group II: defect involves the soft palate and the hard palate to the incisive foramen.
- Group III: unilateral defect extending through the entire palate and alveolus.
- Group IV: bilateral complete cleft.

PATIENT ASSESSMENT
Multidisciplinary Care

A multidisciplinary approach should be used when addressing these patients to achieve optimal outcomes. The team includes initial evaluations by a pediatrician, geneticist, surgeon, feeding specialist, social worker, and possibly others. The children also need to be seen by audiology, otolaryngology, dental, oral surgery, and speech

pathology after the initial visit. Prenatal surgical consultation with the surgeon, geneticist, and speech pathologist before birth is recommended to alleviate some of the anxiety parents may be experiencing.

Surgical Assessment

A thorough physical examination is necessary soon after birth. This should include special attention to the upper lip, alveolar arches, nostrils, primary and secondary palates, nasal alar symmetry, tip projection, alar base position, and width, and any signs of dysmorphia that may lead to identification of additional congenital anomalies or syndromes. Any concern for cardiac or airway issues must be identified and assessed before surgical intervention. Specific evaluation for microform cleft lip and submucosal cleft palate, even considering ultrasound evaluation,[9,10] is important because their presentation is overlooked due to subtle findings on examination. Regular clinic visits after birth allow proper counseling and guidance to the patient's caretakers and the surgeon may need to place several referrals to any necessary specialists.

PRIMARY REPAIR OF CLEFT PALATE
Preoperative Planning and Considerations

The preoperative evaluation is the same as for a child with a cleft lip, although it is particularly important that the caretakers understand proper feeding methods. Cleft palate may also lead to airway obstruction, therefore any airway concerns must be addressed before surgery.[11] The type and width of the cleft must be accurately determined to select the appropriate surgical technique. Of note, patients with a submucous cleft palate may be closely monitored without intervention and only surgically repaired if they develop speech, feeding, or otologic difficulties.[12]

Timing of Repair

The customary timing of cleft palate repair is before 18 months, with the ideal time being 10 to 12 months of age[12] to avoid poor speech and language development associated with delayed repair. Early palate repair must be weighed against the concern of negatively affecting the patient's maxillary growth that may occur with an earlier repair.[13]

Patient Positioning

Positioning is similar for all techniques described next. The patient is placed supine on the operating table usually on a shoulder roll for gentle cervical extension, unless the patient has a syndrome associated with spinal abnormalities. Intubation is with either a standard endotracheal tube or a right angle endotracheal tube that is secured in the midline to the chin. Patients with midface hypoplasia and micrognathia may be difficult to intubate before surgery and experience postoperative airway obstruction; therefore, it is important for the surgical team to communicate concerns and discuss postoperative airway management. Tegaderms are used for eye protection. The surgical bed is rotated at least 90° from the anesthesiologist. Intravenous antibiotics are administered, surgical site is draped, a Dingman mouth retractor (**Fig. 1**) is used to achieve adequate visualization, and the palate is injected with 1% lidocaine with 1:100,000 epinephrine.

Surgical Techniques

The main principles of palatoplasty consist of a tension-free and multilayered closure with repositioning of the velar muscle sling. Several techniques along with modifications exist, and the most commonly performed options are described next.

Two-flap palatoplasty

The two-flap palatoplasty is a widely used technique that is indicated for the closure of complete unilateral and bilateral clefts of the primary and secondary palate. This technique permits easy exposure of the soft tissue musculature that allows release of anomalous attachments of the levator veli palatini to complete an intravelar veloplasty and reorient the levator sling horizontally. Incisions are marked from the tip of the uvula medially along the cleft margin toward midline of the alveolus. The alveolar ridge is then followed posteriorly to the end of the alveolus where a small releasing incision is made. When making the incision along the cleft margin medially it is important to stay 1 mm to 2 mm toward the oral mucosa to ensure a suitable mucosal flap for a tension-free nasal closure. After the incision is complete attention is turned to raising palatal flaps in a subperiosteal plane until there is complete exposure of the hard-soft palate junction, taking care to identify and preserve the greater palatine artery (**Fig. 2**). The greater palatine neurovascular bundle that supplies each flap is encountered and preserved while the foramina fascia should be released to assist with medial advancement of the flap. Osteotomies may also be made through the posterior foramina of the hard palate in significantly wide cleft palates (>20 mm) while meticulously avoiding injury to the bundle itself. Starting medially the abnormal levator muscle attachments are released from their attachment at the posterior edge of the hard palate and cleft margin. The nasal mucosa is also raised off of the superior surface of the hard palate and extended into the soft palate. Muscle fibers are released laterally until the hamulus and tensor veli palatini muscle are seen. One must check all flaps (nasal mucosa, musculature, and oral layer) for adequate length. Vomer flaps are elevated on one side only in a unilateral cleft palate but bilaterally in bilateral cleft palates to decrease the tension on the nasal layer closure.

The nasal layer of the uvula is then closed with horizontal mattress sutures using a 4–0 Vicryl on a TF needle. The remainder of the nasal layer is then closed with simple interrupted sutures using a 4–0 Vicryl on a PS-4c needle burying the knots on the nasal layer (**Fig. 3**). If there is excessive tension on the nasal closure, the central sutures are placed after the muscle layer is approximated to decrease tension. The levator muscle is sutured to create an intravelar veloplasty with a 3–0 Vicryl

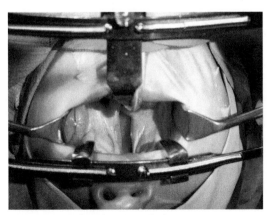

Fig. 1. View of cleft palate before incision using a Dingman mouth retractor.

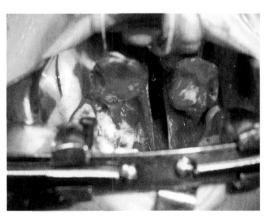

Fig. 2. Two-flap palatoplasty: raised palatal flaps in the subperiosteal plane with preserved greater palatine neurovascular bundles bilaterally.

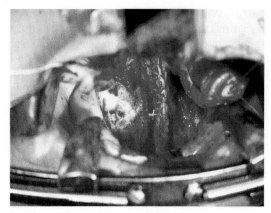

Fig. 3. Two-flap palatoplasty: closed nasal layer.

on an RB1 needle in an interrupted mattress fashion. Once the nasal layer and levator sling are closed, the oral layer is closed with simple interrupted sutures starting at the base of the uvula and moving anteriorly with 4–0 Vicryl on a TF needle. When the hard palate is reached a switch is made to horizontal mattress sutures and to capture some of the nasal mucosa to obliterate the dead space (**Fig. 4**). Once completely closed, hemostasis is achieved and microfibrillar collagen hemostatic agent is placed in the open defects laterally. If there is concern for airway obstruction, one may place a tongue traction stitch. Also, if the cleft is more than 2 cm acellular dermal matrix may be used between the nasal and oral layers at the junction of the soft palate and hard palate as reinforcement to reduce fistula formation.

Furlow double-opposing Z-palatoplasty

The Furlow palatoplasty involves transposing two opposing Z-plasties of the oral and nasal mucosal layers, respectively, with attached levator muscle.

This favorably changes the muscle fibers into a more anatomic position while lengthening the palate and retropositioning the levator sling.[14] This technique is primarily used for clefts isolated to the velum and submucous clefts, although some centers routinely incorporate this procedure with most cleft palate repairs. On the oral layer the mucosa is marked, incised, and the Z-plasty flaps are raised with a left posteriorly based myomucosal flap and a right anteriorly based thick mucosal flap (**Fig. 5**). The nasal layer then needs to have a left anteriorly based mucosal flap and a right posteriorly based myomucosal flap to create the opposing Z-plasty (**Fig. 6**). The nasal mucosal layer incisions should be made with surgical scissors.[15]

Closure is done with a 4–0 Vicryl on a PS-4c needle starting with the nasal layer. To avoid tension one may further release the flap segments with a back cut onto the hard palate. Once the nasal layer is closed (**Fig. 7**), the oral left myomucosal flap is rotated and secured with a 3–0 Vicryl through the levator muscle, and the rest of the oral layer is closed (**Fig. 8**). The uvula is approximated with a horizontal mattress suture. As with the two-flap palatoplasty, a tongue stitch may be used if there is concern for airway obstruction.

The Children's Hospital of Philadelphia modification of this technique involves bilateral relaxing incisions similar to the von Langenbeck method described next, which results in bipedicled mucoperiosteal flaps. The Z-plasty incisions are shortened to avoid intersection with the relaxing incisions. Also, the right anteriorly based mucosal flap has a more variable angle and length with its tip anterior to the uvula and base just posterior to the hamulus. It has been shown to facilitate a tension-free closure and decrease fistula rates while improving speech outcomes.[16]

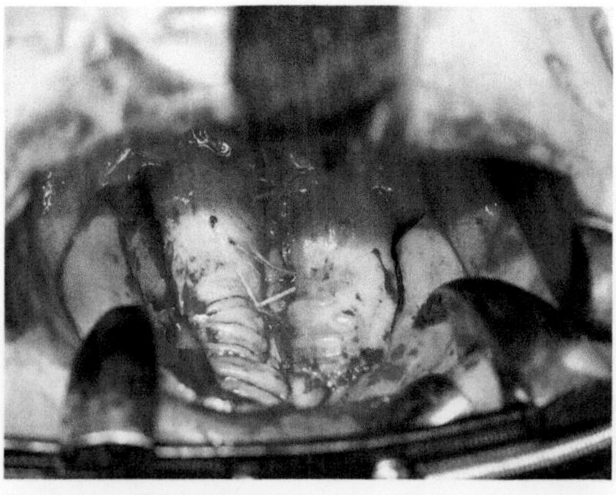

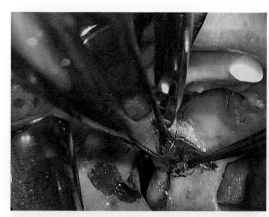

Fig. 4. Two-flap palatoplasty: view of closed oral layer of the hard palate. Horizontal mattress sutures that capture the nasal layer to obliterate dead space.

Fig. 5. Z-palatoplasty: incisions marked. Left posteriorly based myomucosal flap and a right anteriorly based thick mucosal flap.

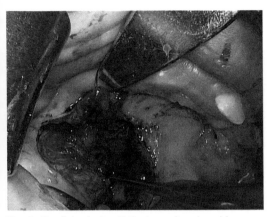

Fig. 6. Z-palatoplasty: distinct nasal and oral layers.

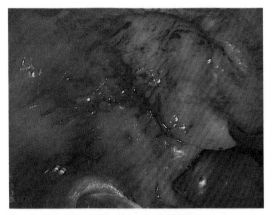

Fig. 8. Z-palatoplasty: closed oral layer.

Von Langenbeck palatoplasty

Von Langenbeck introduced the concept of lateral-releasing incisions to decrease tension. These incisions are made around the alveolar ridge and preserve anteriorly and posteriorly based flaps while sparing the gingiva laterally. The medial cleft edge incisions at the oral/nasal mucosa junction are carried posteriorly to the uvular apex. If necessary, vomer flaps may be designed and elevated to the skull base to compensate for short nasal flaps to ensure a tension-free closure. The hard palate flaps are elevated in a subperiosteal plane laterally to medially. As with previously described techniques, the greater palatine neurovascular bundles need to be identified and preserved. The subperiosteal dissection is carried along the lateral nasal wall to the undersurface of the inferior turbinate bilaterally. Nasal submucosal dissection is completed along the posterior edge of the hard palate, releasing the levator veli palatini from its insertion at the junction of the hard and soft palate.

Closure is done with a 4–0 Vicryl starting with the nasal layer in a simple interrupted fashion, incorporating vomer flaps anteriorly. The apex of the uvula is closed with a single horizontal mattress suture. Next, the intravelar veloplasty is completed. Interrupted or horizontal mattress sutures are used to reorient the levator veli palatini along the posterior velum to create the levator sling. Oral closure is then done with simple interrupted sutures using a 4–0 Vicryl working posteriorly to anteriorly. Finally, the relaxing incisions are stabilized with interrupted sutures through the medial gingival edge and microfibrillar collagen hemostatic agent is placed in the open defects laterally.

Oxford/three-flap technique

The Oxford/three-flap technique is used in incomplete clefts that extend into the hard palate, but do not penetrate the alveolar margin. The flaps are designed as described previously for a two-flap, except the incision is carried from the apex of the cleft to the lateral incisor on each side and then around the alveolar margin (**Fig. 9**). Two flaps are raised in a similar way as the two-flap technique (**Fig. 10**), but when the flaps are sewn together anteriorly, they are sewn to the remaining anterior mucosa, which is the third flap (**Figs. 11–13**).

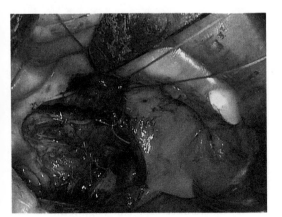

Fig. 7. Z-palatoplasty: closed nasal layer.

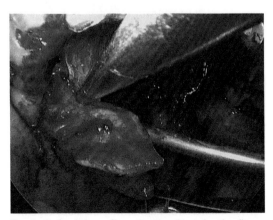

Fig. 9. Oxford/three-flap: starting to make the flaps.

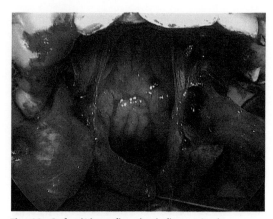

Fig. 10. Oxford/three-flap: both flaps raised.

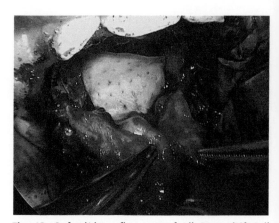

Fig. 12. Oxford/three-flap: use of AlloDerm (LifeCell Corporation, Bridgewater, NJ) between the nasal and oral layers.

Postprocedural Care

Primary goals in the postoperative period include preventing wound complications, providing adequate pain relief, and ensuring the patient is taking in satisfactory nutrition. Every child should stay as an inpatient for at least 1 night to monitor for airway obstruction and ability to tolerate oral intake. Arm restraints that prevent the child from putting their hands and fingers in their mouths should be used for 2 weeks. Bottle-feeding and straws should also be avoided. Antibiotics are prescribed for 1 week, and pain control is achieved with acetaminophen and ibuprofen. A follow-up appointment is scheduled in 3 weeks, and the family is told to call with any additional questions or concerns.

Outcomes/Potential Complications and Management

A successful cleft palate repair includes complete closure of the oral and nasal layers without fistula formation, velopharyngeal competence with

speech and feedings, minimal impact on facial growth, and improved eustachian tube function. Oronasal fistulas typically occur in up to 10% of cases and are usually located at the junction of the hard and soft palate. They may result in hypernasality, nasal emission, and nasal regurgitation. The factors that influence fistula formation all have an impact on the principles of wound closure and include forming robust tissue flaps, maintaining a tension-free closure, and creating a multilayered closure. Velopharyngeal insufficiency (VPI) may occur in up to one-fourth of patients and manifests as hypernasal speech, increased nasal resonance, nasal regurgitation, and nasal emission during phonation.[17] Because several surgical and nonsurgical treatment options exist for VPI[18] a multispecialty team composed of a speech-language pathologist, otolaryngologist, and prosthodontist could assist in choosing the most appropriate option. Of the surgical options listed previously, the Children's Hospital of Philadelphia modification of double-opposing Z-palatoplasty

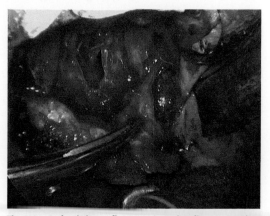

Fig. 11. Oxford/three-flap: sewing the flaps together starting posteriorly.

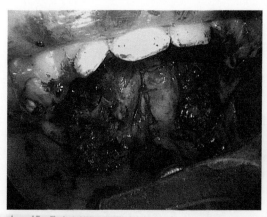

Fig. 13. Oxford/three-flap: oral flaps sewn to the anterior mucosa.

has been associated with low rates of VPI, with only 5.7% of patients demonstrating a clearly incompetent velopharyngeal mechanism.[16] Eustachian tube dysfunction affects nearly all cleft palate patients. It has been demonstrated that patients undergoing a multilayer closure with intravelar veloplasty have significantly improved speech and eustachian tube function outcomes than those undergoing a multilayer closure without the intravelar veloplasty.[19]

MANAGEMENT OF THE ALVEOLAR CLEFT

One of the most controversial topics in cleft care is the management of the alveolar cleft, specifically the indications for primary GPP. Alveolar clefts exist when there is deficient or absence of bone in the primary palate from the nasal sill to the incisive foramen. When an alveolar cleft is present one must weigh the risks and benefits of potentially sparing the patient an additional surgery against iatrogenic restriction of facial growth and malocclusion.

Gingivoperiosteoplasty

GPP has been described as a "boneless bone graft."[20] GPP encourages bone formation in an alveolar cleft through surgical repositioning of the mucosal edges. Goals of the procedure include bony continuity of the alveolar arch, improving alignment and stabilization of the anterior maxilla, nasal symmetry, closing oronasal fistulae, spontaneous eruption of permanent teeth within and next to the cleft, and avoidance of secondary bone grafting. In 1965, Skoog[20] was the first to describe this technique, which involves forming a mucoperiosteal bridge across the bridge to promote osseous formation within the subperiosteal tunnel. At that time the lingual and labial aspects of the cleft were approximated with a large transpositioned flap from a widely undermined maxillary periosteum, which unfortunately subjected the patient to possible iatrogenic facial growth restriction because of extensive subperiosteal dissection. Since then presurgical infant orthopedics and nasoalveolar molding have been used to narrow the cleft and improve alignment of the alveolar segments before surgical repair.

Furthermore, GPP may be broken down into direct and indirect approaches. A direct approach involves using adjacent gingiva, which requires a relatively narrow cleft. Alternatively, during an indirect approach a distant periosteal flap is used as previously described. Current data on the use of nasoalveolar molding/GPP are favorable, although long-term outcome studies are required.[21] Prerequisites for a GPP include appropriate cleft anatomy to allow alveolar bony approximation, an optimally molded alveolar cleft and intact mucosa, and no dental eruption. Once these criteria are met, the GPP can usually be scheduled at the time of the primary lip repair, often between 3 and 5 months. Isolated clefts of the primary palate are often not ideal candidates because the alveolar segments of the primary palate are more resistant to parallel presurgical molding. Also in bilateral clefts, consideration is made as to close both or one alveolar cleft at a time to prevent devascularization of the premaxilla.

Alveolar Bone Grafting

Introduction

The initial descriptions of alveolar bone grafting date back to the start of the twentieth century[22] and the most commonly used procedure today was described in 1972 by Boyne and Sands.[23] The goals of alveolar cleft repair include closing nasolabial/palatal fistulae using local mucoperiosteal flaps, restoring maxillary arch continuity, including stabilization of premaxilla in bilateral clefts with cleft bone grafting, providing bone and support for teeth near the cleft, supporting the nasal ala, and providing bone for dental implants.

Timing

Timing of alveolar cleft repair should aim at minimizing the adverse effects that early repair (<5–6 years old) may have on maxillary growth and avoiding grafting delay until the canine starts to erupt (>10–12 years old). Timing of repair may be classified as primary, early secondary, secondary, and late. Primary alveolar grafting is done before age 2 and is usually done with the primary lip repair typically with a bone graft harvest from the rib. Advantages include early stabilization of the alveolar segments and improved arch form, although midface growth disturbances have led to abandonment of primary grafting in several cleft centers.[24] Early secondary alveolar grafting falls between 2 and 5 years of age using autogenous bone graft typically from the hip. It has been found that 75% to 90% of maxillary adult dimensions are achieved by age 5. Therefore, it is possible that maxillary growth would not be significantly altered if grafting was performed at that time.[25] Secondary alveolar grafting is done between ages 5 and 13 and specific timing is usually based on dental eruption. Several cleft centers repair between 6 and 10 years of age after orthodontic preparation and maxillary expansion have been completed based on the historical recommendation to proceed with repair once the permanent canine root is one-half to two-thirds formed. This concept fails to consider the development and position of the permanent incisor, which is often fully erupted by 7 or 8 years of age and may therefore have compromised periodontal support. Vertical alveolar bone height after grafting is determined by the alveolar bone height of this adjacent incisor, and bone height is only optimized if grafting is completed before completion of the incisor eruption. Preservation of alveolar bone height not only improves function and health of future teeth and implants, but also improves overall cosmesis.[26] Timing within this age range may also be influenced by the eruption of the maxillary permanent first molar, which usually occurs between 6 and 7 years of age. Because many clefts require palatal expansion before repair the presence of this first molar allows an orthodontist to place the palatal expansion device. Finally, late alveolar grafting is done after 13 years of age because this is associated with a greater risk of complications, such as infection, wound breakdown, and graft loss.[27] With all factors considered optimal cleft repair is usually done between the ages of 5 and 7.

Patient evaluation

The patient evaluation should start with a well-documented history of all prior cleft surgeries and thorough physical examination, which includes taking note of all dentition adjacent to and within the cleft along with the size of the cleft and fistulae present. It is important to also appreciate dental arch form, degree of arch collapse, crossbite malocclusion, and position of the premaxilla in a bilateral cleft. Imaging is essential and typically a panoramic radiograph is satisfactory. A medical-grade computed tomography is not recommended in children at the optimal age for alveolar cleft repair given the higher radiation exposure, although cone beam computed tomography is becoming popular. Mobile primary teeth, exposed supernumerary teeth, and exposed permanent lateral incisors should all be removed 6 to 8 weeks before repair because their presence may make palatal closing difficult or impossible. Palatal expansion devices that contact the palate should be removed 3 to 4 weeks before repair to allow resolution of any palatal inflammation if it is present. Expansion may be maintained with a removable device to allow proper oral hygiene and cleaning.

Presurgical orthodontic preparation

The goal of presurgical orthodontic preparation is palatal expansion to improve dental arch relationships before grafting and surgical access to the alveolar cleft itself. Expansion may also reduce

crossbite and improve access during closure of the nasal floor. The degree of expansion should be limited in those with a bilateral cleft and a large palatal fistula. It normally occurs over a time period of 4 to 6 months[28] and the device should be left in place for 3 additional months after the grafting has been completed during grafting consolidation. Presurgical expansion is typically preferred, although postsurgical expansion also is an option, especially with bilateral clefts to allow greater ease of closure of the palatal mucosa. In these cases, grafting consolidation is allowed for 8 weeks before use of the expansion appliance. There is belief among some that postsurgical expansion places the grafting site under a dynamic load during healing, which may lead to improved bone consolidation.[29]

Surgical technique

Repair of the alveolar cleft involves closure of the oronasal fistula and reconstruction of the alveolus with bone graft between the nasal and oral layers. Complete coverage of the graft is critical to its overall success and is achieved by advancing a keratinized buccal mucoperiosteal flap from the lesser maxillary segment on the cleft side. The anticipated bone height is only as high as the alveolar bone level of the patient's adjacent teeth. Bone graft beyond this point leads to unnecessary increased tension on the closure and does not result in additional alveolar bone height. The gold standard involves using an autogenous graft usually harvested from the anterior iliac crest. Autogenous bone offers several advantages over other options, such as osteogenic activity and osteoinductive capability given the presence of viable cells and growth factors while not causing an immunologic reaction. Downsides involve the donor site morbidity and increased operative time. Calvarial bone has been advocated in the past, although it has been shown to have a decreased success rate when compared with the iliac crest (80% vs 93%).[30]

Alternative bone graft products

There are several alternative bone graft products one may use including allogenic, alloplastic, and most recently bone morphogenetic proteins (BMP). Allogenic bone from a cadaveric source has no osteogenic properties, although results have been comparable with autogenous bone.[31] Allogenic bone may also be mixed with autogenous bone to enhance the graft volume in large clefts, which may spare the patient bilateral iliac crest harvesting. Recombinant human BMP is an emerging alternative that is involved in maintenance of the mature skeleton. Three BMPs have the ability to independently induce bone formation,[32] although the oncogenic potential and severe inflammatory response in select populations remains unknown therefore limiting its widespread use. BMP does not have Food and Drug Administration approval for the age group most likely to undergo alveolar cleft grafting because of possibilities of uncertain effects on the immature skeleton, influence on developing dentition, or role in malignant tumor formation.[33] Currently BMP may play a role in the skeletally mature patient but is not approved for use in the typical skeletally immature cleft patient.

Complications

The most common complication after alveolar cleft grafting is mucosal wound dehiscence, which occurs in 1% of prepubertal children[34] and this percentage increases with age.[35] This may lead to a persistent fistula. In general, with good surgical technique and appropriate timing wound breakdown should be rare. Graft loss that requires repeat grafting is also unusual, although more common in the adolescent and young adult. Finally, failure of canine eruption through the grafted alveolus may require surgical exposure and ligation in approximately 1% of cases.[34]

SUMMARY

Appropriate selection, evaluation, management, preparation, and education done by a multidisciplinary team are all essential when caring for a patient with orofacial clefting. Associated congenital anomalies, developmental delay, neurologic conditions, and psychological needs must be recognized and addressed. Because of morphologic variability of various cleft types there are several options for the surgical team to choose from as previously described. Despite the technique used, a multilayer, tension-free closure with velar sling restoration remains the fundamental goal of surgical correction. Presence of an alveolar cleft offers an additional challenge with various management and treatment options. GPP remains controversial and has the attraction of an inductive surgical procedure that provides an opportunity for improving form and function early in life while potentially sparing additional surgery, although the concern of iatrogenic facial growth restriction remains. Alveolar bone grafting also has several considerations including timing, material used, consideration of dentition, and the use of presurgical expansion devices. Overall there are a multitude of factors to consider and decisions to make, which requires a large team of approach when providing care to patients with orofacial clefting.

REFERENCES

1. Genisca AE, Frias JL, Broussard CS, et al, National Birth Defects Prevention Study. Orofacial Clefts in the National Birth Defects Prevention Study, 1997-2004. Am J Med Genet A 2009;149A(6):1149–58.

2. Schutte BC, Murray JC. The many faces and factors of orofacial clefts. Hum Mol Genet 1999;8(10):1853–9.

3. Marginean C, Brinzaniuc K, Muhlfay G, et al. The three-dimensional ultrasonography of the fetal face: history and progress. Rev Med Chir Soc Med Nat Iasi 2010;114(4):1058–63.

4. Ramos GA, Romine LE, Gindes L, et al. Evaluation of the fetal secondary palate by 3-dimensional ultrasonography. J Ultrasound Med 2010;29(3):357–64.

5. Demircioglu M, Kangesu L, Ismail A, et al. Increasing accuracy of antenatal ultrasound diagnosis of cleft lip with or without cleft palate, in cases referred to the North Thames London Region. Ultrasound Obstet Gynecol 2008;31(6):647–51.

6. Tessier P. Anatomical classification facial, craniofacial and latero-facial clefts. J Maxillofac Surg 1976;4:69–92.

7. Mulliken JB. Double unilimb Z-plastic repair of microform cleft lip. Plast Reconstr Surg 2005;116:1623.

8. Veau V. Bec-de-Lievre. Formes Cliniques-Chirurgie. Avec la collaboration de J Recamier. Paris: Masson et Cie; 1938.

9. Meier JD, Banks CA, White DR. Ultrasound imaging to identify occult submucous cleft palate. Otolaryngol Head Neck Surg 2011;145:249–50.

10. Weinberg SM, Brandon CA, McHenry TH, et al. Rethinking isolated cleft palate: Evidence of occult lip defects in a subset of cases. Am J Med Genet A 2008;146A(13):1670–5.

11. Antony AK, Sloan GM. Airway obstruction following palatoplasty: analysis of 247 consecutive operations. Cleft Palate Craniofac J 2002;39:145–8.

12. American Cleft Palate-Craniofacial Association. Standards for cleft palate and craniofacial teams. Available at: http://acpa-cpf.org/team_care/standards/. Accessed January 13, 2016.

13. Liao YF, Mars M. Hard palate repair timing and facial growth in cleft lip and palate: systematic review. Cleft Palate Craniofac J 2006;43:563–70.

14. Pet MA, Marty-Grames L, Blount-Stahl M, et al. The Furlow palatoplasty for velopharyngeal dysfunction: velopharyngeal changes, speech improvements, and where they intersect. Cleft Palate Craniofac J 2015;52(1):12–22.

15. Furlow LT. Cleft palate repair done by opposing Z-plasty. Plast Reconstr Surg 1986;78:724–36.

16. LaRossa D, Jackson OH, Kirschner RE, et al. The Children's Hospital of Philadelphia modification of the Furlow double-opposing z-palatoplasty: long

term speech and growth results. Clin Plast Surg 2004;31(2):243–9.

17. Woo AS. Velopharyngeal dysfunction. Semin Plast Surg 2012;26:170–7.

18. Ruda JM, Krakovitz P, Rose AS. A review of the evaluation and management of velopharyngeal insufficiency in children. Otolaryngol Clin North Am 2012;45:653–69.

19. Hassan ME, Askar S. Does palatal muscle reconstruction affect the functional outcome of cleft palate surgery? Plast Reconstr Surg 2007;119(6):1859–65.

20. Skoog T. The use of periosteal flaps in the repair of clefts of the primary palate. Cleft Palate J 1965;2: 332–9.

21. Hopper RA, Al-Mufarrej F. Gingivoperiosteoplasty. Clin Plast Surg 2014;41(2):233–40.

22. Kazemi A, Stearns JW, Fonseca RJ. Secondary grafting in the alveolar cleft patient. Oral Maxillofac Surg Clin North Am 2002;14(4):477–90.

23. Boyne PJ, Sands NR. Secondary bone grafting of residual alveolar and palatal clefts. J Oral Surg 1972;30(2):87–92.

24. Brattstrom V, McWilliam J. The influence of bone grafting age on dental abnormalities and alveolar bone height in patients with unilateral cleft lip and palate. Eur J Orthod 1989;11(4):351–8.

25. Laowansiri U, Behrents RG, Araujo E, et al. Maxillary growth and maturation during infancy and early childhood. Angle Orthod 2013;83(4):563–71.

26. Enemark H, Sindet-Pedersen S, Bundgaard M. Long-term results after secondary bone grafting of alveolar clefts. J Oral Maxillofac Surg 1987;45(11): 913–9.

27. Trinade-Suedam IK, Da Silva Filho OG, Carvalho RM, et al. Timing of alveolar bone grafting determines different outcomes inpatients with unilateral cleft palate. J Craniofac Surg 2012;23(5): 1283–6.

28. Daw JL Jr, Patel PK. Management of alveolar clefts. Clin Plast Surg 2004;31(2):303–13.

29. Boyne PJ. Bone grafting in the osseous reconstruction of alveolar and palatal clefts. Oral Maxillofac Surg Clin North Am 1991;3(3):589–97.

30. Sadove AM, Nelson CL, Eppley BL, et al. An evaluation of calvarial and iliac donor sites in alveolar cleft grafting. Cleft Palate J 1990;27(3):225–8 [discussion: 229].

31. Maxson BB, Baxter SD, Vig KW, et al. Allogenic bone for secondary alveolar cleft osteoplasty. J Oral Maxillofac Surg 1990;48(9):933–41.

32. Termaat MF, Den Boer FC, Bakker FC, et al. Bone morphogenetic proteins. Development and clinical efficacy in the treatment of fractures and bone defects. J Bone Joint Surg Am 2005;87(6):1367–78.

33. Woo EJ. Adverse events reported after the use of recombinant human bone morphogenetic protein 2. J Oral Maxillofac Surg 2012;70(4):765–7.

34. Hall HD, Werther JR. Conventional alveolar bone grafting. Oral Maxillofac Surg Clin North Am 1991; 3(3):609–16.

35. Dickinson BP, Ashley RK, Wasson KL, et al. Reduced morbidity and improved healing with bone morphogenic protein-2 in older patients with alveolar cleft defects. Plast Reconstr Surg 2008; 121(1):209–17.

Velopharyngeal Dysfunction Evaluation and Treatment

Jeremy D. Meier, MD, Harlan R. Muntz, MD*

KEYWORDS

- Velopharyngeal dysfunction • Hypernasality • Speech endoscopy • Sphincter pharyngoplasty
- Pharyngeal flap • Double-opposing Z-plasty

KEY POINTS

- Perceptual speech analysis and nasal endoscopy are essential for the evaluation of children with velopharyngeal dysfunction.
- The double-opposing Z-plasty technique reorients the levator veli palatini muscle fibers and lengthens the palate, and may be the ideal approach to children with a cleft of the soft palate, a submucous cleft palate, or a shortened palate with a small velopharyngeal gap.
- The sphincter pharyngoplasty creates a dynamic flap that is preferred for patients with a coronal or circular closure pattern. With a large velopharyngeal gap, this can be used in combination with the double-opposing Z-plasty.
- The pharyngeal flap operation can be used to obturate a large velopharyngeal port in patients with sagittal closure.

INTRODUCTION

All sounds in the English language, other than /n/, /m/, and /ng/, are produced via oral airflow. Normal speech, therefore, relies on appropriate closure of the velopharyngeal port. Inadequate closure of the velopharynx during speech production results in velopharyngeal dysfunction (VPD). VPD can arise from structural, neurogenic, or iatrogenic causes. This article reviews the normal functional anatomy of the velopharynx, discusses the evaluation of children with VPD, and outlines treatment options for children with VPD.

VELOPHARYNGEAL ANATOMY

Velopharyngeal closure during speech occurs through the action of several muscles. The levator veli palatini, innervated by the pharyngeal plexus, provides the main muscle mass to the velum.[1] This muscle arises from the inferior surface of the petrous temporal bone and the cartilaginous eustachian tube. The muscle fibers fan out within the soft palate to interdigitate with the contralateral levator veli palatini muscle. The levator veli palatini functions as a sling to pull the velum in a posterosuperior direction. The tensor veli palatini, innervated by cranial nerve V, originates from the medial pterygoid plate, spine of the sphenoid, and eustachian tube. This muscle's tendon wraps around the hamular process and functions to tense and stabilize the soft palate while also opening and closing the eustachian tube. The musculus uvulae serve to add bulk to the dorsal surface of the soft palate and assist in elevating the uvula.[2] The palatoglossus and palatopharyngeus muscles constrict the anterior and posterior tonsillar pillars, respectively. The action of the palatopharyngeus

Division of Otolaryngology, University of Utah School of Medicine, 50 North Medical Drive, Room 3C120 SOM, Salt Lake City, UT 84132, USA
* Corresponding author.
E-mail address: Harlan.muntz@imail.org

Facial Plast Surg Clin N Am 24 (2016) 477–485
http://dx.doi.org/10.1016/j.fsc.2016.06.016

muscle stretches the velum laterally to increase the velar area.[3] The uppermost fibers of the superior pharyngeal constrictor muscle contribute to lateral and posterior pharyngeal wall movement, helping to narrow the velopharyngeal port.

CAUSES OF VELOPHARYNGEAL DYSFUNCTION

VPD includes an array of disorders and often confusing nomenclature has been used to distinguish the origin. Historically, velopharyngeal insufficiency includes any structural defect, such as a cleft palate, that results in insufficient tissue to achieve velopharyngeal closure.[4] Velopharyngeal incompetence represents causes related to neurologic dysfunction or impaired motor control. To simplify, VPD can result from anatomic or neuromuscular causes.

Anatomic
- Cleft palate
- Submucous cleft palate
- Palatal fistula
- Short palate
- Tonsillar hypertrophy or other condition tethering the palate
- Previous adenoidectomy

Neuromuscular
- Acute neurovascular injury (stroke)
- Intracranial process (brain tumor)
- Neurologic deterioration of pharyngeal plexus (amyotrophic lateral sclerosis, Parkinson disease, cerebral palsy, Moebius syndrome)
- Tumor of cranial nerve

EVALUATION OF VELOPHARYNGEAL DYSFUNCTION

The initial evaluation of any child with possible VPD includes a complete history and physical examination. The onset when symptoms were noted, any exacerbating factors, and severity of speech difficulty along with family members' perceptions can help with the initial assessment. In a patient with a history of cleft lip or palate, understanding the technique used to repair the cleft is essential. Asking about any additional pharyngeal procedures, particularly adenoidectomy and/or tonsillectomy, is imperative.

Early in the examination, an informal perceptual speech evaluation can be obtained if the examiner can successfully get the patient talking. If the child is shy or will not communicate in the presence of the physician, the parents may have a recording of their child speaking that can be used to assess speech. Evaluating the length and the mobility of the palate, palpating for a notch at the hard and soft palate junction, and using a mirror to detect fogging with non-nasal sounds are all important aspects of the physical examination.

VPD significantly affects both the child's and the family's quality of life. The Velopharyngeal Incompetence Effects on Life Outcomes (VELO) survey measures speech problems, swallowing problems, situational difficulty, perception by others, emotional impact, and caregiver impact and has been validated as an effective measure of quality of life for children with VPD.[5]

Perceptual Speech Analysis

A formal speech evaluation by an experienced speech-language pathologist is essential for any child with suspected VPD. Language level, articulation, resonance, and the absence or presence of nasal airway emissions are all important aspects of the examination. Nasalized consonants include /m/, /n/, and /ng/, whereas all other consonants and most vowels in the English language are non-nasal. Fogging of a mirror under the nostril can confirm normal air escape with nasal sounds or abnormal air escape with non-nasal sounds. Speech analysis evaluates for evidence of hypernasal resonance, nasal emissions, and nasal turbulence. Facial grimacing during speech may be a clue to the presence of VPD as patients narrow the external nares to decrease nasal airflow.[6] Fogging of a mirror under the nostril during the production of non-nasal speech also suggests abnormal air escape.

Nasometry

Nasometry assesses nasal resonance during speech by measuring the ratio of sound intensity between the mouth and the nose. Nasometry provides objective measurements that help in the initial evaluation and also provide feedback after therapy and surgical intervention.[7] During this test, focus must be placed on appropriately articulated phonemes. Standardized scores for specific phonemic sets exist, and the degree of nasalance can be estimated by calculating the number of standard deviations away from normative values. However, discrepancies in the severity of hypernasality may exist between nasometry scores and the perceptual speech analysis.[8]

Speech Endoscopy

Speech endoscopy is a critical component of any child being considered for VPD surgery.[9–11] Ideally, the procedure is performed with both a physician and speech-language pathologist present. The flexible endoscope should be passed through the nose in the middle meatus region rather than along the floor of the nose so that the endoscope is positioned higher in the naso-pharynx, thereby avoiding parallax or fish-eye distortion views.[4] The patient then repeats a series of words, phrases, or sentences while the velo-pharynx is visualized. The closure pattern of the velopharynx (coronal, sagittal, circular, or circular with Passavant ridge contribution) and the size of velopharyngeal gap remaining during non-nasal speech are assessed. These findings can be used by the surgeon to tailor the appropriate surgi-cal procedure for the patient's needs.

Speech Videofluoroscopy

In speech videofluoroscopy, a small amount of barium is placed in the nose to coat the velophar-ynx. The child repeats a set of phoneme-specific speech tasks while fluoroscopic images are recorded. Many centers no longer use speech vid-eofluoroscopy because of limitations, including ra-diation exposure and the need for multiple views because of the two-dimensional images obtained.

MRI

MRI has recently been investigated as a tool for assessing VPD.[12–14] MRI avoids ionizing radiation and may be useful in uncooperative children. How-ever, cost and the inability to correlate dynamic velopharyngeal function with speech limit its prac-tical application.

TREATMENT
Nonsurgical Treatment

Speech therapy
A speech-language pathologist experienced in the management of children with VPD is essential. Speech therapy alone may be appropriate for children with mild VPD who show improvement af-ter appropriate stimulation, phoneme-specific or intermittent VPD, or VPD with significant articula-tion issues. A time-limited trial of speech therapy is reasonable to consider in many children with VPD. However, in some children, therapy has no chance to cure the problem and surgical interven-tion should not be delayed. Postsurgical therapy is almost always necessary, often to overcome mal-adaptive articulation errors that developed before surgical intervention.

Prosthesis
In some cases the use of a prosthesis may be indi-cated to allow normalization of speech. Prosthe-ses are commonly used in adults after palatal resection for tumor. The use of a palatal lift or obturator may be advantageous in children who have failed surgical intervention or who are at sig-nificant risk of extreme airway obstruction if surgi-cal means are used for VPD. The prosthesis may be removed for sleep, allowing a better airway. If there is adequate palatal length, a palatal lift pros-thesis or obturator may be used. If it is thought that the palate is too short, the lift is often not the ideal prosthesis and an obturator should be considered. Fabrication requires a prosthodontist with experi-ence in maxillary prostheses. The size may be esti-mated and the final fit may be done with flexible endoscopy to help define any gaps in the obtura-tion. Using the mobility of each of the walls of the velopharyngeal port may allow nasal respiration at the same time as improved speech and eating. The prosthesis is attached to stable teeth, so it is not used in mixed dentition or during active ortho-dontia. However, this restriction alone limits its util-ity in most of the pediatric population.

Surgical Treatment

The optimal surgical approach is uniquely tailored to the individual and dependent on what is found in the preoperative assessment. Each approach has distinct advantages and potential disadvantages and the recommended option for one patient may not be ideal for another. It is imperative that surgeons managing VPD become facile with all techniques so that the appropriate procedure can be performed when indicated. A review of the commonly used techniques for each proce-dure is presented later.

Double-opposing Z-plasty palatoplasty
The double-opposing Z-plasty for primary palato-plasty was first described by Leonard Furlow[15] in 1986. This procedure transposes the sagittally ori-ented levator palatini muscle fibers into a more anatomic transverse direction while lengthening the palate and narrowing the nasopharyngeal port.[16] Typically, with right-handed surgeons, a posteriorly based oral myomucosal flap is elevated on the patient's left palate (**Fig. 1**). The flap begins laterally at the hook of the hamulus and extends anteromedially to the midline just posterior to the hard-soft palate junction. An anteriorly based oral mucosa flap is elevated on the right side beginning from the base of the uvula medially and extending posterolaterally to the hook of the hamulus. Nasal mucosal flaps are elevated as mirror images of the oral flaps with the lateral incisions extending near the eustachian tube bilaterally. Closure is accom-plished by rotating the left nasal mucosal flap across the midline and suturing the flap to the right hard palate. The right nasal myomucosal flap is rotated so that the levator muscle is oriented in

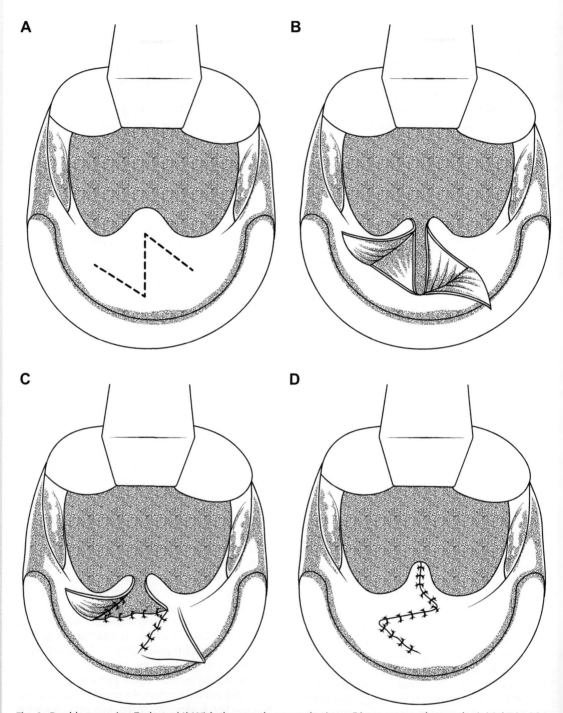

Fig. 1. Double-opposing Z-plasty. (*A*) With the mouth exposed using a Dingman mouth gag, the initial Z incision is marked out on the soft palate and the palate injected with topical anesthetic and epinephrine for hemostasis. (*B*) Typically, with right-handed surgeons, a posteriorly based oral myomucosal flap is elevated on the left and an anteriorly based oral mucosa-only flap is raised on the right. Opposing incisions in the deep layers are marked with the straight line. (*C*) The left nasal mucosal flap is rotated and sutured to the posterior edge of the right hard palate. The right nasal myomucosal flap is rotated to transversely reorient the levator palatini muscle and sutured to the posterior edge of the left nasal mucosal flap. (*D*) The right oral mucosal flap is rotated and sutured to the free oral mucosa along the original incision line. The right oral myomucosal flap is rotated to again reorient the levator fibers and the uvula is reapproximated.

the transverse plane and sutured to the posterior edge of the left nasal mucosal flap anteriorly and the free margin of the left soft palate posteriorly. The right oral mucosal flap is rotated and sutured to the posterior edge of the left hard palate and the left myomucosal flap is rotated to again orient the muscle fibers in the horizontal plane. The uvula is reapproximated.

Double-opposing Z-plasty is the ideal procedure for children with VPD in the following situations:

1. Unrepaired soft palate cleft
2. Submucous cleft palate
3. Noncleft child with a sagittal closure pattern with a shortened palate or decreased palatal elevation

In patients with a history of double-opposing Z-plasty at the time of palatoplasty and minimal residual VPD, redo double-opposing Z-plasty is a viable option. Although repeating the technique could disrupt the levator sling, velopharyngeal function improved in a series of 13 patients with this approach.[17] Much debate remains regarding the ideal technique to repair the soft palate at the time of primary palatoplasty. A systematic review compared speech outcomes and fistula rates between the double-opposing Z-plasty and straight-line intravelar veloplasty (IVPP). No difference in oronasal fistula rates was identified (7.87% in double-opposing Z-plasty compared with 9.81% in IVPP). However, in patients with unilateral cleft lip and palate, those who underwent straight-line closure were 1.64 times more likely to undergo a secondary procedure than those who underwent double-opposing Z-plasty.[18] Although intravelar veloplasty may be appropriate in some patients, more surgeons are turning to double-opposing Z-plasty at the time of initial palate repair.

Sphincter pharyngoplasty

Sphincter pharyngoplasty is a commonly used procedure for VPD,[19,20] and the ideal technique for patients with a coronal or circular closure pattern. This procedure is thought to have a decreased risk of postoperative airway obstruction compared with a pharyngeal flap[4] and theoretically creates a dynamic flap. Sphincter pharyngoplasty is performed by rotating superiorly based myomucosal flaps containing lateral and posterior pharyngeal wall mucosa with the underlying palatopharyngeus and pharyngeal constrictor muscles (**Fig. 2**). A horizontal incision through the posterior pharyngeal wall connects the medial vertical incisions of each flap. The flaps are then rotated and sutured into the posterior

pharyngeal wall. The more superior the flaps and horizontal incision can be made, the better. Slight nuances to this technique include not extending the lateral incision as superiorly as the medial incision, allowing the flap rotation to help narrow the velopharyngeal port laterally. The inferior edges of the flaps can be sutured together in the midline, or 1 flap can be sewn to the superior edge of the horizontal incision and the other flap secured to the inferior border of the horizontal incision. Previously removing the adenoids can allow for easier inset and attachment of the flap in the nasopharynx. The width of the flaps is based on the amount of palatal motion identified in the preoperative assessment as well as the size of the residual nasopharyngeal gap. Wider flaps with greater overlap are used if the port needs to be significantly narrowed. If the velopharyngeal gap is large, the sphincter pharyngoplasty can be performed in conjunction with the double-opposing Z-plasty.

Pharyngeal flap

The pharyngeal flap has historically been the workhorse operation for treatment of VPD.[21–24] This technique is appropriate for patients with poor coronal movement but adequate lateral wall movement. A myomucosal flap is elevated from the posterior pharyngeal wall and inserted into the palate. The flap obturates the central portion of the velopharyngeal port, leaving 2 smaller lateral ports.

Typically, a superiorly based flap is preferred to avoid inferior tethering of the palate and to ensure adequate placement of the flap at the site of velopharyngeal closure (**Fig. 3**). Initially, the palate is divided in the midline and back cuts are made in the nasal mucosa near the posterior edge of the hard palate. The myomucosal flap is elevated off the prevertebral fascia. The flap is inset into the soft palate with simple interrupted sutures. The width of the flap is determined preoperatively based on the degree of lateral wall movement noted during speech endoscopy, with a wider flap used for minimal movement. Catheters passed through the lateral ports are used to maintain patency and assist in appropriate sizing of the ports. These catheters are removed on postoperative day 1.

Inset of the pharyngeal flap can also be performed by creating a through-and-through transverse incision in the soft palate just posterior to the edge of the hard palate.[25,26] The flap is passed through this incision and sutured to the oral mucosal edge of the soft palate, ensuring placement of the flap high in the nasopharynx.

Many surgeons remain concerned about the risks of airway obstruction and obstructive sleep

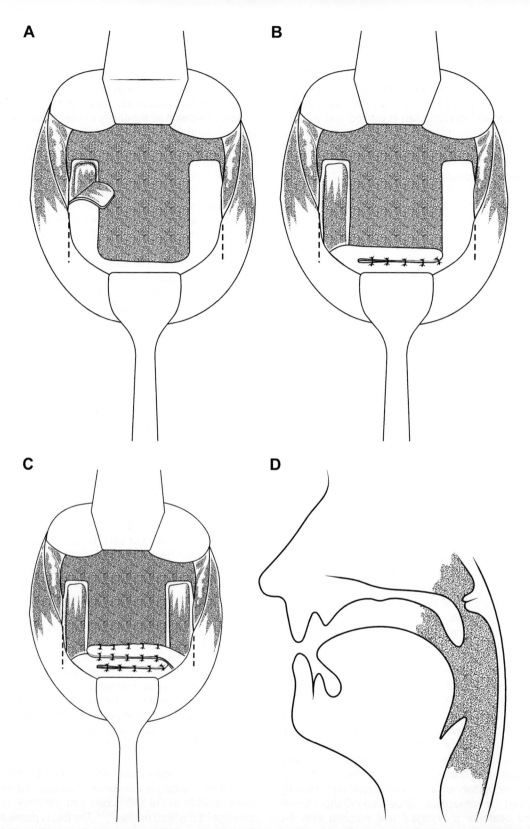

Fig. 2. Sphincter pharyngoplasty. (*A*) The myomucosal flaps are outlined on the lateral pharyngeal wall. These flaps are taken from the posterior tonsillar pillar and/or the tissue along the posterior pharyngeal wall just behind the pillar. The flap is elevated deep to the muscular layer. A horizontal incision through the mucosa in the nasopharynx joins the medial edges of each flap. (*B*) The left myomucosal flap is rotated and sutured to the edge of the horizontal incision in the nasopharynx at the site of velopharyngeal closure. A common error is inserting these flaps too low along the posterior pharyngeal wall. (*C*) The right myomucosal flap is elevated, rotated, and inset with the raw edge opposing the left flap. (*D*) Sagittal view showing the mass effect of the flaps in the nasopharynx.

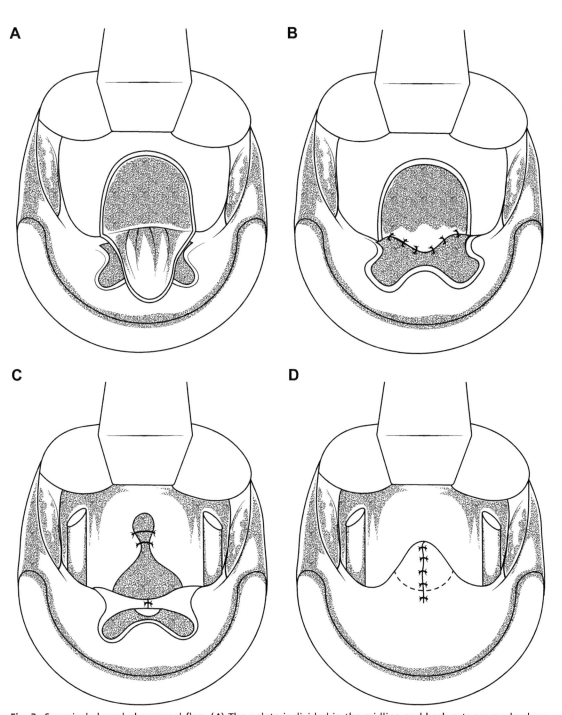

Fig. 3. Superiorly based pharyngeal flap. (*A*) The palate is divided in the midline and back cuts are made along the nasal mucosa at the posterior border of the hard palate. A superiorly based myomucosal flap is then elevated from the posterior pharyngeal wall. The width of the flap is determined based on the amount of sagittal closure seen on nasal endoscopy. (*B*) The nasal mucosa is elevated off the palate at the site of the back cut and the pharyngeal flap is sutured to the divided palate. The catheters are placed to determine the size of the lateral ports and to maintain postoperative patency. (*C*) The nasal mucosal flaps on the palate are then closed over the raw surface of the pharyngeal flap to reduce contraction and scarring of the pharyngeal flap. (*D*) The palate is then reapproximated. The dotted line signifies the location of the pharyngeal flap.

apnea with a pharyngeal flap. However, results in a series of 222 patients undergoing the pharyngeal flap operation suggested that the procedure may be a safe and effective option for patients with VPD.[27]

Posterior wall augmentation

In patients with a small central gap of the velopharynx, augmentation of the posterior pharyngeal wall may be an effective treatment.[28,29] Autogenous posterior pharyngeal wall augmentation using a rolled superiorly based pharyngeal myomucosal flap has been described but did not show improved speech outcomes in a small series.[30] Autologous and nonautologous materials have been implanted into the posterior pharyngeal wall either through injection or a mucosal incision. Implant materials include autologous fat injection.[31,32] Rolled acellular dermis has been used by the authors. However, a recent study evaluating the long-term impact of this technique in pigs showed no residual implant after 6 months.[33]

SUMMARY

The ultimate goal in surgical treatment of VPD is achieving functional closure of the velopharyngeal port during non-nasal speech and limiting the impact on nasal airflow and airway obstruction. Understanding the appropriate assessment and using a multidisciplinary approach is critical to successfully managing children with this challenging problem. Having the full armamentarium of treatment options and knowing the appropriate indication for each approach is essential for surgeons to effectively treat VPD.

REFERENCES

1. Shprintzen RJ, Lencione RM, McCall GN, et al. A three dimensional cinefluoroscopic analysis of velopharyngeal closure during speech and nonspeech activities in normals. Cleft Palate J 1974;11:412–28.
2. Pigott RW, Bensen JF, White FD. Nasendoscopy in the diagnosis of velopharyngeal incompetence. Plast Reconstr Surg 1969;43(2):141–7.
3. Huang MHS, Lee ST, Rajendran K. Anatomic basis of cleft palate and velopharyngeal surgery: implications from a fresh cadaveric study. Plast Reconstr Surg 1998;101:613.
4. Muntz H, Smith ME, Sauder C, Meier JD. Velopharyngeal dysfunction. In: Flint PW, Haughey BH, Lund VJ, et al, editors. Cummings otolaryngology head and neck surgery. 6th edition. Philadelphia: Saunders, Elsevier; 2015. p. 2933–43.
5. Skirko JR, Weaver EM, Perkins JA, et al. Validity and responsiveness of VELO: a velopharyngeal insufficiency quality of life measure. Otolaryngol Head Neck Surg 2013;149(2):304–11.
6. Ruda JM, Krakovitz P, Rosa AS. A review of the evaluation and management of velopharyngeal insufficiency in children. Otolaryngol Clin North Am 2012;45:653–69.
7. Dalston RM, Warren DW, Dalston ET. Use of nasometry as a diagnostic tool for identifying patients with velopharyngeal impairment. Cleft Palate Craniofac J 1991;28(2):184–8.
8. Karenell MP. Nasometric discrimination of hypernasality and turbulent nasal airflow. Cleft Palate Craniofac J 1995;32:145–8.
9. Pigott RW. An analysis of the strengths and weaknesses of endoscopic and radiological investigations of velopharyngeal incompetence based on a 20 year experience of simultaneous recording. Br J Plast Surg 2002;55(1):32–4.
10. Stringer DA, Witzel MA. Comparison of multi-view videofluoroscopy and nasopharyngoscopy in the assessment of velopharyngeal insufficiency. Cleft Palate J 1989;26(2):88–92.
11. D'Antonio LL, Muntz HR, Marsh JL, et al. Practical application of flexible fiberoptic nasopharyngoscopy for evaluating velopharyngeal function. Plast Reconstr Surg 1988;82:611–8.
12. Atik B, Bekerecioglu M, Tan O, et al. Evaluation of dynamic magnetic resonance imaging in assessing velopharyngeal insufficiency during phonation. J Craniofac Surg 2008;19(3):566–72.
13. Kao DS, Soltysik DA, Hyde JS, et al. Magnetic resonance imaging as an aid in the dynamic assessment of the velopharyngeal mechanism in children. Plast Reconstr Surg 2008;122(2):572–7.
14. Perry JL, Kuehn DP. Magnetic resonance imaging and computer reconstruction of the velopharyngeal mechanism. J Craniofac Surg 2009;20(Suppl 2):1739–46.
15. Furlow LT. Cleft palate repair by double opposing Z-plasty. Plast Reconstr Surg 1986;78(6):724–38.
16. Gart MS, Gosain AK. Surgical management of velopharyngeal insufficiency. Clin Plast Surg 2014;41:253–70.
17. Hsu PJ, Wang SH, Yun C, et al. Redo double-opposing Z-plasty is effective for correction of marginal velopharyngeal insufficiency. J Plast Reconstr Aesthet Surg 2015;68(9):1215–20.
18. Timbang MR, Gharb BB, Rampazzo A, et al. A systematic review comparing Furlow double-opposing Z-plasty and straight-line intravelar veloplasty methods of cleft palate repair. Plast Reconstr Surg 2014;134(5):1014–22.
19. Sie KC, Tampakopoulou DA, de Serres LM, et al. Sphincter pharyngoplasty: speech outcome and complications. Laryngoscope 1998;108:1211–7.
20. Georgantopoulou AA, Thatte MR, Razzell RE, et al. The effect of sphincter pharyngoplasty on the

range of velar movement. Br J Plast Surg 1996; 49(6):358–62.

21. Cable BB, Canady JW, Karnell MP, et al. Pharyngeal flap surgery: long-term outcomes at the University of Iowa. Plast Reconstr Surg 2004;113(2):475–8.

22. Hofer SO, Dhar BK, Robinson PH, et al. A 10-year review of perioperative complications in pharyngeal flap surgery. Plast Reconstr Surg 2002;110(6): 1393–7.

23. Levine PA, Goode RL. The lateral port control pharyngeal flap: a versatile approach to velopharyngeal insufficiency. Otolaryngol Head Neck Surg 1982;90:310–4.

24. Morris HL, Bardach J, Jones D, et al. Clinical results of pharyngeal flap surgery: the Iowa experience. Plast Reconstr Surg 1995;95(4):652–62.

25. Emara TA, Quriba AS. Posterior pharyngeal flap for velopharyngeal insufficiency patients: a new technique for flap inset. Laryngoscope 2012;122(2): 260–5.

26. Arneja JS, Hettinger P, Gosain AK. Through-and-through dissection of the soft palate for high pharyngeal flap inset: a new technique for the treatment of velopharyngeal incompetence in velocardiofacial syndrome. Plast Reconstr Surg 2008;122(3):845–52.

27. Cole P, Benerji S, Hollier L, et al. Two hundred twenty-two consecutive pharyngeal flaps: an analysis of postoperative complications. J Oral Maxillofac Surg 2008;66(4):745–8.

28. Perez CF, Brigger MT. Posterior pharyngeal wall augmentation. Adv Otorhinolaryngol 2015;76:74–80.

29. Lypka M, Bidros R, Rizvi M, et al. Posterior pharyngeal augmentation in the treatment of velopharyngeal insufficiency: a 40-year experience. Ann Plast Surg 2010;65(1):48–51.

30. Witt PD, O'Daniel TG, Marsh JL, et al. Surgical management of velopharyngeal dysfunction: outcome analysis of autogenous posterior pharyngeal wall augmentation. Plast Reconstr Surg 1997;99(5): 1287–96.

31. Piotet E, Beguin C, Broome M, et al. Rhinopharyngeal autologous fat injection for treatment of velopharyngeal insufficiency in patients with cleft palate. Eur Arch Otorhinolaryngol 2015;272(5):1277–85.

32. Leuchter I, Schweizer V, Hohlfeld J, et al. Treatment of velopharyngeal insufficiency by autologous fat injection. Eur Arch Otorhinolaryngol 2010;267(6):977–83.

33. O'Reilly AG, Powell BD, Garcia JJ, et al. In vivo durability and safety of rolled acellular dermis in a submucosal pocket in pigs. Cleft Palate Craniofac J 2015;52(2):198–202.

Intermediate and Definitive Cleft Rhinoplasty

Celeste Gary, MD, Jonathan M. Sykes, MD*

KEYWORDS

- Cleft • Rhinoplasty • Cleft nasal deformity • Cleft rhinoplasty • Definitive cleft rhinoplasty
- Intermediate cleft rhinoplasty • Treatment of cleft nasal deformity • Cartilage graft

KEY POINTS

- Understanding of the anatomy of a cleft nose deformity is crucial for definitive treatment of this clinical problem.
- Timing of intermediate and definitive cleft rhinoplasty.
- Preoperative evaluation of aesthetic and functional deficits.
- Goals of the secondary rhinoplasty include relief of nasal obstruction, creation of symmetry and definition of the nasal base and tip, and management of nasal scarring and webbing.
- Rhinoplasty techniques.

 Video content accompanies this article at http://www.facialplastic.theclinics.com.

INTRODUCTION

The cleft nasal deformity associated with cleft lip is a complex deformity. The nose is often the most noticeable aspect of the patient's face once the congenital cleft lip is repaired. This deformity can also cause functional nasal obstruction, which affects the patient throughout his or her development. The cleft nasal deformity involves all tissue layers of the nose including the bony platform, the inner lining, the cartilaginous infrastructure, and the external skin. The degree of the associated deformity is dependent upon the degree of the original lip abnormality.[1] The cleft nasal deformity is also affected by scarring from previous surgeries on the lip and nose and changes resulting from patient growth.[2,3] The ultimate goal of intermediate and definitive cleft rhinoplasty is to minimize functional problems and to maximize the appearance of the nose.[1]

DEVELOPMENT OF THE CLEFT NASAL DEFORMITY

Within normal development, the paired median nasal processes fuse to form the premaxilla, philtrum, columella, and nasal tip. The bilateral maxillary processes form the lateral aspects of the upper lip.[4,5] If the median nasal process fails to fuse with the maxillary process, a cleft lip deformity results. The extent of the cleft lip deformity also determines the extent of the cleft nasal deformity, which falls along a spectrum.

Anatomy of the Unilateral Cleft Lip Nasal Deformity

When a complete, unilateral cleft lip occurs, the maxilla on the cleft side is deficient, which does not allow the alar base on the cleft side to fuse in the midline. The alar base on the cleft side is,

Disclosure Statement: Neither author has any financial or other disclosures with regard to this article.
Division of Facial Plastic and Reconstructive Surgery, Department of Otolaryngology, University of California Davis, 2521 Stockton Boulevard, Suite 6203, Sacramento, CA 95817, USA
* Corresponding author.
E-mail address: jmsykes@ucdavis.edu

therefore, positioned more posterior, lateral, and inferior than the alar base on the noncleft side.[5,6] The cleft nasal septum has attachments to the maxilla on the noncleft side, which cause a caudal septal deviation to the noncleft side, while the posterior septum bows toward the cleft side. The lower lateral cartilage (LLC) on the cleft side has a lengthened lateral crus and shortened medial crus. The weakened and malpositioned cleft-side LLC produces a nostril that is wide and horizontally oriented. This change in position of the lower lateral cartilage also affects the attachment to the upper lateral cartilage, which weakens the scroll region and therefore causes a compromise of the internal nasal valve. The middle third of the nose in the unilateral cleft lip nasal deformity is also characterized by weakness of the upper lateral cartilage and malposition of these cartilages.[7] Again, this weakness results from inadequate skeletal support and often results in a concave upper lateral cartilage, which affects the internal nasal valve on the cleft side. The nasal floor is often absent (**Box 1**, **Fig. 1**).

Anatomy of the Bilateral Cleft Lip Nasal Deformity

When a complete bilateral cleft lip occurs, the maxilla is deficient on both sides. The prolabium is therefore allowed unopposed anterior growth. Both alar bases are located in a more posterior, lateral, and inferior position than in a noncleft nose. The columella is shortened. There is no alteration in the anterior septum. The lateral crura of both lower lateral cartilages are lengthened, and the bilateral medial crura are shortened and splayed.[8] The extent of columellar shortening is related to the size, shape, and position of the prolabium.[5] The entire nasal tip is underprojected, broad, and flattened (**Box 2**, **Fig. 2**).

TIMING OF CLEFT RHINOPLASTY

There is controversy regarding primary cleft rhinoplasty and its ultimate effects. However, regardless of early intervention, definitive rhinoplasty is usually necessary. Definitive rhinoplasty is typically delayed until the patient has completed facial growth. In female patients, secondary rhinoplasty is generally performed around 15 to 17 years of age, and in male patients at approximately 16 to 18 years of age.[5]

Intermediate Rhinoplasty

Intermediate rhinoplasty is defined as any nasal surgery performed between the time of initial cleft lip repair and the time at which the patient reaches facial skeletal maturity. These procedures are becoming less frequent as primary rhinoplasty

---

Box 1
Characteristics of unilateral cleft lip nasal deformity

Nasal tip

Medial crus of lower lateral cartilage shorter on cleft side

Lateral crus of lower lateral cartilage longer on cleft side (total length of lower lateral cartilage is same)

Lateral crus of lower lateral cartilage may be caudally displaced and may produce hooding of alar rim

Alar dome on cleft side is flat and displaced laterally

Columella

Short on cleft side

Base directed to noncleft side (secondary to contraction of orbicularis oris muscle)

Nostril

Horizontal orientation on cleft side

Alar base

Displaced laterally, posteriorly, and inferiorly

Nasal floor

Usually absent

Nasal septum

Caudal deflection to the noncleft side and posterior deviation to the cleft side

From Sykes JM, Jang YJ. Cleft lip rhinoplasty. Facial Plast Surg Clin North Am 2009;17(1):133–44; with permission.

---

becomes more common.[9] Intermediate rhinoplasty procedures are aimed at correcting severe functional abnormalities and minimizing the social stigmata associated with a more noticeable nasal deformity.[10]

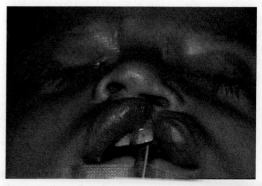

Fig. 1. Unilateral cleft lip nasal deformity. Base view.

Definitive Rhinoplasty

Definitive septorhinoplasty can be performed once the patient has reached facial skeletal maturity. Structural reconstruction of the cleft nose often requires cartilage grafting material from the rib, ear, or septum to achieve adequate support. The goals of the secondary rhinoplasty are the creation of symmetry and definition of the nasal base and tip, relief of nasal obstruction, and management of nasal scarring and webbing.[1]

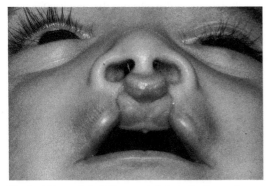

Fig. 2. Bilateral cleft lip nasal deformity. Base view.

PREOPERATIVE EVALUATION OF THE CLEFT NASAL DEFORMITY

It is important to clearly identify the key factors contributing to the nasal deformity in order to select the most appropriate surgical plan. Functional deficits can be assessed through a thorough history involving nasal symptoms. A physical examination, including anterior rhinoscopy, a Cottle maneuver, a modified Cottle maneuver, and possibly an endoscopic examination is imperative to fully assess the functional deficits of the patient.[11] A full set of preoperative photographs should be taken prior to any planned rhinoplasty procedure (**Fig. 3**, Video 1).

The overall goals include:

- Septal reconstruction
- Internal valve rehabilitation
- Nasal tip correction
- Alar appearance
- Alar base symmetry
- Columellar length
- Nasal sill symmetry
- Dorsal augmentation

RHINOPLASTY TECHNIQUES
Approaches

The preference of the senior author (JMS) is to use an open, or external, approach. In most instances, the traditional inverted-V columellar incision is used. When there is significant lack of columellar soft tissue in a bilateral cleft nose deformity, the incision can be modified onto the cleft lip with a V-to-Y closure to increase columellar soft tissue length[1] (**Fig. 4**).

Some authors argue for an endonasal approach, citing the advantages of maintaining an intact skin–soft tissue envelope and maintenance of the vascular supply of the skin.[1]

Graft Harvest

Cleft rhinoplasty often involves the use of graft material from the septum, auricular cartilage, and/or costal cartilage (Videos 2 and 3).

Septal Reconstruction

Repair of the cleft septum is a challenge and the foundation of the definitive cleft rhinoplasty. Complete septal reconstruction requires adequate exposure and complete breakdown of the ligamentous attachments that contribute to the septal deviation.[1] The senior author feels this is best accomplished through an open approach, in which the ligamentous attachments of the medial crura to the septum are completely separated. If an endonasal approach is used, a complete transfixion incision connected to

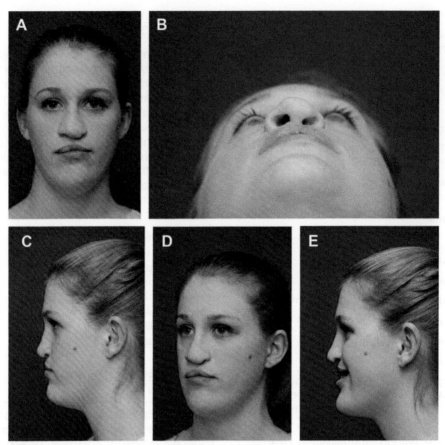

Fig. 3. Preoperative photo documentation. (*A*) AP view. (*B*) Base view. (*C*) Right lateral view. (*D*) Right oblique view. (*E*) Right lateral view with smile.

bilateral intercartilaginous incisions can be used to obtain adequate exposure.

Returning the caudal septum to midline

This can be accomplished by resecting a portion of the inferior caudal septum to swing the caudal septum to the nasal spine in a technique known as the swinging door. The caudal septum is then secured in its new position with a suture.[12] The senior

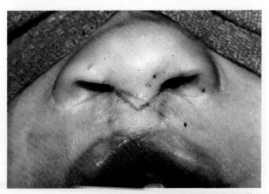

Fig. 4. Modified incision to allow for columellar lengthening when closed in a V-Y fashion.

author prefers to use 5-0 polydioxanone suture to secure the septum back onto the nasal spine (**Fig. 5**).

Cartilage grafting is often necessary to accomplish adequate central segment support. Cartilage can be obtained from a few sources including the nasal septum, auricular cartilage, and costal cartilage.

Adding to the existing septal support

The important concept is that indeterminate of whichever technique is used, the end result is a caudal aspect of the septum that is straight and well supported.

Caudal septal extension graft This is a straight cartilage graft that is affixed to the existing caudal septum in an end-to-end or end-to-side technique.[13]

Caudal batten graft This graft is placed in the same orientation as the caudal septum below the junction of the septum and the upper lateral cartilage to stabilize and reinforce the caudal septum.[14]

Extended spreader grafts These are cartilage grafts placed in between the dorsal septum and

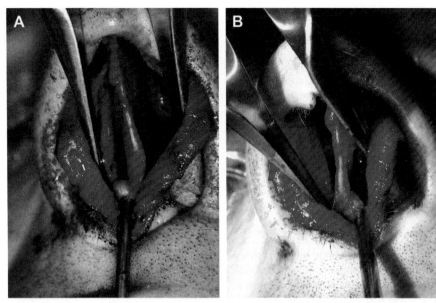

Fig. 5. (*A*) Caudal septal deflection. (*B*) After swinging-door maneuver. (*From* Sykes JM, Tasman A, Suarez GA. Cleft lip nose. Clin Plastic Surg 2016;43:223; with permission.)

the upper lateral cartilages, which extend past the existing caudal septum and can help stabilize the existing caudal septum and/or septal extension grafts. These grafts can help correct dorsal external deviations and can be placed only on 1 side to correct asymmetries in the middle third of the nose.[15]

Extracorporeal septoplasty This technique involves explanation of the septal cartilage, reshaping of this cartilage on the operative field (out of the patient), and reimplantation of the septum with fixation caudally and dorsally[16,17] (**Fig. 6**, Video 4).

Internal Valve Rehabilitation

Spreader grafts
These are grafts placed in between the dorsal septum and the upper lateral cartilage and run from the inferior edge of the bony pyramid to the inferior edge of the upper lateral cartilage (20–35 mm in length). Spreader grafts create a

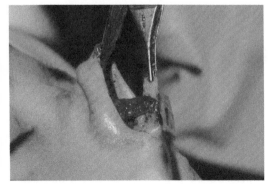

Fig. 6. Columellar strut graft.

widened superior angle of the internal nasal valve, therefore increasing airflow.[18] These can be placed via an endonasal or open rhinoplasty approach.[19] Spreader grafts can also be placed asymmetrically to correct asymmetric middle third deficiencies as in unilateral cleft lip nasal deformities.

Autospreader technique
The redundant dorsal portion of the upper lateral cartilage is scored and folded into the space between the dorsal septum and the lateral upper lateral cartilage to augment the superior angle of the internal nasal valve.[20,21]

Nasal Tip Correction

Nasal tip correction should focus on improving tip symmetry, definition, and projection. The main deficiency of the nasal tip in the cleft nose deformity is a lack of support. In most clefts, the cleft side nasal tip needs projection and rotation, because the secondary nasal deformity typically has underprojection and hooding of the cleft tip.

Tongue-in-groove
This entails suture fixation of the medial crura of the lower lateral cartilages to the caudal end of the nasal septum or septal extension graft, which allows the tip to be projected, deprojected, lengthened, or shortened.[22]

Columellar strut graft
Columellar strut graft is a cartilage graft placed in between the existing medial crura, which can increase projection and reinforce the strength of the existing medial crura.[23]

Lateral crural steal

The lateral crura are advanced medially in a curvilinear fashion, which increases the length of the medial crura at the expense of the lateral crura. The tip is therefore relocated in a superior and anterior direction.[24] This can be done asymmetrically in the unilateral cleft deformity to correct the pathologic deformity of the cleft side lower lateral cartilage.

Tip graft

Many forms of cartilage and soft tissue can be used to camouflage irregularities and improve tip definition.

Alar Appearance

The lateral crus of the cleft side LLC is often misshapen, with excess length and a concavity as compared with the noncleft side. This deformity causes compromise and collapse of the external nasal valve.

Alar rim graft

Alar rim graft is a nonanatomic graft placed inferior to the existing lower lateral cartilage in a precise pocket that helps to strengthen and support the alar rim.[25]

Lateral crural strut graft (alar strut graft)

This is a cartilage graft affixed to the deep surface of the existing lower lateral crura with the lateral edge place in a pocket developed at the pyriform aperture, which elevates, reshapes, and supports the lower lateral crura and nasal ala.[26]

Lower lateral cartilage turn-in flap (alar turn-in flap)

The cephalic end of the lower lateral cartilage is scored, turned down, and sutured to the undersurface of the caudal portion of the lower lateral cartilage, which strengthens and supports the lower lateral cartilage and helps to improve the preexisting concavity.[27]

Turnover of the lower lateral crura (flip-flop technique)

The lateral crura is dissected off the underlying vestibular skin, excised, turned over, and resutured to the vestibular lining, which changes the shape of the alar rim from concave to convex[28] (**Fig. 7**, Video 5).

Alar Base Symmetry

Secondary to poor skeletal support and previous surgery, the alar base is often asymmetric. This can be one of the most difficult aspects of the cleft nasal deformity to fix. Techniques other than definitive rhinoplasty (eg, nasoalveolar molding, primary rhinoplasty, and alveolar bone grafting) may result in augmentation of this portion of the cleft nasal deformity.[29,30]

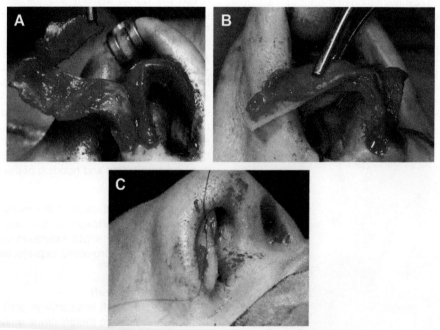

Fig. 7. (*A*) Alar turn-in flap of the cephalic aspect of LLC. (*B*) Lateral crural strut graft. (*C*) Alar batten graft (*From* Sykes JM, Tasman A, Suarez GA. Cleft lip nose. Clin Plastic Surg 2016;43:225; with permission.)

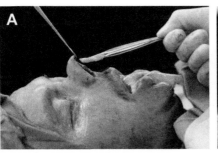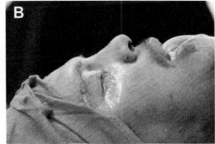

Fig. 8. Chopped cartilage and tissue glue dorsal augmentation graft. (*A*) Graft prior to insertion. (*B*) Lateral view after graft placement.

Columellar Length

When there is significant lack of columellar soft tissue in a bilateral cleft nose deformity, the external rhinoplasty incision can be modified onto the cleft lip with a V-to-Y closure to increase columellar soft tissue length.[1,31]

Nasal Sill Symmetry

A common secondary deformity that is a result of the original cleft lip repair is a lack of complete closure of the sill of the nose. This defect occurs when the superior portion of the orbicularis oris muscle is incompletely closed. This can be addressed with both surgical and nonsurgical methods, which include

- Reopening of the superior aspect of the lip with realignment of the muscle
- Dermal flap to fill the defect
- Fat augmentation
- Injectable fillers

Dorsal Augmentation

When addressing the dorsum during a definitive rhinoplasty for a congenital cleft patient, the senior author prefers augmentation grafting to reduction techniques in order to minimize trauma to the upper third of the nose, including conservative osteotomies for deviated nasal bones and diced cartilage onlay grafting.

Diced cartilage solidified with tissue sealant (Tasman technique) is molded into an onlay graft for dorsal augmentation[32] (**Figs. 8** and **9**, Video 6).

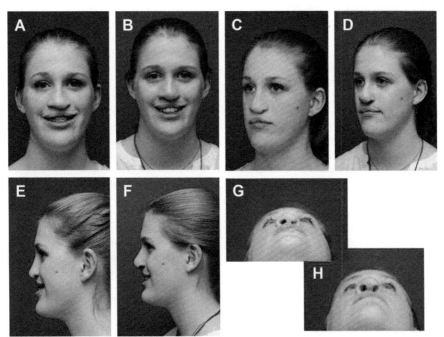

Fig. 9. Preoperative and 1 month postoperative photos. (*A*) Preoperative AP view. (*B*) Postoperative AP view. (*C*) Preoperative oblique view. (*D*) Postoperative oblique view. (*E*) Preoperative lateral view. (*F*) Postoperative lateral view. (*G*) Preoperative base view. (*H*) Postoperative base view. AP, anterior-posterior.

SUMMARY

Because the nose on a patient with a congenital cleft is noticeable to the observer, intermediate rhinoplasty and definitive cleft rhinoplasty are important and challenging parts of definitive cleft care. Successful reconstruction of cleft nasal deformities requires a detailed understanding of the normal and pathologic anatomy, attention to function and aesthetics, and thorough knowledge of advanced rhinoplasty techniques.

SUPPLEMENTARY DATA

Supplementary data related to this article can be found at http://dx.doi.org/10.1016/j.fsc.2016.06.017.

REFERENCES

1. Sykes JM, Tasman A, Suarez GA. Cleft lip nose. Clin Plast Surg 2016;43:223–35.
2. Sykes JM. Surgical management of the cleft lip nasal deformity. Current Opinion in Otolaryngology and Head and Neck Surgery 2000;8(1):54–7.
3. Sykes JM, Senders CW. Pathologic anatomy of cleft lip, palate, and nasal deformities. In: Meyers AD, editor. Biological basis of facial plastic surgery. New York: Thieme Medical Publishers; 1993. p. 57–71.
4. Capone R, Sykes J. Evaluation and management of cleft lip and palate disorders. In: Papel ID, editor. Facial plastic and reconstructive surgery. 3rd edition. Stuttgart (NY): Thieme; 2009. p. 1059–60.
5. Sykes JM, Jang YJ. Cleft lip rhinoplasty. Facial Plast Surg Clin North Am 2009;17(1):133–44.
6. Blair VP. Nasal deformities associated with congenital cleft of the lip. JAMA 1925;84:185–7.
7. Jablon JH, Sykes JM. Nasal airway problems in the cleft lip population. Facial Plast Surg Clin North Am 1999;7:391–403.
8. Coleman J, Sykes J. Cleft lip rhinoplasty. In: Papel ID, editor. Facial plastic and reconstructive surgery. 3rd edition. Stuttgart (NY): Thieme; 2009. p. 1082.
9. Gudis DA, Patel KG. Update on primary cleft lip rhinoplasty. Curr Opin Otolaryngol Head Neck Surg 2014;22(4):260–6.
10. Shih CW, Sykes JM. Correction of the cleft-lip nasal deformity. Facial Plast Surg 2002;18(4):253–62.
11. Cannon DE, Rhee JS. Evidence-based practice: functional rhinoplasty. Otolaryngol Clin North Am 2012;45(5):1033–43.
12. Metzenbaum M. Replacement of the lower end of the dislocated septal cartilage vs. submucous resection of the dislocated end of the septal cartilage. Arch Otolaryngol 1929;9:282–92.
13. Byrd HS, Andochick S, Copit S, et al. Septal extension grafts: a method of controlling tip projection shape. Plast Reconstr Surg 1997;100(4):999–1010.
14. Byrd HS, Salomon J, Flood J. Correction of the crooked nose. Plast Reconstr Surg 1998;102(6):2148–57.
15. Toriumi DM. Subtotal septal reconstruction: an update. Facial Plast Surg 2013;29:492–501.
16. Most SP. Anterior septal reconstruction: outcomes after a modified extracorporeal septoplasty technique. Arch Facial Plast Surg 2006;8(3):202–7.
17. Gubisch W. The extracorporeal septum plasty: a technique to correct difficult nasal deformities. Plast Reconstr Surg 1995;95(4):672–82.
18. Sheen JH. Spreader graft: a method of reconstructing the roof of the middle nasal vault following rhinoplasty. Plast Reconstr Surg 1984;73(2):230–9.
19. Rohrich RJ, Hollier LH. Use of spreader grafts in the external approach to rhinoplasty. Clin Plast Surg 1996;23(2):255–62.
20. Lerma J. The "lapel" technique. Plast Reconstr Surg 1998;102(6):2274–5.
21. Oneal RM, Berkowitz RL. Upper lateral cartilage spreader flaps in rhinoplasty. Aesthet Surg J 1998;18(5):370–1.
22. Kridel RW, Scott BA, Foda HM. The tongue-in-groove technique in septorhinoplasty. A 10-year experience. Arch Facial Plast Surg 1999;1(4):246–56.
23. Dibbell DG. A cartilaginous columellar strut in clift lip rhinoplasties. Br J Plast Surg 1976;29(3):247–50.
24. Kridel RW, Konior RJ, Shumrick KA, et al. Advances in nasal tip surgery: the lateral crural steal. Arch Otolaryngol Head Neck Surg 1989;115(10):1206–12.
25. Troell RJ, Powell NB, Riley RW, et al. Evaluation of a new procedure for nasal alar rim and valve collapse: nasal alar rim reconstruction. Otolaryngol Head Neck Surg 2000;122(2):204–11.
26. Toriumi DM. New concepts in nasal tip contouring. Arch Facial Plast Surg 2006;8(3):156–85.
27. Apaydin F. Lateral crural turn-in flap in functional rhinoplasty. Arch Facial Plast Surg 2012;14(2):93–6.
28. Ballert JA, Park SS. Functional rhinoplasty: treatment of the dysfunctional nasal sidewall. Facial Plast Surg 2006;22(1):49–54.
29. Li J, Shi B, Liu K, et al. A photogrammetric study of the effects of alveolar bone graft on nose symmetry among unilateral cleft patients. J Plast Reconstr Aesthet Surg 2011;64(11):1436–43.
30. Chang CS, Por YC, Liou EJ, et al. Long-term comparison of four techniques for obtaining nasal symmetry in unilateral complete cleft lip patients: a single surgeon's experience. Plast Reconstr Surg 2010;126(4):1276–84.
31. Carlino F. Modified forked flap for controlling columella length in cleft lip open rhinoplasty. J Craniomaxillofac Surg 2008;36(3):131–7.
32. Baker SR. Diced cartilage augmentation: early experience with the Tasman technique. Arch Facial Plast Surg 2012;14(6):451–5.

Craniofacial Microsomia

Kathleyn A. Brandstetter, MD*, Krishna G. Patel, MD, PhD

KEYWORDS

- Craniofacial microsomia • Hemifacial microsomia • Oculoauriculovertebral syndrome
- Distraction osteogenesis • Costochondral grafting

KEY POINTS

- There are several classification systems for craniofacial microsomia that group patients based on their degree of asymmetry. The most recent and comprehensive of these is the OMENS PLUS (Orbit, Mandible, Ear, Nerve, Soft tissue) system.
- Treatment of craniofacial microsomia is based on the severity of the deformity.
- Timing of surgical repair remains controversial.
- Mandibular distraction osteogenesis is a well-accepted method of correction of mandibular asymmetry but there is evidence of relapse if patients undergo distraction before completion of growth.
- Treatment includes not only correction of skeletal deformities but also soft tissue deficits (by means of free tissue flaps, fat grafting, and implants).

INTRODUCTION

Craniofacial microsomia (CFM) is a term used to describe a spectrum of craniofacial abnormalities caused by abnormal development of the first and second pharyngeal arch derivatives. The term CFM is often used interchangeably with several other terms, including otomandibular dysostosis, lateral facial dysplasia, malformation syndrome of the first and second arches, temporal oculoauricular dysplasia, and hemifacial microsomia (HFM). In addition, Goldenhar syndrome is considered a variant of CFM, which also includes epibulbar dermoids and vertebral anomalies. It is thought that the entities mentioned earlier represent several different phenotypical presentations that exist within a continuum, and thus the term oculoauriculovertebral spectrum (OAVS) was proposed by Cohen and colleagues[1] in 1989 to encompass all of these variants. Each of the variants includes some degree of developmental abnormality of the facial skeleton (mandible, maxilla, zygoma, and/or temporal bone), ear, and soft tissues.

EPIDEMIOLOGY

CFM is the second most common craniofacial birth defect after cleft lip and palate. It affects an estimated 1 in 3600 to 5600 live births in the United States each year. Literature reviews suggest that it is 50% more prevalent in boys (3:2 ratio). Ten percent of cases are bilateral, and most unilateral cases occur on the right.[2]

CAUSE/PATHOGENESIS

The mechanism behind CFM is thought to be related to the development of the pharyngeal arch structures. The pharyngeal arches start to form around the fourth week of embryologic development and are composed of mesenchymal cells that give rise to various facial structures (including skeletal, muscular, and neural elements). The morphogenesis of these structures depends on continuous and reciprocal tissue-tissue interactions, and any disruption of these interactions can lead to developmental abnormalities.[3,4] There

Disclosures: Neither author has any conflicts of interest or disclosures.
Department of Otolaryngology Head and Neck Surgery, Medical University of South Carolina, 135 Rutledge Avenue, MSC 550, Charleston, SC 29425, USA
* Corresponding author.
E-mail address: brandste@musc.edu

Facial Plast Surg Clin N Am 24 (2016) 495–515
http://dx.doi.org/10.1016/j.fsc.2016.06.006
1064-7406/16/© 2016 Elsevier Inc. All rights reserved.

are 2 leading theories to explain the pathogenesis of CFM:

1. Vascular disruption of the stapedial artery during development of the first and second pharyngeal arch derivatives leads to hematoma formation and subsequent abnormal growth and malformation of the mandible.[5]
2. Death, failure of development, or failure of migration of cells from the neural crest to the pharyngeal arches, causing dysmorphology of the arches.[6]

GENETICS

The causes of CFM include both extrinsic and genetic risk factors. Most documented cases are sporadic with no relevant family history. However, there is growing evidence for a genetic predisposition. Previously, a positive family history was documented in about 2% of patients who were within the OAVS spectrum. However, recent studies have shown significantly larger numbers of familial cases. It is also hypothesized that the reported percentage of familial involvement is underestimated given the broad phenotypic spectrum, with some family members having mild presentations that go undetected.[7,8] In a study by Kaye and colleagues,[9] 44% of cases of CFM had a positive family history of facial malformation, with an overall recurrence rate of 2% to 3% in first-degree relatives. Their data favored an autosomal dominant mode of inheritance with incomplete penetrance rather than a recessive or polygenetic mode of transmission.

Several chromosomal abnormalities have been identified in patients with CFM (**Table 1**). Studies reveal that the 22q11 locus may harbor genes important for regulation of craniofacial symmetry and first and second pharyngeal arch development, because craniofacial skeletal and soft tissue asymmetries have been observed in patients with genomic imbalances on the 22q11 locus.[40] The Crkl gene (in the 22q11 region) regulates signaling events in developing pharyngeal arches, again supporting its potential contribution to craniofacial dysmorphism.[41] The OTX2 gene was also identified as a very likely causal gene in CFM. This gene encodes a transcription factor that plays a critical role in craniofacial development and anterior brain morphogenesis. Zielinski and colleagues[13] investigated the largest CFM pedigree to date and found that a duplication in chromosome 14q22.3 (coding for OTX2) was present in all affected individuals.

Environmental factors are also thought to play a causative role in CFM. It is hypothesized that gestational diabetes, exposure to teratogens such as thalidomide, vasoactive drug use, smoking, and multiple gestation pregnancies cause disruption of embryonic blood flow during fetal development, leading to several structural congenital anomalies.[42–44]

PRESENTATION

There are no established criteria for diagnosis of CFM. However, several studies have indicated that either mandibular or auricular defects are mandatory for diagnosis. Cousley[45] proposed in his 1993 article the following minimum diagnostic criteria:

1. Ipsilateral mandibular and ear defects (external/middle)
2. Asymmetrical mandibular or ear defects (external/middle) in association with:
   a. Two or more indirectly associated anomalies, or
   b. A positive family history of HFM

There are varying degrees of severity within the spectrum of CFM. Mandibular deficiency can range from missing the condylar cartilage and disc to complete developmental failure of the ramus. The maxilla, temporal bone, and orbit can also be affected as a result of primary malformation. However, CFM is not characterized by bony dysmorphism alone, because there is soft tissue, neural, and muscular involvement as well. **Table 2** outlines the anomalies that are seen and their incidence.

CLASSIFICATION SYSTEMS

The heterogeneity of phenotypic presentations in CFM has led to difficulty developing a reproducible classification system to distinguish between varying degrees of deformity and to help aid in surgical planning.[49] The first accepted classification was proposed by Pruzansky[50] in 1969, and focused on the size and shape of the mandible and glenoid fossa. Kaban and colleagues[51,52] modified this classification system in 1988, proposing further stratification of the type II mandible based on the relationship of the mandibular condyle and glenoid fossa (**Fig. 1**). Another classification system described in the literature is the SAT (skeletal malformations, auricular involvement, and soft tissue defects) system, proposed by David and colleagues[53] in 1987. Vento and colleagues[46] took this one step further, defining the OMENS (Orbit, Mandible, Ear, Nerve, Soft tissue) classification system, which expanded the SAT system to include other affected structures: orbital distortion, mandibular hypoplasia, ear

Table 1
Chromosomal abnormalities seen in CFM

Abnormality	Gene	Type	Reference
22q11.2	Crkl	Deletion	Xu et al,[10] 2008; Digilio et al,[11] 2009; Tan et al,[12] 2011
14q22.3	OTX2		Zielinki et al,[13] 2014
3q29		Deletion	Guida et al,[14] 2015
14q32	GCS		Kelberman et al,[15] 2001
15q26.2–3			Huang et al,[16] 2010
1p22.2-p31.1		Deletion	Callier et al,[17] 2008
12p13.33		Deletion	Rooryck et al,[7] 2010; Adbelmoity et al,[18] 2011
Trisomy 22			Kobrynski et al,[19] 1993
14q23.1		Duplication	Ballesta-Martinez et al,[20] 2013; Ou et al,[21] 2008
15q24		Deletion	Brun et al,[22] 2012
5q13.2		Deletion	Huang et al,[16] 2010
5p15.33-pter		Deletion	Descartes et al,[23] 2006; Josifova et al,[24] 2004; Ladekarl et al,[25] 1968; Ala-Mello et al,[26] 2008
10p14-p15		Duplication	Dabir et al,[27] 2006
14q31.1–3		Deletion	Gimelli et al,[28] 2013
15q24.1		Deletion	Brun et al,[22] 2012
Trisomy 18			Verloes et al,[29] 1991
Deletion 22qter		Deletion	Herman et al,[30] 1988
22q11.1–.21		Duplication	Quintero-Rivera,[31] 2013; Torti et al,[32] 2013
X chromosome aneuploidies			Garavelli et al,[33] 1999; Poonawalla et al,[34] 1980
t(9;18) (p23;q12.2)		Translocations	Rooryck et al,[7] 2010
inv9(p11;q13)		Inversion	Stanojevic et al,[35] 2000
inv14(p11.2;q22.3)		Inversion	Northup et al,[36] 2010
Mosaicism trisomy 7		Mosaic	Hodes et al,[37] 1981
Mosaicism trisomy 9		Mosaic	de Ravel et al,[38] 2001; Wilson et al,[39] 1983
Mosaicism trisomy 22		Mosaic	de Ravel et al,[38] 2001
8q13			Cousley et al,[2] 1997

deformities, nerve defects, and soft tissue deficiencies. A modified version has since been published (OMENS PLUS), which is used when noncraniofacial structures are also involved.[48] The hope with these classification systems (outlined in **Table 3**) is that better differentiation of key phenotypical elements will lead to improved diagnosis, treatment planning, prognostic predictions, data evaluation, and case correlation.[4]

TREATMENT OVERVIEW

Treatment of CFM poses a challenging issue because there are both soft tissue and skeletal deficiencies that need to be addressed. Before surgical intervention, computed tomography (CT) with three-dimensional (3D) reconstruction is becoming an increasingly popular imaging modality to better delineate asymmetries. However, the posteroanterior (PA) cephalogram is still the gold standard method for assessing facial asymmetry. With these images, clinicians can measure maxillary and mandibular deviations from midline, differences in ramus height, and occlusal cant. These measures are important in objectively assessing improvements in asymmetry caused by surgical intervention.

The major goals in treating CFM include improvements in facial symmetry, functional jaw movement, occlusion, and patient satisfaction. Kaban and colleagues[54] outlined 4 main treatment objectives:

1. Increase size of mandible and associated soft tissue
2. Create temporomandibular joint (TMJ) if one is lacking
3. Foster vertical maxillary growth
4. Obtain stable occlusion

Table 2
Clinical presentation of CFM

Site	Percentage of Patients (%)
Mandibular deficiency	89–100
Other Bony Anomalies	
Maxillary hypoplasia	—
Temporal bone deformity	—
Orbit	15–43
Ear anomalies	65–99
Microtia/anotia	66–99
Preauricular skin tags	34–67
Conductive hearing loss	50–66
Ossicular chain defects	—
Pinna abnormalities	—
External auditory canal atresia	—
Soft tissue defects	17–95
Masticatory/facial muscle hypoplasia	85–95
Parotid gland hypoplasia	—
Deficiency of subcutaneous tissue	—
Transverse oral cleft	18–61
Cranial nerve involvement	10–45
Anomalies Outside Head and Neck	
Vertebral/rib defects	16–60
Cardiac defects	4–33
Renal/genitourinary defects	4–15
Central nervous system anomalies	5–18

Data from Refs.[45–48]

SURGICAL TIMING

Defining the timing of surgical intervention is challenging, because of the controversy as to whether facial asymmetry in these patients progresses over time or remains fixed. In reviewing the literature, there are 2 separate fields of thought:

1. Clinicians who think that the asymmetry is progressive favor early surgical intervention.
2. Clinicians who think that the asymmetry is fixed propose delayed intervention once the children reach skeletal maturity.

Note that both fields of thought agree on early surgical intervention in children at risk for airway compromise because of their mandibular deformity.

Those surgeons who support early correction of asymmetry (before skeletal maturity) believe

A
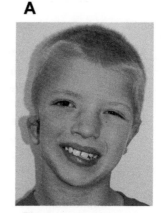

B
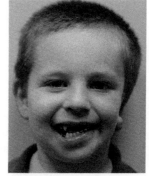 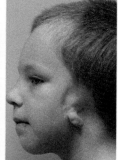

C
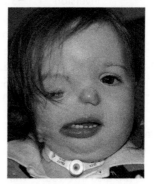

Fig. 1. Examples of Pruzansky-Kaban type IIa (*A*), IIb (*B*), and III (*C*) deformities. (*A, B*) Both mandibular and auricular anomalies are present. (*C*) Multiple additional anomalies, including orbital asymmetry and lateral oral clefting.

that mandibular skeletal asymmetry worsens with time, because the affected side has little or no growth. They argue that early intervention allows improved growth potential and functionality of structures by minimizing secondary skeletal deformities caused by limited growth of adjacent structures. In addition, they think that early intervention improves masticatory muscle hypoplasia,

Table 3
Grading systems for CFM

Pruzansky Classification of CFM (1969)[50]

Grade I	Mandible with mild hypoplasia
Grade II	Mandible with more severe hypoplasia in addition to malformation of common bony landmarks
Grade III	Mandible with complete effacement of common mandibular landmarks (absent ramus, condyle, TMJ)

Pruzansky-Kaban Classification (1988)[51]

Grade I	Mandible with mild hypoplasia
Grade II	
IIa	Mandibular ramus, condyle, and TMJ are present, normal in shape, but hypoplastic
IIb	Mandibular ramus is hypoplastic and markedly abnormal in form and location (medial and anterior) without articulation with temporal bone
Grade III	Mandible with complete effacement of common mandibular landmarks (absent ramus, condyle, TMJ)

SAT Classification System (1987)[53]

Skeletal malformations	S1	Small mandible of normal shape
	S2	Mandible very different in size and shape than normal. Condyle, ramus, and sigmoid notch identifiable but distorted
	S3	Mandible severely malformed: ranges from poorly identifiable ramal component to complete agenesis of ramus
	S4	S3 mandible with orbital involvement: posterior recession of lateral and posterior orbital rims
	S5	S4 defect with orbital dystopia, hypoplasia and asymmetric neurocranium, flat temporal fossa
Auricular involvement	A0	Normal
	A1	Small malformed auricle but all features are retained
	A2	Rudimentary auricle with hook at cranial end corresponding with helix
	A3	Malformed lobule and absent remainder of pinna
Soft tissue defects	T1	Minimal contour defect without cranial nerve involvement
	T2	Moderate defect
	T3	Major defect, obvious facial scoliosis, severe hypoplasia of cranial nerves, parotid, muscles of mastication, eye involvement; facial clefts

OMENS Classification (1991)[46]

Orbit (orbital distortion)	O_0	Normal orbital size and position
	O_1	Abnormal orbital size
	O_2	Abnormal orbital position
	O_3	Abnormal orbital size and position
Mandible (mandibular hypoplasia)	M_0	Normal mandible
	M_1	Small mandible and glenoid fossa
	M_{2a}	Short mandibular ramus but good position of glenoid fossa
	M_{2b}	Short mandibular ramus; TMJ is inferiorly, medially and anteriorly displaced; condyle is hypoplastic
	M_3	Complete absence of mandibular ramus, glenoid fossa and TMJ
Ear (ear anomaly)	E_0	Normal ear
	E_1	Mild hypoplasia and cupping but all structures present
	E_2	Absence of external auditory canal with hypoplasia of concha
	E_3	Malpositioned lobule with absent auricle; lobular remnant inferiorly and anteriorly displaced

(continued on next page)

Table 3 (continued)		
Nerve (nerve involvement)	N_0	No facial nerve involvement
	N_1	Upper facial nerve involvement (temporal, zygomatic branches)
	N_2	Lower facial nerve involvement (buccal, mandibular, and cervical branches)
	N_3	All branches of facial nerve involved
Soft tissue (soft tissue deficiency)	S_0	No obvious soft tissue or muscle deficiency
	S_1	Minimal subcutaneous/muscle deficiency
	S_2	Moderate subcutaneous/muscle deficiency
	S_3	Severe soft tissue deficiency caused by subcutaneous and muscular hypoplasia

Abbreviation: TMJ, temporomandibular joint.

optimizes dental development, and affords improved patient aesthetic appearance and body image development.[55]

Those investigators in favor of waiting to correct mandibular asymmetry think that the most favorable aesthetic results come from reconstruction at an age closer to skeletal maturity (age 13–15 years in girls, 15–16 years in boys). They argue that relapse of asymmetry occurs during growth phases, leading to a need for multiple additional procedures. They highlight technical reasons for delaying surgical reconstruction until the permanent dentition phase, noting that procedures performed later have decreased blood loss and other surgical risk factors. Patient compliance also improves in these cases compared with early distraction osteogenesis.

Studies of the outcomes following early and late skeletal correction of CFM vary greatly in terms of results, and most of these studies are small and retrospective, consisting of level IV evidence. Several larger systematic reviews have been conducted to address this issue, and these studies concluded that there was a lack of evidence supporting early skeletal correction in these children. However, some institutions still support early distraction. This article discusses the evolution of surgical treatment of CFM chronologically.

HISTORY OF TREATMENT

In the days before mandibular distraction osteogenesis (MDO), early mandibular reconstruction was achieved by mandibular osteotomy and autogenous grafting, most frequently using costochondral cartilaginous rib grafting.[54,56–59] Dating back to the 1970s, the degree of the deformity in CFM was used to guide treatment. Those children with more severe defects (Pruzansky Kaban types IIb and III) underwent surgery prepubertally to

reconstruct the mandible, whereas treatment of children with milder deformities tended to be more variable. Many were not treated until adolescence or received functional orthodontic appliances, whereas others underwent early mandibular osteotomies to keep up with vertical midfacial growth.[60] Soft tissue deficiencies were usually not addressed until after restoration of bony symmetry.[60]

MODERN APPROACH TO TREATMENT

Regardless of timing of skeletal repair, the choice of procedure is based on the severity of the defect and degree of deficit of mandibular bone stock. In the meta-analysis by Pluijmers and colleagues,[61] patients with type I deformities were most often treated with MDO. However, elongation and rotation with osteotomy was also used to treat type I and IIa patients. Those with type IIa deformities most commonly underwent MDO and those with IIb deformities most commonly underwent reconstruction with grafts. Type III deformities were most often treated with iliac or costochondral grafting to recreate the TMJ, sometimes followed by MDO.[61]

GRAFTS

Gillies[62] first described the use of cartilage and bone from the rib cage to address the hypoplastic mandible in the 1920s. Along with providing adequate bony length, the cartilaginous portion of the graft serves as a neocondyle. The most popular graft material used is the costochondral cartilaginous rib graft, followed by iliac crest, interposed temporal bone, and fibula. Its popularity stems from the potential for growth along with its adaptability and workability. However, studies have suggested unpredictable growth patterns and the potential for overgrowth on the treated side. Grafting also has risks, including infection, donor site morbidity, reankylosis, fracture, and resorption.[63]

Follow-up studies of mandibular grafting showed high rates of resorption of graft material and recurrence of asymmetry.[64] Thus, with the advent of MDO, grafts became used mainly in conjunction with distraction or in patients with Pruzansky type IIb and III deformities requiring construction or reconstruction of the TMJ and ramus. Occasionally, grafts were used in type IIa patients as interposed bone to lengthen the affected mandible. However, the normal side outgrew the affected side after elongation in 50% of patients.[64] In addition, patients with costochondral grafting before MDO tended to have higher rates of postoperative complications (44%–68%).[64,65]

DISTRACTION OSTEOGENESIS

Several cases of mandibular corpus distraction were reported in the literature during the first half of the twentieth century,[66–69] but the technique of MDO did not gain popularity until the early 1990s when McCarthy's group at New York University began to perform the procedure.[70] The technique was slowly adopted over the following years but became widely accepted with the advent of bidirectional distraction (described by Klein and Howaldt[130] in 1995).[60] The principal aims of MDO are to provide stable expansion of the mandible with concurrent lengthening and expansion of surrounding muscle and soft tissue. Initially, mandibular distraction devices were only external. These devices offered excellent mechanical strength but had some complications, including unsightly pin site scars, pin site infections, and dislodgement of the device. These complications led surgeons to design internal mandibular devices. These devices are inserted through either an oral or external approach and provide excellent mechanical strength. The downsides include the need for removal at the end of the distraction and bony overgrowth on the device, making removal difficult.[65,71]

Initial studies of MDO revealed some significant advantages compared with costochondral grafting. MDO increased the vertical length of the mandible,[72] produced greater bone stock,[73] improved soft tissue asymmetry by encouraging hypertrophy of the muscles lying parallel to the distraction vector,[74–76] and had less relapse than costochondral cartilage grafting.[76,77] In addition, operative times were generally shorter; the complications were fewer; the postoperative course was simpler; and there was less blood loss, greater

vector control of advancement,[78] no donor site morbidity, and an ability to lengthen the mandible at a younger age.[76,79]

STABILITY OF DISTRACTION

In the decade following the advent of MDO, studies began to note the need for repeated distraction to maintain symmetry during growth.[80–83] Molina and colleagues[84] published one of the first of these studies in 1995, of 65 patients with CFM who were treated with early MDO and followed for an average of 19 months postoperatively. Facial development on the unaffected side proceeded normally, whereas the distracted side showed delayed growth, leading to some return of asymmetry. Thus the investigators proposed overcorrection and second-stage distraction.

The concept of overcorrection has since been suggested in multiple additional studies as a method to combat the need for repeated distraction.[51,54,82,83,85–87] However, overcorrection has its downsides as well, including creating a dental crossbite on the contralateral side, leading to so-called occlusal disasters.[88,89] Overcorrection also increases the abnormal form and position of bone and soft tissues, creating a secondary chin malformation, making future genioplasty more difficult.[85,90] In addition, overcorrection did not reduce the number of surgeries these children underwent.[80–83]

INCREASING SUPPORT FOR DELAYED SURGICAL INTERVENTION

Several systematic reviews have been conducted over the past decade of long-term stability of the distracted mandible in patients with CFM.[60,61,91] The investigators all commented on the lack of evidence-based data supporting early versus delayed surgical intervention. All of the studies consist of level IV evidence, and many of the studies are flawed in their design, making their data questionable in terms of validity. **Table 4** outlines these studies. Conclusions were similar for all 3 systematic reviews:

- MDO performed before skeletal maturation leads to relapse of asymmetry, despite overcorrection.
- The earlier the correction, the more likely the procedure will need to be repeated.[60]
- In addition, there was evidence suggesting adverse effects of MDO on growth of the affected mandible.

Table 4
Overview of literature

Stability Following Surgery

Publication Author	Study Design	Therapy	Follow-up Period	Long-term Outcomes	Conclusions	Level of Evidence
Kaban et al,[51] 1988	Retrospective case series (n = 17)	Elongation and rotation by osteotomy vs grafting	4 y	Stable occlusion with E&R, 50% of grafted mandibles outgrown by normal side		IV
Kearns et al,[55] 2000	Retrospective case series (n = 67)	Untreated	>13 y	Statistically significant progression of asymmetry from the deciduous to mixed dentition phase in all measurements in group II patients (mandible type IIB or III)	Hemifacial microsomia is progressive; early surgical intervention is warranted	IV
Padwa et al,[86] 1998	Retrospective case series (n = 33)	Grafting	5.5 y	16% of patients had significant return of asymmetry as determined by occlusal cant	Proposed overcorrection	IV
Molina et al,[84] 1995	Retrospective case series (n = 65)	Early MDO	19 mo	Younger patients had faster growth on the unaffected side compared with the treated mandible	Proposed overcorrection and second-stage distraction	IV
Molina et al,[88] 2004	Prospective case series (n = 4)	Early MDO	12 y	Stable symmetry. In patients <5 y old, secondary occlusal disaster and need for reoperations seen	Stable symmetry	IV
Hollier et al,[81] 1999	Prospective case series (n = 8)	Early MDO	32.6 mo	Growth of affected vertical ramus slower than the unaffected side in all patients	Proposed overcorrection	IV
Grayson et al,[92] 1997	Retrospective case series (n = 5)	Early MDO	1–6 y	Increase in height over 5 y of growth is greater on the side that is not distracted	Proposed overcorrection	IV
Baek et al,[90] 2005	Retrospective case series (n = 19)	Early MDO	2.7 y	Type I and IIa mandibles stable, type IIb and III mandibles with relapse		IV

Study	Study design	Intervention	Follow-up	Results	Comments	Level of evidence
Cavaliere et al,[93] 2002	Prospective case series (n = 2)	Early MDO	1–2 y	Type III mandibles: improvement in contour of affected side, full range of jaw motion. No mention of relapse at end of follow-up		IV
Altug-Atac et al,[94] 2008	Retrospective case series (n = 11)	Early MDO	6 mo	Significant improvement in hard and soft tissue asymmetry, no mention of relapse		IV
Kulewicz et al,[95] 2004	Prospective case series (n = 28)	Early MDO	3 mo to 1 y	Stable results in lengthening and occlusion after 1 y. Coordinated growth of maxillomandibular complex	Proponent of early correction	IV
Shetye et al,[96] 2006	Retrospective case series (n = 12)	Early MDO	5–10 y	No alteration in growth pattern. 1 y after MDO, 26.6% relapse in ramus height, 40% relapse in occlusal and bigonial plane canting	Small amount of relapse but, by 1 y, asymmetry stabilized	IV
Jansma et al,[85] 2004	Retrospective case series (n = 2)	Early MDO	2.5 y	Stable results until end of follow-up	No evidence of relapse following MDO	IV
Ortiz Monasterio et al,[97] 1982	Retrospective case series (n = 6)	Iliac and costochondral grafts	3.5–5 y	Overcorrection used and, by end of follow-up, slight decrease in overcorrection but no relapse or increase in asymmetry	Proposed overcorrection	IV
Trahar et al,[98] 2003	Prospective case series (n = 6)	Early MDO	1–2 y	Stable mandibular length without relapse	Proponent of early correction	IV
Gui et al,[99] 2011	Retrospective case series (n = 21)	MDO + graft	3 y	Greatly improved 3D facial symmetry with minimal relapse. 18 of 21 patients very satisfied with results		IV
Scolozzi et al,[100] 2006	Retrospective case series (n = 5)	MDO	2.2 y	Horizontal improvement in symmetry, stable		IV
Satoh et al,[101] 2002	Prospective case series (n = 10)	MDO	1.3–3.3 y	Stable results with 2 of 10 patients showing slight occlusal change		IV

(continued on next page)

Table 4
(continued)

Publication Author	Study Design	Therapy	Follow-up Period	Long-term Outcomes	Conclusions	Level of Evidence
Huang et al,[102] 1999	Prospective case series (n = 5)	MDO	1 y	Stable symmetry. More downward movement of chin than forward movement		IV
Munro et al,[103] 1989	Retrospective case series (n = 22)	Grafting	1–9 y	16 of 18 with facial growth, 2 of 18 with overgrowth (and relapse of asymmetry)		IV
Vargervik et al,[57] 1986	Prospective case series (n = 14)	Grafting	5.2 y	11 of 14 stable with minimal relapse/return of asymmetry		IV
Ousterhout et al,[104] 1987	Prospective case series (n = 14)	Grafting	5.2 y	11 of 14 stable with minimal relapse/return of asymmetry		IV
Converse et al,[105] 1973	Retrospective case series (n = 12)	Grafting	3–12 y	Residual asymmetry present but stable (no relapse)		IV
Relapse of Asymmetry						
Mommaerts et al,[60] 2002	Meta-analysis (8 studies included)	Early MDO	NA	Results revealed high percentage of overcorrection, repeated osteodistraction procedures and soft tissue complications	Despite initial correction, there is relapse of facial asymmetry. The earlier the correction, the more likely that the procedure will have to be repeated. MDO may have possible adverse effect on growth of affected mandible. MDO does not lead to lateral augmentation of soft tissue	I
Nagy et al,[91] 2009	Meta-analysis (13 studies included)	Early MDO	3 m to 10 y	7 studies with stable results at end of follow-up (short-term or nonobjective evaluation), 6 studies with unstable results. Type IIb, type III deformities showed relapse with need for reoperation	No convincing evidence supporting effectiveness of early mandibular osteodistraction	I

Study	Study type	Intervention	Follow-up	Results	Conclusion	Level
Pluijmers et al,[61] 2014	Meta-analysis (19 studies included)	Early MDO, graft + MDO, graft alone, E&R		Most common intervention was bone grafting (CCG, rib, iliac). Good results in short term but increased asymmetry over time with MDO and graft patients (type II, III mandible). Most stable results in milder deformities	Single-stage correction should be postponed until permanent dentition phase or skeletal maturity. Treatment of severely hypoplastic mandible should include multistage treatment protocol	I
Kusnoto et al,[106] 1999	Retrospective case series (n = 6)	Early MDO	1.5 y	Unoperated patients have fairly stable asymmetry over time. Most favorable results found in body rather than ramus of mandible. Slight decrease in mandible length noted (~5%)	Mild relapse noted. Recommend 3D evaluation for improved surgical planning	IV
Marquez et al,[107] 2000	Case report (n = 1)	Early MDO	2 y	Relapse of 87% of vertical distraction length, AP gain was stable. Soft tissue matrix decreased with MDO	Distraction osteogenesis does not accelerate growth and does not predictably increase length of mandible	IV
Meazzini et al,[108–110] 2012, 2008, 2005	Prospective case series (n = 14, 17, 8)	Early MDO	11 y, 5 y, 5.8 y	Excellent postoperative results but symmetry obtained was lost at completion of growth (nearly 100% loss of vertical correction)	MDO is not stable over time	IV
Batra et al,[111] 2006	Retrospective case series (n = 3)	Early MDO	7 y	30%–60% relapse in ramus height		IV
Gursoy et al,[112] 2008	Retrospective case series (n = 2)	Early MDO	5 y	No relapse in vertical or horizontal mandibular length. Relapse of mandibular/skeletal profile and form to predistraction state		IV
Polley et al,[80] 1997	Retrospective case series (n = 26)	Unoperated patients	13 y	No significant change in asymmetry over the 13 y of growth. This finding was not influenced by grade and side of mandibular deformity	Skeletal mandibular asymmetry in HFM is not progressive in nature. Growth on affected side parallels that of the nonaffected side	IV

(continued on next page)

Table 4
(continued)

Publication Author	Study Design	Therapy	Follow-up Period	Long-term Outcomes	Conclusions	Level of Evidence
Rachmiel et al,[113] 1995	Retrospective case series (n = 11)	MDO	1 y	Some relapse in vertical mandibular height noted based on PA cephalograms		IV
Huisinga-Fischer et al,[114] 2003	Prospective case series (n = 8)	Early MDO	1–3 y	After 1 y, relapse in 50% of patients. Relapse is progressive 3 y after MDO and all patients showed relapse		IV
Ko et al,[115] 2004	Retrospective case series (n = 10)	Early MDO	13 mo	30% relapse in ramus height, 16% relapse in chin position. Occlusal plane stable		IV
Wan et al,[116] 2011	Retrospective case series (n = 47)	MDO, graft alone, graft + MDO	13 y	MDO patients with minimal relapse, 4 of 27 with increased asymmetry), 9 of 27 graft patients with increased asymmetry (and 2 of 27 with overgrowth), 3 of 16 graft + MDO patients with bone resorption and relapse	Relapse seen more frequently with graft-only patients, most stable results in graft + MDO patients	IV
Santamaria et al,[117] 2008	Retrospective case series (n = 8)	Graft alone (fibular free flap), graft + MDO	3.8 y	6 of 8 graft patients with partial improvement in occlusion, 2 of 8 with total improvement; 3 of 8 patients with increased asymmetry long term; 2 of 2 graft + MDO patients with partial improvement, no mention of relapse		IV

Chow et al,[118] 2008	Retrospective case series (n = 4)	MDO	7 y	Outgrowth of normal side after 2 y. Relapse of asymmetry noted	IV
Cerajewska et al,[119] 2002	Prospective case series (n = 14)	Grafting	4 y	Bilateral growth of ramus, minimal relapse of mandibular body length	IV
Hay et al,[120,121] 2000, 2000	Prospective case series (n = 15)	Grafting	3.5 y	Bilateral growth of ramus, minimal relapse of mandibular body length	IV
Singh et al,[122] 1999	Prospective case series (n = 14)	Grafting	3 y	Bilateral growth of ramus, minimal relapse of mandibular body length	IV
Padwa et al,[86] 1998	Retrospective case series (n = 33)	Grafting	5 y	42% successful (<5° occlusal cant), 42% acceptable (5°–8°), 16% unsuccessful (>8°); 50% of grafted mandibles outgrown by normal side	IV
Mulliken et al,[123] 1989	Retrospective case series (n = 8)	Grafting	4.5 y	42% successful (<5° occlusal cant), 42% acceptable (5°–8°), 16% unsuccessful (>8°); 50% of grafted mandibles outgrown by normal side	IV

Abbreviations: AP, anteroposterior; CCG, costocartilaginous rib graft; E&R, elongation and rotation; NA, not available; PA, posteroanterior.

With respect to soft tissue deficits, they concluded that soft tissue management is best performed separately from skeletal surgery.[60]

Based on the results of their analysis, Nagy and colleagues[91] proposed their own treatment timeline for patients with CFM, emphasizing postponement of definitive reconstruction of type I, IIa, and IIb deformities until the permanent dentition phase (**Box 1**). Several additional investigators have proposed treatment timelines, including Cousley and Calvert,[2] who stratified their protocol based on patient age (**Box 2**).

The most recent meta-analysis of long-term stability following treatment of CFM was published in 2014 by Pluijmers and colleagues.[61] It assessed 285 patients who underwent surgical treatment of mandibular asymmetry in HFM, including MDO, elongation and rotation by osteotomy, grafting, and the combination of grafting plus MDO. Their results are summarized in **Table 5**. They concluded that more stable results were seen in patients with milder deformities (types I–IIa) and the best results for both mild and severe cases were seen with the combination of grafting followed by MDO. Based on their analysis, Pluijmers and colleagues[61] recommended postponing single-stage skeletal correction until the permanent dentition phase or completion of growth.[61]

TEMPOROMANDIBULAR JOINT RECONSTRUCTION

In type III cases in which patients have unstable occlusion, a TMJ has to be created in addition to lengthening the affected mandibular ramus. Even with multidirectional distraction osteogenesis, it is impossible to induce formation of the joint at the right location given the medially displaced, hypoplastic remnant structures. Total joint reconstruction (often combined with orbitozygomatic reconstruction) is often performed during the mixed dentition phase. Surgical options include costochondral grafting, cranial bone grafts, total TMJ prostheses, and/or microvascular free tissue transfers. Costochondral grafting has been the gold standard technique for most type III deformities and studies have found that mandibular symmetry and occlusion improved considerably with this procedure. However, studies have again shown that the later it is performed the more stable the result. Regardless of timing of initial TMJ reconstruction, the final facial rotation surgery is done in the permanent dentition phase.[60] Some investigators, such as Polley and Figueroa,[80] prefer interim distraction in type III mandibles to help improve (but not correct) facial symmetry before reconstruction of the TMJ. However, they do not reconstruct the lateral temporozygomatic deficiency and condylar abutment at that time.

SOFT TISSUE CORRECTION

The soft tissue deficits in patients with CFM are multidimensional, with varying degrees of deficiency noted in skin, subcutaneous tissue, muscles of mastication, and the parotid gland. Supporters of MDO initially claimed that the surrounding soft tissues increased in volume during lengthening secondary to muscle hypertrophy.[80,83,88,89,124–126] However, the issue remains controversial because multiple other studies have shown a decrease in soft tissue volume in response to skeletal enlargement by MDO.[54,107] In cases in which the soft tissue correction is warranted, experts support proceeding with skeletal realignment before correction of soft tissue deficits to avoid the need of additional soft tissue procedures in the future. Options for surgical correction include microvascular free tissue transfer (including fasciocutaneous and osseocutaneous options, with the parascapular flap being one of the most popular), serial autologous fat grafting, and implants.[81,127]

Tanna and colleagues[127] compared serial autologous fat grafting with microvascular free flap and concluded that serial fat grafting was a useful

---

Box 1
Nagy and colleagues'[91] proposed treatment outline

Type I, IIa patients

Presurgical orthodontics

Standard 3D orthognathic correction during permanent dentition phase

Type IIb

Standard 3D orthognathic advancement with positional correction during permanent dentition phase

If bone stock limited, extra volume can be obtained with unidirectional corpus distraction 1 year before facial rotational surgery or with interpositional bone grafting

Type III

Reconstruction of TMJ during mixed dentition phase

Data from Nagy K, Kuijpers-Jagtman AM, Mommaerts MY. No evidence for long-term effectiveness of early osteodistraction in hemifacial microsomia. Plast Reconstr Surg 2009;124(6):2061–71.

Box 2
Cousley and Calvert's[2] timeline of treatment of CFM

I. Infancy

Correction of soft tissue defects such as preauricular tags, cleft lip/palate, and gross macrostomia

Nerve graft repair of facial palsy

Hearing augmentation (hearing aids)

Osteotomies to correct clinically significant orbital dystopia and plagiocephaly

Elongation of mandible by bone distraction or costochondral grafting in cases with severe skeletal defects leading to respiratory or feeding problems

II. Mixed dentition (approximately 6–12 years of age)

Reconstruction of malformed auricles using either autogenous rib cartilage grafts or osseointegrated implants (for prosthetic ears)

Middle ear reconstruction (predominantly bilateral cases)

Composite nerve and muscle grafts repair of facial palsy

Promotion of mandibular and maxillary growth, and masticatory function using 1 or more of the following techniques:

Orthodontic functional appliances

Costochondral grafts to reconstruct the condyle-ramus unit and TMJ

Mandibular distraction or interpositional rib grafts

III. Adolescence and adulthood

Final orthodontic and orthognathic surgical correction of facial skeleton and occlusion, including adjunctive use of bone recontouring, onlay bone graft techniques, and vascularized bone grafts

Soft tissue augmentation, including vascularized free tissue transfer, to redress any significant asymmetry persisting after bony reconstruction

Definitive correction of auricular morphology, position, and secondary defects

Data from Cousley RR, Calvert ML. Current concepts in the understanding and management of hemifacial microsomia. British J Plast Surg 1997;50(7):536–51.

---

alternative to the microvascular flap after skeletal reconstruction. The mean number of procedures was less for the free-flap group versus the fat-grafting group, but the combined surgical time was much greater for the free-flap group. The volume of soft tissue implanted and the symmetry rating were 20% to 25% higher in microvascular group than the fat-grafting group, but the complication rate was also higher for this group. No statistically significant difference in patient or physician satisfaction was noted.[127] Thus, either option is reasonable, and the investigators recommended basing decisions on whether the patient will be returning to the operating room for other procedures during childhood, making it possible to coordinate serial fat grafting during these times.

Several studies have investigated the use of implants, such as high-density porous polyethylene, to augment the hypoplastic mandible in HFM.[128,129] In addition, alloplastic material such as Medpor (Stryker Craniomaxillofacial, Portage, MI) can be used to augment areas of soft tissue deficiency. These synthetic implants can be preformed or custom designed from 3D CT image guidance. However, there are limited data for the outcomes of such implants.

CORRECTION OF EAR ANOMALIES

The ear anomalies associated with CFM can involve the outer ear, external auditory canal, and middle ear structures and range from mild hypoplasia to anotia. The surgical treatment of these anomalies parallels treatment of isolated ear deformities. Patients with mild hypoplasia and cupping can be treated with simple reshaping of the existing cartilage in many cases. As the deformity worsens and the bony deficiency becomes more severe, treatment is more extensive and achieving a good aesthetic outcome becomes more challenging. Various materials have been used for ear reconstruction, each with its risks

Table 5
Pluijmers and colleagues'[61] long-term outcomes results based on treatment type and mandibular classification

Treatment Type	Pruzansky-Kaban Classification	Long-term Results
MDO (n = 104)	Type I (n = 14)	Minimal relapse
	Type I and IIa (n = 39)	Slight increase in asymmetry in first year, 43% of patients with relapse at 5 y
	Type II (n = 4)	Slight decrease in mandibular length
	Type IIa (n = 24)	46% of patients with relapse of asymmetry
	Type IIb (n = 12)	>50% of patients with relapse (exact numbers not included)
	Type III (n = 11)	>50% of patients with relapse (exact numbers not included)
Elongation and rotation (n = 6)	Type I (n = 6)	Stable results
	Type IIa (n = 1)	Stable results, mild chin point deviation
Iliac/rib graft (n = 19)	Type IIa (n = 19)	Minimal relapse
Fibular free flap (n = 8)	Type IIb (n = 1)	Minimal relapse
	Type III (n = 7)	Increased asymmetry
Costochondral graft (n = 44)	Type IIb (n = 19) Type III (n = 25)	75% of patients with relapse of asymmetry
Mandibular cortex graft + MDO (n = 21)	Type I (n = 11)	Minimal relapse
	Type II (n = 4)	Minimal relapse
	Type III (n = 6)	Minimal relapse
Fibular free flap + MDO (n = 2)	Type III (n = 2)	No relapse
Costochondral graft + MDO (n = 16)	Type III (n = 16)	12.5% of patients with relapse

Data from Pluijmers BI, Caron CJ, Dunaway DJ, et al. Mandibular reconstruction in the growing patient with unilateral craniofacial microsomia: a systematic review. Int J Oral Maxillofac Surg 2014;43(3):286–95.

and benefits. Autologous reconstruction is multistaged and generally involves the use of costal cartilage grafts to recreate the auricular framework. Several groups have also studied the use of alloplastic materials such as porous polyethylene, which would avoid donor site morbidity; allow reconstruction in younger, smaller patients; and typically provide stable rigidity. However, use of these materials is still controversial. Furthermore, the details of these procedures are beyond the scope of this article.[113]

SURGICAL COMPLICATIONS

As with any surgical procedures, the techniques discussed earlier have risks. Grafting procedures (most notably mandibular grafting) can be unpredictable because of the risk for undesirable resorption (described earlier), leading to decreased volume and strength of the reconstructed area. These patients also experience morbidity at the donor site. In terms of MDO, risks include pin-track infections, tooth germ injury, pain, hypertrophic facial scars, device fracture,

limited mouth opening, and open-bite deformity, as well as the tendency for external fixation pins to loosen.[64,81,91,130–132] With MDO in type IIb and III patients, there is risk for posterosuperior movement of the proximal jaw segment (small and easier to move) causing uncontrolled displacement and relapse of facial asymmetry after removal of the device.[133,134]

SUMMARY

CFM is characterized by anomalies of the first and second pharyngeal arch structures and includes a wide spectrum of phenotypes ranging in severity. Treatment of these patients depends on the degree of deformity of the facial framework. Classification systems have emerged over the years to better stratify these patients and develop a standardized treatment algorithm based on patient class. There are still debates regarding the timing of surgical correction for these patients, because some individuals support early intervention and others encourage providers to wait until completion of growth to surgically correct their bony asymmetries. Three systematic reviews in the past decade have supported the latter argument. Regardless, treatment includes lengthening of the mandible (by traditional osteotomy and elongation/rotation, grafting, or MDO), recreation of the TMJ (in more severe cases), and correction of soft tissue deformities and ear anomalies. Despite modifications in surgical technique and timing over the years, many of these children require multiple surgeries during childhood and adolescence to correct their facial asymmetries.

REFERENCES

1. Cohen MM Jr, Rollnick BR, Kaye CI. Oculo-auriculo-vertebral spectrum: An updated critique. Cleft Palate J 1989;26:276–86.
2. Cousley RR, Calvert ML. Current concepts in the understanding and management of hemifacial microsomia. Br J Plast Surg 1997;50(7):536–51.
3. Ohtani J, Hoffman WY, Vargervik K, et al. Team management and treatment outcomes for patients with hemifacial microsomia. Am J Orthod Dentofacial Orthop 2012;141(4 Suppl):S74–81.
4. Fariña R, Valladares S, Torrealba R, et al. Orthognathic surgery in craniofacial microsomia: treatment algorithm. Plast Reconstr Surg Glob Open 2015;3(1):e294.
5. Poswillo D. The pathogenesis of 1st and 2nd branchial arch syndrome. Oral Surg Oral Med Oral Pathol 1973;35:301–28.
6. Johnston MC, Bronsky PT. Animal models for human craniofacial malformations. J Craniofac Genet Dev Biol 1991;11:277–91.
7. Rooryck C, Souakri N, Cailley D, et al. Array-CGH analysis of a cohort of 86 patients with oculoauriculovertebral spectrum. Am J Med Genet A 2010;152A:1984–9.
8. Rollnick BR, Kaye CI. Hemifacial microsomia and variants: pedigree data. Am J Med Genet 1983;15:233–53.
9. Kaye CI, Martin AO, Rollnick BR, et al. Oculoauriculovertebral anomaly: segregation analysis. Am J Med Genet 1992;43:913–7.
10. Xu J, Fan YS, Siu VM. A child with features of Goldenhar syndrome and a novel 1.12 Mb deletion in 22q11.2 by cytogenetics and oligonucleotide array CGH: is this a candidate region for the syndrome? Am J Med Genet A 2008;146A(14):1886–9.
11. Digilio MC, McDonald-McGinn DM, Heike C, et al. Three patients with oculo-auriculo-vertebral spectrum and microdeletion 22q11.2. Am J Med Genet A 2009;149A(12):2860–4.
12. Tan TY, Collins A, James PA, et al. Phenotypic variability of distal 22q11.2 copy number abnormalities. Am J Med Genet A 2011;155A(7):1623–33.
13. Zielinski D, Markus B, Sheikh M, et al. OTX2 duplication is implicated in hemifacial microsomia. PLoS One 2014;9(5):e96788.
14. Guida V, Sinibaldi L, Pagnoni M, et al. A de novo proximal 3q29 chromosome microduplication in a patient with oculo auriculo vertebral spectrum. Am J Med Genet A 2015;167A(4):797–801.
15. Kelberman D, Tyson J, Chandler DC, et al. Hemifacial microsomia: progress in understanding the genetic basis of a complex malformation syndrome. Hum Genet 2001;109(6):638–45.
16. Huang XS, Li X, Tan C, et al. Genome-wide scanning reveals complex etiology of oculo-auriculo-vertebral spectrum. Tohoku J Exp Med 2010;222:311–8.
17. Callier P, Faivre L, Thauvin-Robinet C, et al. Array-CGH in a series of 30 patients with mental retardation, dysmorphic features, and congenital malformations detected an interstitial 1p22.2-p31.1 deletion in a patient with features overlapping the Goldenhar syndrome. Am J Med Genet A 2008;146A(16):2109–15.
18. Abdelmoity AT, Hall JJ, Bittel DC, et al. 1.39 Mb inherited interstitial deletion in 12p13.33 associated with developmental delay. Eur J Med Genet 2011;54(2):198–203.
19. Kobrynski L, Chitayat D, Zahed L, et al. Trisomy 22 and facioauriculovertebral (Goldenhar) sequence. Am J Med Genet 1993;46(1):68–71.
20. Ballesta-Martínez MJ, López-González V, Dulcet LA, et al. Autosomal dominant oculoauriculovertebral spectrum and 14q23.1 microduplication. Am J Med Genet A 2013;161A(8):2030–5.
21. Ou Z, Martin DM, Bedoyan JK, et al. Branchiootorenal syndrome and oculoauriculovertebral spectrum features associated with duplication of SIX1, SIX6, and OTX2 resulting from a complex chromosomal rearrangement. Am J Med Genet A 2008;146A(19):2480–9.
22. Brun A, Cailley D, Toutain J, et al. 1.5 Mb microdeletion in 15q24 in a patient with mild OAVS phenotype. Eur J Med Genet 2012;55(2):135–9.
23. Descartes M. Oculoauriculovertebral spectrum with 5p15.33-pter deletion. Clin Dysmorphol 2006;15(3):153–4.
24. Josifova DJ, Patton MA, Marks K. Oculoauriculovertebral spectrum phenotype caused by an unbalanced t(5;8)(p15.31;p23.1) rearrangement. Clin Dysmorphol 2004;13(3):151–3.
25. Ladekarl S. Combination of Goldenhar's syndrome with the Cri-Du-Chat syndrome. Acta Ophthalmol (Copenh) 1968;46(3):605–10.
26. Ala-Mello S, Siggberg L, Knuutila S, et al. Further evidence for a relationship between the 5p15 chromosome region and the oculoauriculovertebral

anomaly. Am J Med Genet A 2008;146A(19): 2490–4.

27. Dabir TA, Morrison PJ. Trisomy 10p with clinical features of facio-auriculo-vertebral spectrum: a case report. Clin Dysmorphol 2006;15(1):25–7.

28. Gimelli S, Cuoco C, Ronchetto P, et al. Interstitial deletion 14q31.1q31.3 transmitted from a mother to her daughter, both with features of hemifacial microsomia. J Appl Genet 2013;54(3):361–5.

29. Verloes A, Seret N, Bernier V, et al. Branchial arch anomalies in trisomy 18. Ann Genet 1991;34(1): 22–4.

30. Herman GE, Greenberg F, Ledbetter DH. Multiple congenital anomaly/mental retardation (MCA/MR) syndrome with Goldenhar complex due to a terminal del(22q). Am J Med Genet 1988;29(4): 909–15.

31. Quintero-Rivera F, Martinez-Agosto JA. Hemifacial microsomia in cat-eye syndrome: 22q11.1-q11.21 as candidate loci for facial symmetry. Am J Med Genet A 2013;161A(8):1985–91.

32. Torti EE, Braddock SR, Bernreuter K, et al. Oculo-auriculo-vertebral spectrum, cat eye, and distal 22q11 microdeletion syndromes: a unique double rearrangement. Am J Med Genet A 2013;161A(8): 1992–8.

33. Garavelli L, Virdis R, Donadio A, et al. Oculo-auriculo-vertebral spectrum in Klinefelter syndrome. Genet Couns 1999;10(3):321–4.

34. Poonawalla HH, Kaye CI, Rosenthal IM, et al. Hemifacial microsomia in a patient with Klinefelter syndrome. Cleft Palate J 1980;17(3):194–6.

35. Stanojević M, Stipoljev F, Koprcina B, et al. Oculo-auriculo-vertebral (Goldenhar) spectrum associated with pericentric inversion 9: coincidental findings or etiologic factor? J Craniofac Genet Dev Biol 2000;20(3):150–4.

36. Northup JK, Matalon D, Hawkins JC, et al. Pericentric inversion, inv(14)(p11.2q22.3), in a month old with features of Goldenhar syndrome. Clin Dysmorphol 2010;19(4):185–9.

37. Hodes ME, Gleiser S, DeRosa GP, et al. Trisomy 7 mosaicism and manifestations of Goldenhar syndrome with unilateral radial hypoplasia. J Craniofac Genet Dev Biol 1981;1(1):49–55.

38. de Ravel TJ, Legius E, Brems H, et al. Hemifacial microsomia in two patients further supporting chromosomal mosaicism as a causative factor. Clin Dysmorphol 2001;10(4):263–7.

39. Wilson GN, Barr M Jr. Trisomy 9 mosaicism: another etiology for the manifestations of Goldenhar syndrome. J Craniofac Genet Dev Biol 1983; 3(4):313–6.

40. Beleza-Meireles A, Clayton-Smith J, Saraiva JM, et al. Oculo-auriculo-vertebral spectrum: a review of the literature and genetic update. J Med Genet 2014;51:635–45.

41. Miller KA, Tan TY, Welfare MF, et al. A mouse splice-site mutant and individuals with atypical chromosome 22q11.2 deletions demonstrates the crucial role for crkl in craniofacial and pharyngeal development. Mol Syndromol 2014;5(6):276–86.

42. Robinson LK, Hoyme HE, Edwards DK, et al. Vascular pathogenesis of unilateral craniofacial defects. J Pediatr 1987;111:236–9.

43. Van Allen MI. Structural anomalies resulting from vascular disruption. Pediatr Clin North Am 1992; 39:255–77.

44. Werler MM, Sheehan JE, Hayes C, et al. Vasoactive exposures, vascular events and hemifacial microsomia. Birth Defects Res A Clin Mol Teratol 2004; 70:389–95.

45. Cousley RRJ. A comparison of two classification systems for hemifacial microsomia. Br J Oral Maxillofac Surg 1993;3(1):78–82.

46. Vento AR, LaBrie RA, Mulliken JB. The O.M.E.N.S. classification of hemifacial microsomia. Cleft Palate Craniofac J 1991;28:68–76.

47. Gorlin RJ, Cohen MM Jr, Levin LS. Branchial arch and oro-acral disorders. Syndromes of the head and neck. 3rd edition. Oxford (united Kingdom): Oxford University Press; 1990. p. 641–9.

48. Tuin AJ, Tahiri Y, Paine KM, et al. Clarifying the relationships among the different features of the OMENS+ classification in craniofacial microsomia. Plast Reconstr Surg 2015;135(1):149e–56e.

49. Wink JD, Goldstein JA, Paliga JT, et al. The mandibular deformity in hemifacial microsomia: a reassessment of the Pruzansky and Kaban classification. Plast Reconstr Surg 2014;133(2):174–81.

50. Pruzansky S. Not all dwarfed mandibles are alike. Birth Defects 1969;1:120–9.

51. Kaban LB, Moses MH, Mulliken JB. Surgical correction of hemifacial microsomia in the growing child. Plast Reconstr Surg 1988;82:9–19.

52. Takahashi-Ichikawa N, Susami T, Nagahama K, et al. Evaluation of mandibular hypoplasia in patients with hemifacial microsomia: a comparison between panoramic radiography and three-dimensional computed tomography. Cleft Palate Craniofac J 2013;50:381–7.

53. David DJ, Mahatumarat C, Cooter RD. Hemifacial microsomia: a multisystem classification. Plast Reconstr Surg 1987;80:525–35.

54. Kaban LB, Padwa BL, Mulliken JB. Surgical correction of mandibular hypoplasia in hemifacial microsomia: the case for treatment in early childhood. J Oral Maxillofac Surg 1998;56(5):628–38.

55. Kearns GJ, Padwa BL, Mulliken JB, et al. Progression of facial asymmetry in hemifacial microsomia. Plast Reconstr Surg 2000;105(2):492–8.

56. Kaban LB, Mulliken JL, Murray JE. Three dimensional approach to analysis and treatment of hemifacial microsomia. Cleft Palate J 1981;18:90.

57. Vargervik K, Ousterhout D, Farias M. Factors affecting long-term results in hemifacial microsomia. Cleft Palate J 1986;23:53–68.

58. Peltomaki T, Ronning O. Growth of costochondral fragments transplanted from mature to young isogeneic rats. Cleft Palate Craniofac J 1993;30:159–63.

59. Sailer HF. Experience using lyophilized bank cartilage for facial contour correction. J Maxillofac Surg 1976;4:149–57.

60. Mommaerts MY, Nagy K. Is early osteodistraction a solution for the ascending ramus compartment in hemifacial microsomia? A literature study. J Craniomaxillofac Surg 2002;30(4):201–7.

61. Pluijmers BI, Caron CJ, Dunaway DJ, et al. Mandibular reconstruction in the growing patient with unilateral craniofacial microsomia: a systematic review. Int J Oral Maxillofac Surg 2014;43(3):286–95.

62. Gillies HD. Plastic surgery of the face. Lancet 1920;196:177–92.

63. Zanakis NS, Gavakos K, Faippea M, et al. Application of custom-made TMJ prosthesis in hemifacial microsomia. Int J Oral Maxillofac Surg 2009;38(9):988–92.

64. Corcoran J, Hubli EH, Salyer KE. Distraction osteogenesis of costochondral neomandibles: a clinical experience. Plast Reconstr Surg 1997;100:311–5.

65. Stelnicki EJ, Hollier L, Lee C, et al. Distraction osteogenesis of costochondral bone grafts in the mandible. Plast Reconstr Surg 2002;109:925–33.

66. Sonntag E, Rosenthal W. Lehrbuch der Mund-und Kieferchirurgie. Leipzig (Germany): Georg Thieme; 1930. p. 173–5.

67. Wassmund M. Lehrbuch der praktischen chirurgie des mundes und der kiefer. Band 1. Leipzig (Germany): Hermann Meusser; 1935. p. 275.

68. Kazanjian VH. The interrelation of dentistry and surgery in the treatment of deformities of the face and jaws. Am J Orthod Oral Surg 1941;27:10–30.

69. Crawford MJ. Selection of Appliances for Typical Facial Fractures. Oral Surg Oral Med Oral Pathol 1948;1(5):442–51.

70. Klein C, Howaldt HP. Correction of mandibular hypoplasia by means of bidirectional callus distraction. J Craniofac Surg 1996;7(4):258–66.

71. Burstein FD. Resorbable distraction of the mandible: technical evolution and clinical experience. J Craniofac Surg 2008;19(3):637–43.

72. McCarthy JG. The role of distraction osteogenesis in the reconstruction of the mandible in unilateral craniofacial microsomia. Clin Plast Surg 1994;21:625–31.

73. Cakir-Ozkan N, Eyibilen A, Ozkan F, et al. Stereologic analysis of bone produced by distraction osteogenesis or autogenous bone grafting in mandible. J Craniofac Surg 2010;21(3):735–40.

74. Fisher E, Staffenberg DA, McCarthy JG, et al. Histopathologic and biochemical changes in the muscles affected by distraction osteogenesis of the mandible. Plast Reconstr Surg 1997;99(2):366–71.

75. Mackool RJ, Hopper RA, Grayson BH, et al. Volumetric change of the medial pterygoid following distraction osteogenesis of the mandible: an example of the associated soft-tissue changes. Plast Reconstr Surg 2003;111(6):1804–7.

76. McCarthy JG, Katzen JT, Hopper R, et al. The first decade of mandibular distraction: lessons we have learned. Plast Reconstr Surg 2002;110(7):1704–13.

77. van Strijen PJ, Breuning KH, Becking AG, et al. Stability after distraction osteogenesis to lengthen the mandible: results in 50 patients. J Oral Maxillofac Surg 2004;62(3):304–7.

78. Hollier LH, Rowe NM, Mackool RJ, et al. Controlled multiplanar distraction of the mandible. Part III: laboratory studies of sagittal (anteroposterior) and horizontal (mediolateral) movements. J Craniofac Surg 2000;11(2):83–95.

79. Singh DJ, Glick PH, Bartlett SP. Mandibular deformities: single-vector distraction techniques for a multivector problem. J Craniofac Surg 2009;20(5):1468–72.

80. Polley JW, Figueroa AA, Liou EJ, et al. Longitudinal analysis of mandibular asymmetry in hemifacial microsomia. Plast Reconstr Surg 1997;99(2):328–39.

81. Hollier LH, Kim JH, Grayson B, et al. Mandibular growth after distraction in patients under 48 months of age. Plast Reconstr Surg 1999;103(5):1361–70.

82. Gosain AK. Plastic Surgery Educational Foundation DATA Committee. Distraction osteogenesis of the craniofacial skeleton. Plast Reconstr Surg 2001;107(1):278–80.

83. McCarthy JG, Stelnicki EJ, Mehrara BJ, et al. Distraction osteogenesis of the craniofacial skeleton. Plast Reconstr Surg 2001;107(7):1812–27.

84. Molina F, Ortiz Monasterio F. Mandibular elongation and remodeling by distraction: a farewell to major osteotomies. Plast Reconstr Surg 1995;96(4):825–40 [discussion: 841–2].

85. Jansma J, Bierman MW, Becking AG. Intraoral distraction osteogenesis to lengthen the ascending ramus. Experience with seven patients. Br J Oral Maxillofac Surg 2004;42(6):526–31.

86. Padwa BL, Mulliken JB, Maghen A, et al. Midfacial growth after costochondral graft construction of the mandibular ramus in hemifacial microsomia. J Oral Maxillofac Surg 1998;56(2):122–7.

87. Oeltjen JC, Hollier LH, McCarthy JG. Mandibular growth after osteodistraction. In: Samchukov M, Cope J, Cherkashin A, editors. Craniofacial distraction osteogenesis. St Louis (MO): Mosby; 2001. p. 297–304.

88. Molina F. Mandibular distraction: surgical refinements and long-term results. Clin Plast Surg 2004;31(3):443–62, vi–vii.

89. Ortiz Monasterio F, Molina F, Andrade L, et al. Simultaneous mandibular and maxillary distraction in hemifacial microsomia in adults: avoiding occlusal disasters. Plast Reconstr Surg 1997; 100(4):852–61.

90. Baek SH, Kim S. The determinants of successful distraction osteogenesis of the mandible in hemifacial microsomia from longitudinal results. J Craniofac Surg 2005;16(4):549–58.

91. Nagy K, Kuijpers-Jagtman AM, Mommaerts MY. No evidence for long-term effectiveness of early osteodistraction in hemifacial microsomia. Plast Reconstr Surg 2009;124(6):2061–71.

92. Grayson BH, McCormick S, Santiago PE, et al. Vector of device placement and trajectory of mandibular distraction. J Craniofac Surg 1997;8: 473–80.

93. Cavaliere CM, Buchman SR. Mandibular distraction in the absence of an ascending ramus and condyle. J Craniofac Surg 2002;13:527–32.

94. Altug-Atac AT, Grayson BH, McCarthy JG. Comparison of skeletal and soft-tissue changes following unilateral mandibular distraction osteogenesis. Plast Reconstr Surg 2008;121:1751–9.

95. Kulewicz M, Cudzilo D, Hortis-Dzierzbicka M, et al. Distraction osteogenesis in the treatment of hemifacial microsomia (in Polish). Med Wieku Rozwoj 2004;8:761–72.

96. Shetye PR, Grayson BH, Mackool RJ, et al. Long-term stability and growth following unilateral mandibular distraction in growing children with craniofacial microsomia. Plast Reconstr Surg 2006;118:985–95.

97. Ortiz-Monasterio F. Early mandibular and maxillary osteotomies for the correction of hemifacial microsomia. A preliminary report. Clin Plast Surg 1982; 9:509–17.

98. Trahar M, Sheffield R, Kawamoto H, et al. Cephalometric evaluation of the craniofacial complex in patients treated with an intraoral distraction osteogenesis device: A preliminary report. Am J Orthod Dentofacial Orthop 2003;124:639–50.

99. Gui L, Zhang Z, Zang M, et al. Restoration of facial symmetry in hemifacial microsomia with mandibular outer cortex bone grafting combined with distraction osteogenesis. Plast Reconstr Surg 2011;127:1997–2004.

100. Scolozzi P, Herzog G, Jaques B. Simultaneous maxillo-mandibular distraction osteogenesis in hemifacial microsomia: a new technique using two distractors. Plast Reconstr Surg 2006;117:1530–42.

101. Satoh K, Suzuki T, Uemura T, et al. Maxillo-mandibular distraction osteogenesis for hemifacial microsomia in children. Ann Plast Surg 2002;49:572–8.

102. Huang CS, Ko WC, Lin WY, et al. Mandibular lengthening by distraction osteogenesis in children—a one- year follow-up study. Cleft Palate Craniofac J 1999;36:269–74.

103. Munro IR, Phillips JH, Griffin G. Growth after construction of the temporomandibular joint in children with hemifacial microsomia. Cleft Palate J 1989;26: 303–11.

104. Ousterhout DK, Vargervik K. Surgical treatment of the jaw deformities in hemifacial microsomia. Aust N Z J Surg 1987;57:77–87.

105. Converse JM, Horowitz SL, Coccaro PJ, et al. The corrective treatment of the skeletal asymmetry in hemifacial microsomia. Plast Reconstr Surg 1973; 52:221–32.

106. Kusnoto B, Figueroa AA, Polley JW. A longitudinal three-dimensional evaluation of the growth pattern in hemifacial microsomia treated by mandibular distraction osteogenesis: a preliminary report. J Craniofac Surg 1999;10:480–6.

107. Marquez IM, Fish LC, Stella JP. Two-year follow-up of distraction osteogenesis: its effect on mandibular ramus height in hemifacial microsomia. Am J Orthod Dentofacial Orthop 2000; 117(2):130–9.

108. Meazzini MC, Mazzoleni F, Bozzetti A, et al. Comparison of mandibular vertical growth in hemifacial microsomia patients treated with early distraction or not treated: follow up till the completion of growth. J Craniomaxillofac Surg 2012;40:105–11.

109. Meazzini MC, Mazzoleni F, Bozzetti A, et al. Does functional appliance treatment truly improve stability of mandibular vertical distraction osteogenesis in hemifacial microsomia. J Craniomaxillofac Surg 2008;36:384–9.

110. Meazzini MC, Mazzoleni F, Gabriele C, et al. Mandibular distraction osteogenesis in hemifacial microsomia: long-term follow-up. J Craniomaxillofac Surg 2005;33(6):370–6.

111. Batra P, Ryan FS, Witherow H, et al. Long term results of mandibular distraction. J Indian Soc Pedod Prev Dent 2006;24:30–9.

112. Gürsoy S, Hukki J, Hurmerinta K. Five year follow-up of mandibular distraction osteogenesis on the dentofacial structures of syndromic children. Orthod Craniofac Res 2008;11:57–64.

113. Rachmiel A, Levy M, Laufer D. Lengthening of the mandible by distraction osteogenesis: report of cases. J Maxillofac Surg 1995;54:838.

114. Huisinga-Fischer CE, Vaandrager JM, Prahl-Andersen B. Longitudinal results of mandibular distraction osteogenesis in hemifacial microsomia. J Craniofac Surg 2003;14:924–33.

115. Ko EW, Hung KF, Huang CS, et al. Correction of facial asymmetry with multiplanar mandible distraction: A one-year follow-up study. Cleft Palate Craniofac J 2004;41:5–12.

116. Wan DC, Taub PJ, Allam KA, et al. Distraction osteogenesis of costocartilaginous rib grafts and treatment algorithm for severely hypoplastic mandibles. Plast Reconstr Surg 2011;127: 2005–13.

117. Santamaria E, Morales C, Taylor JA, et al. Mandibular microsurgical reconstruction in patients with hemifacial microsomia. Plast Reconstr Surg 2008; 122:1839–49.

118. Chow A, Lee HF, Trahar M, et al. Cephalometric evaluation of the craniofacial complex in patients treated with an intraoral distraction osteogenesis device: a long-term study. Am J Orthod Dentofacial Orthop 2008;134:724–31.

119. Cerajewska TL, Singh GD. Morphometric analyses of the mandible in prepubertal craniofacial microsomia patients treated with an inverted-L osteotomy. Clin Anat 2002;15:100–7.

120. Hay AD, Singh GD. Mandibular transformations in prepubertal patients following treatment for craniofacial microsomia: thin-plate spline analysis. Clin Anat 2000;13:361–72.

121. Hay AD, Ayoub AF, Moos KF, et al. Euclidean distance matrix analysis of surgical changes in prepubertal craniofacial microsomia patients treated with an inverted L osteotomy. Cleft Palate Craniofac J 2000;37:497–502.

122. Singh GD, Hay AD. Morphometry of the mandible in prepubertal craniofacial microsomia patients following an inverted L osteotomy. Int J Adult Orthodon Orthognath Surg 1999;14:229–35.

123. Mulliken JB, Ferraro NF, Vento AR. A retrospective analysis of growth of the constructed condyle-ramus in children with hemifacial microsomia. Cleft Palate J 1989;26:312–7.

124. Takato T, Hikiji H. Distraction and tissue regeneration. Clin Calcium 2002;12(2):207–11.

125. Pensler JM, Goldberg DP, Lindell B, et al. Skeletal distraction of the hypoplastic mandible. Ann Plast Surg 1995;34(2):130–6 [discussion: 136–7].

126. Diner PA, Kollar EM, Vazquez MP. Mandibular distraction. Ann Chir Plast Esthet 1997;42(5):547–55.

127. Tanna N, Broer PN, Roostaeian J, et al. Soft tissue correction of craniofacial microsomia and progressive hemifacial atrophy. J Craniofac Surg 2012; 23(1):2024–6.

128. Rai A, Datarkar A, Arora A, et al. Utility of high density porous polyethylene implants in maxillofacial surgery. J Maxillofac Oral Surg 2014;13(1):42–6.

129. Andrade NN, Raikwar K. Medpor in maxillofacial deformities: report of three cases. J Maxillofac Oral Surg 2009;8(2):192–5.

130. Klein C, Howaldt HP. Lengthening of the hypoplastic mandible by gradual distraction in children. A preliminary report. J Craniomaxillofac Surg 1995; 23:68.

131. Carls FR, Sailer HF. Seven years clinical experience with mandibular distraction in children. J Craniomaxillofac Surg 1998;26(4):197–208.

132. Tharanon W, Sinn DP. Mandibular distraction osteogenesis with multidirectional extraoral distraction device in hemifacial microsomia patients: three-dimensional treatment planning, prediction tracings, and case outcomes. J Craniofac Surg 1999; 10(3):202–13.

133. Rubio-Bueno P, Padrón A, Villa E, et al. Distraction osteogenesis of the ascending ramus for mandibular hypoplasia using extraoral or intraoral devices: a report of 8 cases. J Oral Maxillofac Surg 2000; 58(6):593–601.

134. Takashima M, Kitai N, Mori Y, et al. Mandibular distraction osteogenesis using an intraoral device and bite plate for a case of hemifacial microsomia. Cleft Palate Craniofac J 2003;40(4): 437–45.

Nonsyndromic Craniosynostosis and Deformational Head Shape Disorders

Lisa M. Morris, MD

KEYWORDS

- Craniosynostosis • Deformational plagiocephaly • Positional plagiocephaly
- Nonsyndromic craniosynostosis • Treatment of craniosynostosis • Cranial vault reconstruction
- Minimally invasive • Helmet therapy

KEY POINTS

- The incidence of infant head shape abnormalities is increasing. Physicians should be able to identify these patients and distinguish between deformational plagiocephaly and craniosynostosis.
- Deformational plagiocephaly does not have a known negative impact on the brain; however, early diagnosis and treatment is needed to correct the dysmorphic head.
- Most craniosynostoses are nonsyndromic and include sagittal, metopic, coronal, lambdoid, and multisuture synostosis. Surgeons should be able to make a diagnosis based on clinical findings.
- Surgical indications for craniosynostosis are to correct the abnormal craniofacial appearance, prevent negative effects of increased intracranial pressure on the brain and optic nerves, and protect the globe of the eye.
- Cranial vault reconstruction immediately corrects both the fused suture and cranial abnormality; minimally invasive procedures allow for improvement of the cranial shape over time.

INTRODUCTION

A persistent abnormal head shape is a concerning finding in an infant and can be from craniosynostosis (intrinsic) or deformational plagiocephaly (DP; extrinsic) causes. It is imperative the treating physician can differentiate between the 2 abnormalities to initiate appropriate treatment and avoid any long-term sequela. *Craniosynostosis* is the premature fusion of 1 or more cranial sutures, causing an abnormal head shape. This early fusion of the cranial sutures restricts normal skull growth, causing not only a dysmorphic head shape but also possible increased intracranial pressure leading to neurocognitive impairment. *Deformational plagiocephaly*, in contrast, is an atypical head shape caused by extrinsic forces pushing on the soft, malleable skull bones. The cranial sutures remain open and functional, with no risk for increased intracranial pressure causing impairment to the developing brain.

DEFORMATIONAL PLAGIOCEPHALY

Also termed *positional plagiocephaly* or *nonsynostotic plagiocephaly*, this asymmetric head shape abnormality has increased in incidence over the past 2 decades and is the leading cause for atypical head shapes.[1–5] The cause of DP is asymmetric external forces on the soft infant calvarium, which are typically created by gravity pushing the infants head against the crib mattress

The author has nothing to disclose.
Craniofacial Foundation of Utah, 5089 South 900 East, Suite 100, Salt Lake City, UT 84117, USA
E-mail address: lisa.m.morris5@gmail.com

facialplastic.theclinics.com

with an equal but opposite force pushing back on the head (**Fig. 1**). In 1992, the American Academy of Pediatrics initiated the Back to Sleep Campaign in which infants were placed on their backs during sleep to reduce the risk of sudden infant death syndrome.[6–10] This campaign dramatically deceased the incidence of sudden infant death syndrome, but resulted in a significant increase in DP.[4,5] A recent study in Canada found that nearly 47% of infants between 7 and 12 weeks of age had some degree of DP.[11] Children with torticollis are at increased risk for DP, because they have limited head movement and lie with their head turned to only 1 side. Any preference of head position should be viewed as an early manifestation of torticollis and a high risk for DP.[12] Other risk factors for DP include prematurity, developmental delay, multiple gestation pregnancy, male gender, assisted delivery, primaparity, uterine abnormalities, oligohydramnios, and breech presentation. Each of these factors cause intrauterine deformation and/or increase the risk of limited head movement during the first months of life.[5,7,13] Deformational changes of the skull can lead to various head shapes, depending on what part of the head is positioned against the surface of the bed (**Box 1**).

Treatment of Deformational Plagiocephaly

Parental education about the etiology of DP and the importance of alternating the sleeping position by placing the infant supine and turning the head to either side will help to prevent the deformity from developing.[5,9,13] Infants with torticollis, or any evidence of head position preference, should undergo physical therapy to allow full range of motion of the neck.[13] The underlying goal of repositioning therapy is to keep the infant from lying on the flat part of the head. This includes monitored tummy time during the day, avoiding a car seat when not in a vehicle, and encouraging free and spontaneous movements of the infant.[12] If the infant is young (<3 months) and the deformity is mild, repositioning of the infant to prevent lying on the flattened portion of the head may be all

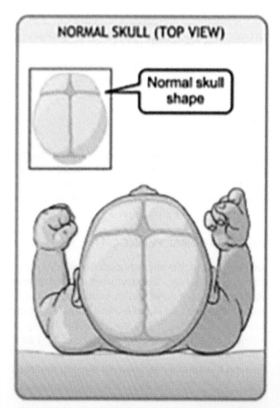
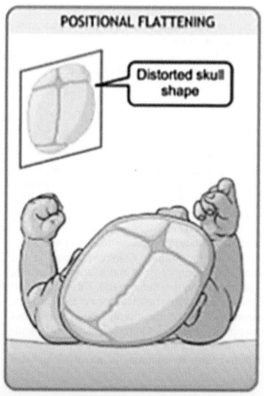

Fig. 1. Normal head shape versus deformational plagiocephaly. This figure depicts the changes that occur to the soft cranium with deformational plagiocephaly. In the illustration on the right, there is flattening of the right occipital region and forward advancement of the right frontal region. (*From* Mortenson P, Steinbok P, Smith D. Deformational plagiocephaly and orthotic treatment: indications and limitations. Childs Nerv Syst 2012;28(9):1408; with permission.)

Box 1
Deformational plagiocephaly, deformational brachycephaly, and deformational dolichocephaly

- *Deformational plagiocephaly* refers to asymmetry of the head, typically with a flattening of 1 side of the occiput. In more severe cases, the ipsilateral ear, forehead and cheek are also deviated forward. From a vertex view, this creates a parallelogram shape to the head[7,9] (see **Fig. 1**).
- *Deformational brachycephaly* denotes flatness of the midline of the occiput with widening of the biparietal region of the skull.[9]
- *Deformational dolichocephaly* results in a long, narrow head with flattening on either side. This deformity is found most commonly in premature infants who spent time in the neonatal intensive care unit and were positioned on the sides of their head because they lacked sufficient neck control to sleep on the back of their head.[7]

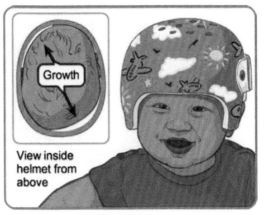

Fig. 2. A customized orthotic helmet for the treatment of deformational plagiocephaly. (*From* Mortenson P, Steinbok P, Smith D. Deformational plagiocephaly and orthotic treatment: indications and limitations. Childs Nerv Syst 2012;28(9):1409; with permission.)

that is required. Often a wedge or rolled up blanket can be placed under the torso on 1 side to appropriately position the child.[5] If the infant is older (>4–6 months) with failed repositioning therapy, orthotic helmets are often required to mold the cranium back to a normocephalic appearance.[8,14] Helmet molding is possible owing to an infant's malleable skull and rapid brain growth.[9] The helmet is custom fit to the infant's head with close approximation at the overexpanded areas of the skull, and the flat areas are left with excess space. As normal cranial growth occurs, the helmet redirects skull growth into the excess spaces to allow normalization of the head shape. There is no restriction of brain expansion. The skull grows into the ideal shape and the rate of correction is proportionate to the rate of head growth. Younger infants will correct faster than older infants. If the deformity is severe in an older child, there may not be sufficient cranial growth remaining to completely normalize the head shape.[13] The helmet is worn 23 hours a day and requires monthly adjustments by an orthotist (**Fig. 2**).

CRANIOSYNOSTOSIS

Craniosynostosis, or early fusion of 1 or more cranial sutures, is typically an intrauterine event. The infant presents with an abnormal head shape at the time of birth or shortly thereafter. A human skull has 6 major cranial sutures, or dense fibrous connections that separate the individual cranial bones

(**Fig. 3**). In the normal skull, these sutures allow for compression of the cranial bones during passage through the birth canal and enable rapid skull growth during the first few years of life as the brain triples in size.[15,16] Craniosynostosis restricts skull growth perpendicular to the affected suture. Continued brain enlargement leads to compensatory overgrowth of the skull at the remaining patent sutures, causing progressive deformity that typically parallels the fused suture. This is known as Virchow's law[17] and allows us to predict the characteristic dysmorphic head shape associated with each type of sutural fusion.

Epidemiology, Etiology, and Diagnosis

The incidence of craniosynostosis is 1 in 2000 to 2500 children.[15,18,19] The etiology of craniosynostosis is multifactorial, involving environmental factors, genetic mutations, and intrinsic bone abnormalities[20–23] with only 8% of cases being familial or syndromic.[24] Diagnosis of most craniosynostosis can be performed typically with physical examination alone owing to Virchow's Law.[21,23] Each type of craniosynostosis will have a characteristic dysmorphic head shape. Three-dimensional computed tomography scanning is reserved for atypical findings, to confirm the diagnosis, and to assist in surgical planning.

Classification

Craniosynostosis can be classified into syndromic or nonsyndromic. Nonsyndromic craniosynostosis is further classified as either isolated or complex fusions. In isolated fusions, a single cranial suture is affected and includes the sagittal, metopic,

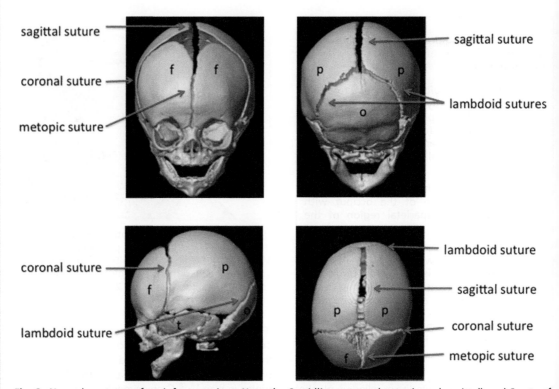

Fig. 3. Normal anatomy of an infant cranium. Note the 2 midline sutures (metopic and sagittal) and 2 sets of paired lateral sutures (coronal and lambdoid). f, frontal bone; o, occipital bone; p, parietal bone; t, temporal bone.

coronal, or lambdoid sutures. Complex craniosynostosis indicates fusion of multiple sutures. Complex craniosynostoses have a higher risk of being associated with a genetic syndrome and an increased risk of elevated intracranial pressure with each additional suture that is fused.[15]

Isolated craniosynostosis

Sagittal craniosynostosis Sagittal craniosynostosis (**Fig. 4**) is the most common type of synostosis,

occurring 1 in 2000 births and has a male-to-female ratio of 3.5 to 1.[23,25–27] The dysmorphic head shape created by fusion of the sagittal suture is termed *scaphocephaly*, meaning boatlike, or *dolichocephaly*, meaning long.[20,27] The overall head shape is long and narrow with a decreased posterior skull width and height compared with the rest of the skull, owing to decreased growth perpendicular to the sagittal suture.[21] Compensatory growth causes elongation of the head,

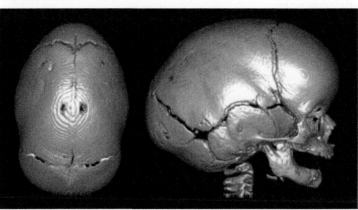

Clinical Findings

- Long, narrow head
- Decreased posterior skull width
- Decreased posterior skull height
- Frontal bossing
- Bitemporal narrowing

Fig. 4. Sagittal craniosynostosis.

through the lambdoid sutures, and variable frontal bossing of the forehead, from the coronal and metopic suture overgrowth.[28,29] These children typically present with an increased head circumference, 98th percentile or greater.[21]

Metopic craniosynostosis Premature fusion of the metopic suture results in a triangular-shaped head, termed *trigonocephaly* (**Fig. 5**). This condition presents with a prominent ridge along the metopic suture associated with narrowing of the bitemporal region and forehead, creating a triangular appearance to the forehead.[15] Hypotelorism is a common finding with supraorbital retrusions and deficient lateral orbital rims. The occipitoparietal region widens with compensatory growth, enhancing the triangular shape of the head. The incidence of premature metopic fusion has been increasing and is now the second most common type of craniosynostosis.[19,22] The current incidence is 1 in 5200 with males more commonly affected than females.[22] The metopic suture is the first suture to close physiologically, occurring between 3 and 8 months of age.[30] Metopic ridging can be encountered without the sequela of trigonocephaly or hypotelorism. In these patients, no surgical intervention is needed and the ridge typically softens as the child grows.

Coronal craniosynostosis Unilateral coronal synostosis creates an asymmetric anterior head shape, or *anterior plagiocephaly*. The affected coronal suture growth is restricted, causing the dysmorphic head shape shown in **Fig. 6**. This synostosis is more common in females than males, and the right side is more often affected than the left.[31]

Lambdoid craniosynostosis *Posterior plagiocephaly* means asymmetry of the posterior skull, which is caused by either unilateral lambdoid synostosis or DP. Unilateral lambdoid fusion is the least common type of isolated craniosynostosis, with an incidence of 1 in 40,000.[32] The deformity will be noted at the time of birth and worsens progressively over time. These infants present with the findings listed in **Fig. 7**. These abnormalities result in a trapezoid appearance when viewed from above, whereas DP has a parallelogram shape (**Fig. 8**).[33]

Complex craniosynostosis

Complex craniosynostosis is the rarest type of synostosis and a syndromic diagnosis should be ruled out in these patients. In addition, multisuture fusions have a more complex surgical treatment than isolated synostoses. Czerwinski and colleagues[34] found that 45% of their complex craniosynostosis patients required more than 1 operative procedure and have a greater incidence of Chiari I malformations. A few of the more common types of complex craniosynostosis are discussed in **Box 2 (Fig. 9)**.

Management of Craniosynostosis

Surgical indications

Surgical management is the required treatment for craniosynostosis. The 2 surgical indications include (1) correction of the abnormal appearance of the cranial deformity and (2) treatment or avoidance of elevated intracranial pressure to prevent negative impacts on neurocognitive development and vision impairment.[18,21,35,36] The dysmorphic head shape that occurs can be severe. Restoring normal craniofacial appearance can improve the parent–child relationship and prevent severe psychosocial sequela resulting from the craniofacial deformity.[18] Elevated intracranial pressure can result from restricted skull growth owing to the

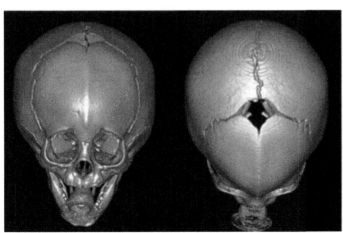

Clinical Findings

- Triangular-shaped forehead
- Bitemporal narrowing
- Supraorbital retrusion
- Deficient lateral orbital rims
- Hypotelorism
- Occiptoparietal widening

Fig. 5. Metopic craniosynostosis.

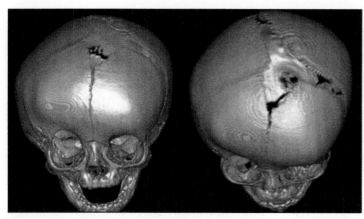

Clinical Findings

- Asymmetric anterior head shape
- Ipsilateral forehead flattening
- Ipsilateral supraorbital rim elevation and retrusion
- Contralateral frontal bossing
- Deviation of nasal root towards affected side

Fig. 6. Right unilateral coronal craniosynostosis.

fused suture(s) leading to insufficient intracranial volume for the growing brain. The body tries to accommodate by compensatory growth in other areas of the skull; however, this is not usually sufficient. This increased pressure has the potential to damage neuropsychological and visual function.[37] Elevated intracranial pressure has been shown to be present in 14% to 24% of patients with isolated craniosynostosis[18,37,38] and increases with each additional fusion.[15] A study by Renier and associates[38] found pressure to be elevated in 47% of patients with multisutural fusions. This same study showed a statistically significant inverse relationship between intracranial pressure and intelligence levels, with increased intracranial pressure associated with lower intelligence.[38] After successful surgical treatment, patients typically fall within the normal range for intelligence based on IQ scores, but are at an increased risk of developing subtle neurocognitive deficits.[18,39,40] Magge and colleagues[41] found patients with surgically corrected sagittal craniosynostosis had an increased incidence of a reading or spelling disability (50%) compared with the general population (5%).

Timing of surgery

The timing of surgery depends on multiple factors including the type and severity of synostosis, surgical technique, comorbidities, and also surgeon preference. Most craniofacial surgeons agree that surgical intervention is ideally performed before 12 months of age.[15] Generally speaking, early intervention occurs between 2 to 3 months of age with minimally invasive procedures. Surgical intervention at this early age takes advantage of the thin, pliable cranial bones, and rapidly growing brain.[15] Early intervention may result in less severe compensatory deformity and early treatment of elevated intracranial pressure. Later surgical intervention (6–12 months old) allows for firmer cranial bones to support the surgical reconstruction, allowing for less relapse and the child also has a greater total blood volume.[21]

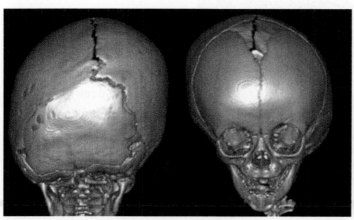

Clinical Findings

- Posterior head asymmetry
- Ipsilateral occipital flattening
- Ipsilateral occipitomastoid bulge
- Reduction of ipsilateral skull height
- Inferior positioning of ipsilateral skull base
- Contralateral frontoparietal bossing

Fig. 7. Left unilateral lambdoid craniosynostosis.

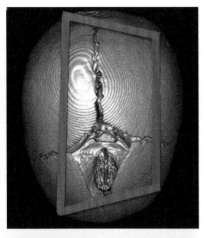

Unilateral Lambdoid Synostosis

-ipsilateral occipital flatness

-contralateral frontal bossing

-trapezoid shape when viewed from above

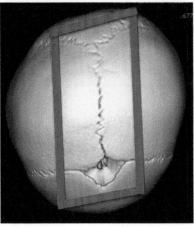

Deformational Plagiocephaly

-ipsilateral occipital flatness

-ipsilateral frontal anterior displacement

-parallelogram shape when viewed from above

Fig. 8. Distinguishing between lambdoid craniosynostosis and deformational plagiocephaly can be done by evaluating the head shape from the vertex view. The figures show the forehead facing inferiorly (as if looking from above with the child facing you). Lambdoid craniosynostosis will have flatness of the occiput on the affected side, however the forehead will show fullness of the contralateral side. This creates a trapezoid appearance. Deformational plagiocephaly will have flatness of the affected side of the occiput, but with fullness of the ipsilateral forehead, causing a parallelogram shape.

Surgical Techniques

Background

Surgical management of craniosynostosis has evolved significantly over the years. In the late 1800s, strip craniectomies, where the first procedures reported for craniosynostosis.[42] The goal was to release the fused suture and allow the area of constriction to expand with the growing brain. In the 1970s, the goals shifted to not only releasing the constrictions, but also addressing the overall aesthetic appearance of the skull by correcting the compensatory cranial deformities as well.[43] Cranial vault reconstructions were introduced, using long incisions with removal and rearrangement of large bone flaps to create a normal head shape. These were prolonged surgical procedures with increased blood loss, but achieved excellent results. Over the past few decades,

less invasive surgical procedures have been reintroduced with the addition of new techniques and applications to achieve the same outcomes realized by more aggressive cranial vault reconstructions with less blood loss and shorter scars.

Cranial vault reconstruction

Cranial vault reconstruction offers the ability to normalize the entire head shape on the operating room table and enlarge the intracranial volume by removing the affected cranial bones, remodeling of the bone flaps, and repositioning the bone flaps into a normal position. It is advocated that overcorrection be performed to counteract any potential relapse at the site of previous synostosis.[21]

Frontoorbital advancement Frontoorbital advancement expands the anterior cranial vault volume

---

Box 2
Bicoronal craniosynostosis, bilateral lambdoid craniosynostosis, and Mercedes Benz pattern craniosynostosis

Bicoronal Craniosynostosis

Bicoronal synostosis (see **Fig. 9**) causes a short head shape, termed *brachycephaly*. The head is short in the anteroposterior dimension and wide in the temporal regions. The head seems to be tall (*turricephaly*) and the forehead flat with both eyebrows seeming to be elevated.[21] These children can often develop exorbitism, with both eyes seeming to be more prominent and proptotic. Some individuals develop acrocephaly (conical-shaped head) if the anterior fontanel is open. This is the most common type of multisuture fusion and is not uncommonly associated with a syndromic diagnosis.

Bilateral Lambdoid Craniosynostosis

The associated deformity consists of a flattened occipital region, widened occipitoparietal region, and elongation of the vertex. These patients have a high risk for developing a Chiari I malformation.[33]

Mercedes Benz Pattern Craniosynostosis

This comprises the fusion of the sagittal and both lambdoid sutures. The patient will present with anterior turricephaly, brachycephaly, decreased posterior skull width, and a flattened occiput with sublambdoidal indentation. These patients carry an increased risk for Chiari I malformations.[33]

---

by moving both the forehead and the superior portion of the orbits forward. This technique is used for any metopic or coronal suture involvement (isolated, complex, or syndromic). The entire anterior skull can be remodeled to treat hypotelorism, frontal bossing, supraorbital malpositioning, and bitemporal narrowing. Performed in the supine position, this technique requires a coronal incision with elevation of the temporalis muscles, supraorbital periosteum, and periorbita of the upper half of the orbit. A frontal bone flap is removed followed by the supraorbital bandeau, which includes the superior aspect of the orbit and approximately 1 cm of the inferior portion of the frontal bone. On the back table, the bandeau is thinned and recontoured to an overcorrected shape. The midline is flattened to 180°, the superior orbital rims are burred to create symmetry, and the lateral tenons are bent 90° at the lateral orbital rim. Fixation is performed typically with absorbable plates, sutures, or reinforcing bone grafts to maintain an overcorrected shape. The supraorbital bandeau is then replaced in a more forward, and overcorrected, position and fixated to the glabella and temporoparietal bones. The frontal bone flap is then recontoured with a combination of burring, barrel staves osteotomies, reshaping with a Tessier bone bender, and rotated 180° before replacing. It is fixated anteriorly to the supraorbital bandeau to recreate a smooth forehead and left unfixated on the sides and posteriorly to allow for brain expansion. There are often bony defects

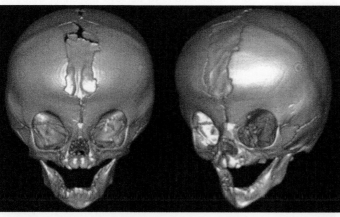

Fig. 9. Bicoronal craniosynostosis.

Clinical Findings

- Wide transverse diameter
- Short in anteroposterior dimension
- Tall forehead (*turricephaly*)
- Flat forehead
- Elevated eyebrows
- Large or bulging eyes

that persist along the posterior edge of the frontal bone flap. Any excess bony pieces can be positioned to help fill the void. The use of bone dust is advocated by some, but is controversial. The bone voids will often fill in if the child is less than 12 months old because the dura is highly osteogenic at this age, but may require a cranioplasty when older, if defects persist (**Fig. 10**).

Posterior cranial vault reconstruction For fusion of the sagittal or lambdoid sutures, a posterior cranial vault reconstruction may be considered when the deformity only involves the posterior skull. The patient is positioned prone and a coronal incision is performed. The occiput and parietal bones are typically removed and recontoured before repositioning into an overcorrected position.[28] The temporal bones may be out-fractured or included with the parietal bone flaps. The bone flaps are then repositioned to achieve the desired shape and fixated, leaving areas of the reconstruction without fixation to allow for brain expansion (**Fig. 11**).

Total cranial vault reconstruction Total cranial vault reconstruction is reserved for patients with severe skull deformities involving both the anterior and posterior skull. This is typically found in sagittal craniosynostosis with severe frontal bossing, some complex craniosynostosis, and syndromic craniosynostosis. Some centers prefer to perform cranial vault reconstruction in 2 stages, but a total cranial vault reconstruction is an option to correct the entire skull deformity in 1 operation. Positioning the patient in the modified prone (sphinx or cobra) position with the patient's neck extended allows for easy access to both the anterior and posterior cranium. The entire calvarium may be removed as multiple bone flaps with subsequent remodeling as described[43] (**Fig. 12**).

Minimally invasive techniques
Minimally invasive procedures offer the option of smaller incisions or surgical dissection to decrease the amount of blood loss and operative time. These procedures are typically performed at a younger age (<3–6 months). The cranial bone at this age is thin and malleable with a small diploic space, allowing for minimal blood loss.[44]

Endoscopic strip craniectomy with helmet therapy Endoscopic strip craniectomy with postoperative orthotic helmet therapy was introduced by Jimenez and Barone in 1996.[44,45] They were the first to introduce the use of the endoscope to avoid a long coronal incision. For sagittal craniosynostosis, the patient is placed in the sphinx position and a large rectangular bone flap is removed from the vertex of the skull extending from the anterior fontanelle to the lambda, thus including the entire sagittal suture and adjacent cranial bone. Lateral wedge and barrel stave osteotomies are performed to allow for lateral expansion of the bitemporal and biparietal regions. Postoperatively, the patient is placed in a customized orthotic helmet to correct the head shape. Owing to the rapid growth of the brain and cranium at this age, the helmet guides further cranial growth by limiting growth in the areas of excessive convexity and allowing expansion of the areas of previous constriction. Helmets are worn 23 hours a day and up to 12 months of age to prevent the relapse back to the initial deformity.[46] Owing to the osteogenic properties of the dura at this age, the bone defect typically fills in completely (**Fig. 13**).

Spring-assisted strip craniectomy Spring-assisted strip craniectomy was first performed by Lauritzen and associates in 1997.[47] This technique can be done with either a vertical scalp incision or through

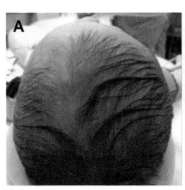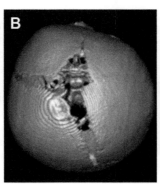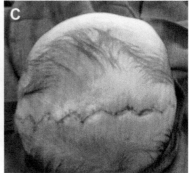

Fig. 10. (*A*) Preoperative and (*C*) postoperative reconstruction of right unilateral coronal craniosynostosis with a unilateral frontoorbital advancement. (*B*) Computed tomography scan showing the fused right coronal suture. Note the overcorrection that is performed of the right forehead in C. This will allow for some regression of the bone and will soften over a few months.

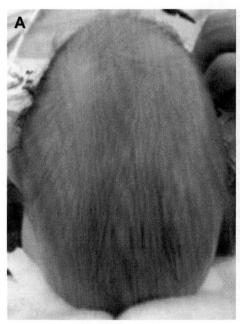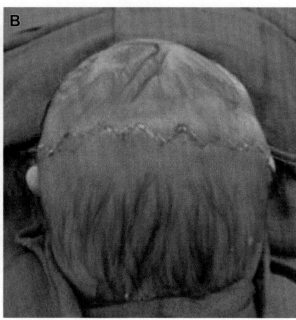

Fig. 11. (*A*) Preoperative and (*B*) postoperative reconstruction of sagittal craniosynostosis. A posterior cranial vault reconstruction was performed with the patient in the prone position. Note the immediate correction of the cranial deformity.

limited transverse incisions.[36,48] In this procedure, a strip craniectomy is performed and a series of dynamic springs are placed with the footplates within the bone defect and the body of the springs in the subgaleal plane. The distractive forces of the springs expand the skull at the locations of previous constriction to achieve normal head shape.[47] Over time, the bone defect reossifies and a short operative procedure is required to remove the springs.

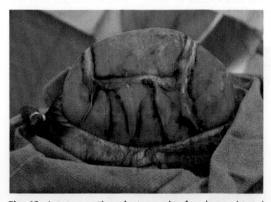

Fig. 12. Intraoperative photograph of a planned total cranial vault reconstruction. Markings have been made to identify the planned osteotomies. The patient is in the sphinx position with the forehead facing to the left in the photo. Note that both the frontal bone and occipital bone are easily accessible.

Cranial vault distraction osteogenesis Cranial vault distraction osteogenesis is another option for minimally invasive surgery (**Fig. 14**). Its use is typically limited to patients with multisuture fusions or syndromic diagnosis when multiple surgeries may be required and increased intracranial volume expansion is of the utmost importance. This has been found to be successful in both younger and older patients. Scalp flaps are elevated via a coronal incision to allow adequate exposure of the cranium. Cranial osteotomies are created, but the flap is left in situ, attached to the underlying dura. Cranial distractors are then placed along the osteotomy site, and the scalp incision is closed. After an initial latency period in which immature bone is formed within the osteotomy site, distraction is initiated by turning of the distraction arms at a specified rate (0.6–1.2 mm/d) depending on the age of the patient. This is continued at a regular rate until the intended distraction distance is reached. The bone is left to consolidate for 2 months before removal of the distractors under general anesthesia. This technique allows for expansion of not only the bone, but also the soft tissue, which is typically the limiting factor in other cranial expansion procedures.[49]

Follow-up

Routine follow-up is indicated until skeletal maturity. Patients should be evaluated for signs of

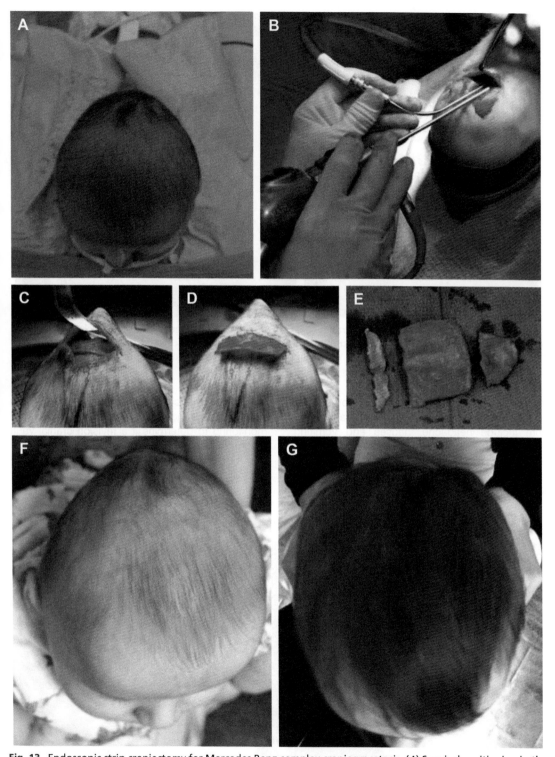

Fig. 13. Endoscopic strip craniectomy for Mercedes Benz complex craniosynostosis. (*A*) Surgical positioning in the sphinx position. (*B*) Endoscopic elevation of dura off the intracranial surface of cranium via anterior incision. (*C*) Visualization of cranial bones before osteotomies. (*D*) Removal of rectangular bone flap from vertex. (*E*) Amount of bone removed with craniectomy extending from anterior fontanelle to fused lambdoid sutures. (*F*) Preoperative photo of dysmorphic head shape. (*G*) Normalized head shape after completing helmet therapy. Note the surgical incisions are well-camouflaged.

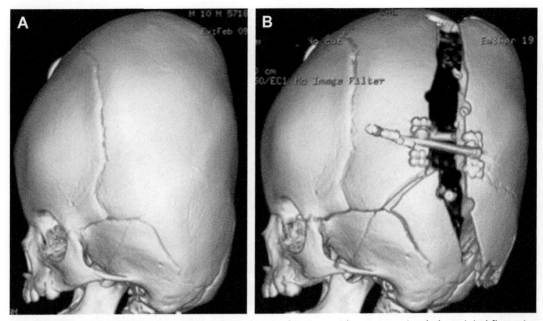

Fig. 14. (*A*) Preoperative computed tomography (CT) scan of patient with severe turricephaly occipital flattening. (*B*) Postoperative CT scan during posterior cranial distraction. CT scans are not used routinely to monitor progress; this CT scan was taken for evaluation of a ventriculoperitoneal shunt (seen in the right frontal bone).

increased intracranial pressure and for esthetic results. Symptoms of increased intracranial pressure include headache, nausea and vomiting, developmental delay, irritability, visual disturbances, declining academic performance, and seizures.[43,50,51] Concerns for intracranial hypertension should be evaluated with fundoscopic examination for papilledema, computed tomography/MRI scan of the head, and possibly invasive intracranial monitoring to determine if a revision cranial vault reconstruction is needed. Secondary cranioplasty may be indicated to repair any persistent bone defects that did not reossify, contour irregularities, or cosmetic abnormality[52] (**Fig. 15**).

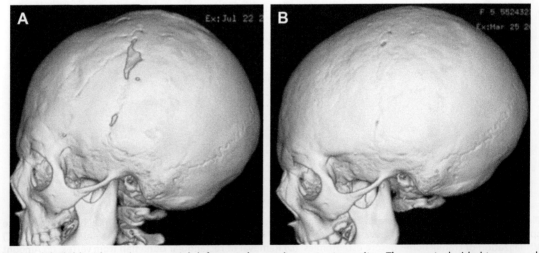

Fig. 15. (*A*) Child with persistent cranial defects at the previous osteotomy sites. The parents decided to proceed with a cranioplasty with hydroxyapatite cement to fill in the defects. (*B*) Computed tomography (CT) scan obtained after cranioplasty. CT scans are not routinely performed to follow results; however, this child suffered an unrelated trauma to the head and demonstrated good coverage of the previous bony defects.

SUMMARY

The majority of abnormal infant head shapes will be a result of DP; however, it is of utmost importance to rule out craniosynostosis at initial presentation to ensure appropriate treatment is implemented. This is essential to ensure unnecessary surgery is avoided and maximize neurocognitive and visual function, as well as achieve acceptable aesthetics in this challenging but rewarding patient population.

REFERENCES

1. Kane AA, Mitchell LE, Craven KP, et al. Observations on a recent increase in plagiocephaly without synostosis. Pediatrics 1996;97(6 Pt 1):877–85.
2. Collett BR, Gray KE, Starr JR, et al. Development at age 36 months in children with deformational plagiocephaly. Pediatrics 2013;131(1):e109–115.
3. O'Broin ES, Allcutt D, Earley MJ. Posterior plagiocephaly: proactive conservative management. Br J Plast Surg 1999;52(1):18–23.
4. Persing J, James H, Swanson J, et al. Prevention and management of positional skull deformities in infants. American Academy of Pediatrics Committee on Practice and Ambulatory Medicine, Section on Plastic Surgery and Section on Neurological Surgery. Pediatrics 2003;112(1 Pt 1):199–202.
5. Kalra R, Walker ML. Posterior plagiocephaly. Childs Nerv Syst 2012;28(9):1389–93.
6. American Academy of Pediatrics AAP Task Force on Infant Positioning and SIDS: Positioning and SIDS. Pediatrics 1992;89(6 Pt 1):1120–6.
7. Rogers GF. Deformational plagiocephaly, brachycephaly, and scaphocephaly. Part I: terminology, diagnosis, and etiopathogenesis. J Craniofac Surg 2011;22(1):9–16.
8. Argenta L, David L, Thompson J. Clinical classification of positional plagiocephaly. J Craniofac Surg 2004;15(3):368–72.
9. Dec W, Warren SM. Current concepts in deformational plagiocephaly. J Craniofac Surg 2011;22(1):6–8.
10. Levi B, Wan DC, Longaker MT, et al. Deformational plagiocephaly: a look into the future. J Craniofac Surg 2011;22(1):3–5.
11. Mawji A, Vollman AR, Hatfield J, et al. The incidence of positional plagiocephaly: a cohort study. Pediatrics 2013;132(2):298–304.
12. Cavalier A, Picot MC, Artiaga C, et al. Prevention of deformational plagiocephaly in neonates. Early Hum Dev 2011;87(8):537–43.
13. Rogers GF. Deformational plagiocephaly, brachycephaly, and scaphocephaly. Part II: prevention and treatment. J Craniofac Surg 2011;22(1):17–23.
14. Mortenson P, Steinbok P, Smith D. Deformational plagiocephaly and orthotic treatment: indications and limitations. Childs Nerv Syst 2012;28(9):1407–12.
15. Persing JA. MOC-PS(SM) CME article: management considerations in the treatment of craniosynostosis. Plast Reconstr Surg 2008;121(Suppl 4):1–11.
16. Twigg SR, Wilkie AO. A genetic-pathophysiological framework for craniosynostosis. Am J Hum Genet 2015;97(3):359–77.
17. Virchow R. Uber den Cretinismus, namentlich in Franken, und uber pathologische Schadelformen. Verh Phys med Gesell Wurzburg 1851;2:230–71.
18. Hankinson TC, Fontana EJ, Anderson RC, et al. Surgical treatment of single-suture craniosynostosis: an argument for quantitative methods to evaluate cosmetic outcomes. J Neurosurg Pediatr 2010;6(2):193–7.
19. Di Rocco F, Arnaud E, Renier D. Evolution in the frequency of nonsyndromic craniosynostosis. J Neurosurg Pediatr 2009;4(1):21–5.
20. Governale LS. Craniosynostosis. Pediatr Neurol 2015;53(5):394–401.
21. Fearon JA. Evidence-based medicine: craniosynostosis. Plast Reconstr Surg 2014;133(5):1261–75.
22. van der Meulen J. Metopic synostosis. Childs Nerv Syst 2012;28(9):1359–67.
23. Massimi L, Caldarelli M, Tamburrini G, et al. Isolated sagittal craniosynostosis: definition, classification, and surgical indications. Childs Nerv Syst 2012;28(9):1311–7.
24. Lajeunie E, Crimmins DW, Arnaud E, et al. Genetic considerations in nonsyndromic midline craniosynostoses: a study of twins and their families. J Neurosurg 2005;103(Suppl 4):353–6.
25. Kolar JC. An epidemiological study of nonsyndromal craniosynostoses. J Craniofac Surg 2011;22(1):47–9.
26. Lajeunie E, Le Merrer M, Bonaiti-Pellie C, et al. Genetic study of scaphocephaly. Am J Med Genet 1996;62(3):282–5.
27. Tatum SA, Jones LR, Cho M, et al. Differential management of scaphocephaly. Laryngoscope 2012;122(2):246–53.
28. Ocampo RV Jr, Persing JA. Sagittal synostosis. Clin Plast Surg 1994;21(4):563–74.
29. Delashaw JB, Persing JA, Broaddus WC, et al. Cranial vault growth in craniosynostosis. J Neurosurg 1989;70(2):159–65.
30. Weinzweig J, Kirschner RE, Farley A, et al. Metopic synostosis: defining the temporal sequence of normal suture fusion and differentiating it from synostosis on the basis of computed tomography images. Plast Reconstr Surg 2003;112(5):1211–8.
31. Lajeunie E, Le Merrer M, Bonaiti-Pellie C, et al. Genetic study of nonsyndromic coronal craniosynostosis. Am J Med Genet 1995;55(4):500–4.

32. Al-Jabri T, Eccles S. Surgical correction for unilateral lambdoid synostosis: a systematic review. J Craniofac Surg 2014;25(4):1266–72.

33. Rhodes JL, Tye GW, Fearon JA. Craniosynostosis of the lambdoid suture. Semin Plast Surg 2014;28(3): 138–43.

34. Czerwinski M, Kolar JC, Fearon JA. Complex craniosynostosis. Plast Reconstr Surg 2011;128(4): 955–61.

35. Wall SA, Thomas GP, Johnson D, et al. The preoperative incidence of raised intracranial pressure in nonsyndromic sagittal craniosynostosis is underestimated in the literature. J Neurosurg Pediatr 2014; 14(6):674–81.

36. Taylor JA, Maugans TA. Comparison of spring-mediated cranioplasty to minimally invasive strip craniectomy and barrel staving for early treatment of sagittal craniosynostosis. J Craniofac Surg 2011; 22(4):1225–9.

37. Thompson DN, Malcolm GP, Jones BM, et al. Intracranial pressure in single-suture craniosynostosis. Pediatr Neurosurg 1995;22(5):235–40.

38. Renier D, Sainte-Rose C, Marchac D, et al. Intracranial pressure in craniostenosis. J Neurosurg 1982; 57(3):370–7.

39. Speltz ML, Kapp-Simon K, Collett B, et al. Neurodevelopment of infants with single-suture craniosynostosis: presurgery comparisons with case-matched controls. Plast Reconstr Surg 2007;119(6):1874–81.

40. Starr JR, Kapp-Simon KA, Cloonan YK, et al. Presurgical and postsurgical assessment of the neurodevelopment of infants with single-suture craniosynostosis: comparison with controls. J Neurosurg 2007; 107(Suppl 2):103–10.

41. Magge SN, Westerveld M, Pruzinsky T, et al. Long-term neuropsychological effects of sagittal craniosynostosis on child development. J Craniofac Surg 2002;13(1):99–104.

42. Mehta VA, Bettegowda C, Jallo GI, et al. The evolution of surgical management for craniosynostosis. Neurosurg Focus 2010;29(6):E5.

43. Seruya M, Tan SY, Wray AC, et al. Total cranial vault remodeling for isolated sagittal synostosis: part I. Postoperative cranial suture patency. Plast Reconstr Surg 2013;132(4):602e–10e.

44. Jimenez DF, Barone CM. Endoscopic technique for sagittal synostosis. Childs Nerv Syst 2012;28(9): 1333–9.

45. Jimenez DF, Barone CM. Endoscopic craniectomy for early surgical correction of sagittal craniosynostosis. J Neurosurg 1998;88(1):77–81.

46. Jimenez DF, Barone CM, Cartwright CC, et al. Early management of craniosynostosis using endoscopic-assisted strip craniectomies and cranial orthotic molding therapy. Pediatrics 2002; 110(1 Pt 1):97–104.

47. Lauritzen CG, Davis C, Ivarsson A, et al. The evolving role of springs in craniofacial surgery: the first 100 clinical cases. Plast Reconstr Surg 2008; 121(2):545–54.

48. van Veelen ML, Mathijssen IM. Spring-assisted correction of sagittal suture synostosis. Childs Nerv Syst 2012;28(9):1347–51.

49. Ong J, Harshbarger RJ 3rd, Kelley P, et al. Posterior cranial vault distraction osteogenesis: evolution of technique. Semin Plast Surg 2014;28(4):163–78.

50. Connolly JP, Gruss J, Seto ML, et al. Progressive postnatal craniosynostosis and increased intracranial pressure. Plast Reconstr Surg 2004;113(5): 1313–23.

51. Thomas GP, Johnson D, Byren JC, et al. The incidence of raised intracranial pressure in nonsyndromic sagittal craniosynostosis following primary surgery. J Neurosurg Pediatr 2015;15(4):350–60.

52. Matushita H, Alonso N, Cardeal DD, et al. Frontal-orbital advancement for the management of anterior plagiocephaly. Childs Nerv Syst 2012;28(9):1423–7.

Syndromic Craniosynostosis

James C. Wang, MD, PhD[a,b], Laszlo Nagy, MD[c], Joshua C. Demke, MD[d,*]

KEYWORDS

- Apert syndrome • Craniofacial syndromes • Crouzon syndrome • FGFR mutations
- Muenke syndrome • Pfeiffer syndrome • Saethre-Chotzen syndrome • Syndromic craniosynostosis

KEY POINTS

- Syndromic craniosynostosis is rare, occurring in 1:30,000 to 1:100,000 live births.
- Fibroblast growth factor receptor and tumor growth factor-β receptor mutations have been reported to be associated with many forms of syndromic craniosynostosis.
- Intracranial hypertension, developmental delays, and strabismus are more frequent in syndromic forms of craniosynostosis than isolated synostosis.
- Distraction osteogenesis is a useful adjunct in syndromic synostosis to increase intracranial volume and is helpful with fronto-orbital and midface advancements.
- Addressing decompression by increasing intracranial volume and decreasing intracranial pressure before 1 year of age is a common goal through an interdisciplinary team approach.

INTRODUCTION

Syndromic craniosynostosis, premature fusion of the cranial sutures in syndromic patients, has been reported to affect from 1:100,000 to 1:30,000[1] live births causing restriction in skull and skull base growth with associated midface hypoplasia and dysmorphisms being common. There are greater than 150 syndromes associated with craniosynostosis.[1–4] Patients with syndromic craniosynostosis are more liable to have ventricular expansion, hydrocephalus, expanded subarachnoid space, and cerebellar tonsillar herniation compared with patients with sporadic single-suture synostoses.[5] Increased intracranial pressure (ICP) is more likely to occur in patients with syndromic craniosynostosis and multisuture synostosis.[5] Cerebrospinal fluid (CSF) flow disturbance may present in one of two ways: ventriculomegaly present before craniofacial surgery, or normal or small ventricles that progressively increase after forehead advancement and cranial suture release. If these conditions are progressive, they can be associated with decreased cognitive function and intelligence quotients. Chronic transependymal fluid transfer, ventriculomegaly causing deformity of long tracks, and periventricular fibrosis are likely to change brain function.[6] In syndromic synostosis, brain developmental anomalies, such as septum pellucidum and corpus callosum dysgenesis, and hypogyria are not infrequent. Brain distortion and local compression causes additional damage. Crouzon syndrome has the highest incidence of hydrocephalus.[7] In Apert syndrome, ventricular dilation occurs frequently,

[a] Department of Otolaryngology—Head and Neck Surgery, Texas Tech University Health Sciences Center, 3601 4th Street, Stop 8312, Lubbock, TX 79430, USA; [b] Department of Otolaryngology—Head and Neck Surgery, University of Cincinnati, Cincinnati, OH, USA; [c] Pediatric Neurosurgery, Department of Pediatrics, West Texas Craniofacial Center of Excellence, Texas Tech University Health Sciences Center, 3601 4th Street, Lubbock, TX 79430, USA; [d] Division of Facial Plastic and Reconstructive Surgery, Department of Otolaryngology—Head and Neck Surgery, West Texas Craniofacial Center of Excellence, Texas Tech University Health Sciences Center, 3601 4th Street, Stop 8312, Lubbock, TX 79430, USA
* Corresponding author.
E-mail address: joshua.demke@ttuhsc.edu

Facial Plast Surg Clin N Am 24 (2016) 531–543
http://dx.doi.org/10.1016/j.fsc.2016.06.008

but usually is nonprogressive in nature.[7] In most cases of syndromic craniosynostosis, venous outflow obstruction and/or chronic tonsillar herniation are found.[7] In cases of venous hypertension, a higher CSF pressure is required to maintain the CSF outflow balance. Cognitive impairment is common in Apert syndrome and cloverleaf deformities presenting 20% of the time in Crouzon, Pfeiffer, and Saethre-Chotzen type I syndromes.[5]

Timing of surgery for patients with syndromic craniosynostosis depends on the presenting symptoms, such as the degree of exorbitism and signs and symptoms of elevated ICP.[5] There is a higher incidence of hydrocephalus following early surgery, which is one consideration for delaying surgery.[8–11] The incidence of hydrocephalus in craniosynostosis is 4% to 10%.[7] There is no clear consensus on the ideal operative window for syndromic craniosynostosis; however, delaying surgery beyond 1 year results in a higher likelihood of elevated ICP, cognitive deficits, and behavioral problems.[8–11] Therefore, decompression, increasing intracranial volume, and addressing ICP before 1 year of age is a common goal.[12,13] One institutional study states that when there is no concern for elevated ICP the ideal operative window for these procedures in the syndromic population seems to be 6 to 9 months of age.[14] Pediatric ophthalmology evaluation of vision, strabismus, and fundoscopic examination to rule out papilledema are important. When papilledema is present, MRI and/or ICP monitoring are often useful in evaluating signs of pressure or hydrocephalus. Proptosis is common as a result of hypoplastic orbits frequently leading to scleral show, lagophthalmos, and dry eyes and may require either temporary tarsorrhaphies or fronto-orbital advancement (FOA) to protect the eyes from exposure keratitis and eventual midface advancement to greater improve orbital volume.[2,12,13,15–18]

Chiari malformation–related central apnea or alteration of cranial nerve nuclei–related muscle tone might contribute to obstructive sleep apnea (OSA). Obstructive airway can lead to brain hypoperfusion and hypoxemia. Chiari malformation can occur because of obstruction of venous outflow and reduced posterior fossa volume. Cinalli and coworkers[2] in 1995 revealed that premature lambdoid suture closure is the main factor for Chiari malformation and proved that this pathologic process is present almost universally in Crouzon syndrome. Based on the authors experience, idiopathic or brain-related multisuture synostosis can present the same way once synostosis is present with increase in brain volume.

There is greater likelihood with syndromic patients to require multiple surgeries, not only to improve cranial volume and shape early on but also to address midface, orbital, and cranial deformities that often persist and/or recur as a result of poor bone growth in early childhood and adolescence.[5] Diagnosing and treating upper airway obstruction and timely decompression and reconstruction of the skull are all crucial in syndromic patients.[19]

EVALUATION AND DIAGNOSIS OF CRANIOSYNOSTOSIS

Detailed pregnancy history, birth history, family history, and medication or drug exposure in utero is crucial to document. Syndromic forms of synostosis are often inherited in an autosomal-dominant (AD) fashion, although spontaneous mutations frequently occur. A review of systems should note any presence of associated headaches, irritability, seizures, or neurodevelopmental or cognitive delays. A timeline of the duration and progression of head shape change is important because progressive unilateral occipital flattening suggests deformational plagiocephaly, whereas bilateral progressive flattening implies positional brachycephaly. Bilateral coronal craniosynostosis is one of the most common findings in syndromic synostosis including Crouzon, Muenke, and Apert with a head that is short in the anteroposterior dimension (brachycephaly) frequently coupled with increased vertical height in the cephalocaudal dimension of the skull (turricephaly). A good history is often all that is needed to distinguish the typical positional brachycephalic skull, a shape that progressively developed, from syndromic types of brachycephaly.

However, deformities present since birth are more suggestive of synostosis, although positional deformities can also be present at birth as a result of malpositioned fetal lie, oligohydramnios, and in utero constraints of pregnancy with twins or multiples. Photographic documentation from a variety of views of the head and face including frontal, left lateral, right lateral, vertex, and oblique views should be obtained (**Fig. 1**).

Meticulous physical examination of the head includes palpation of the sutures and fontanelles, inspection of the orbits and face (noting any asymmetry, ptosis, lagophthalmos, dystopia, hypertelorism, hypotelorism, facial paresis/paralysis), measurement of the fronto-occipital circumference, and calculation of the cephalic index ratio (skull width/skull length). Location, size, and shape of the ears relative to the head should be noted. A head to toe examination is essential for evaluation of syndromic craniosynostosis to detect carpal/pedal anomalies (**Table 1**) that may be present

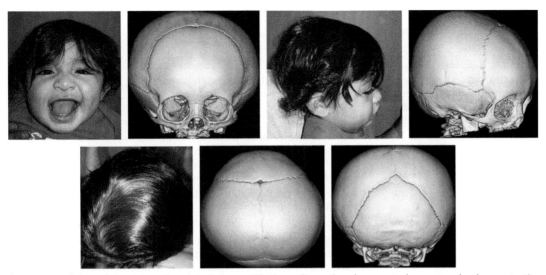

Fig. 1. Frontal, lateral, vertex, and occipital views with three-dimensional computed tomography demonstrating nonsynostotic positional brachycephaly, although mild metopic ridging is evident without significant trigonocephaly.

and the presence of possible cardiac or respiratory difficulties; when there is still uncertainty a three-dimensional (3D) computed tomography (CT) of the head definitively rules in or out craniosynostosis.

Midface or mandibular hypoplasia, and adeno-tonsillar hypertrophy if present, can contribute to sleep-disordered breathing or OSA. CT and MRI of the head are often useful to identify any hydro-cephalus, signs of ICP elevation, or posterior fossa problems, such as Chiari (**Fig. 2**), which could lead to central sleep apnea.

Elevation of ICP can present acutely, subacutely, or chronically from microcephaly, venous anomalies, and hydrocephalus.[5] Nonspecific signs and symptoms such as irritability, lack of appetite, and inconsolable crying are important indicators of increased ICP.[5] More prominent signs are a bulging fontanelle and engorged scalp veins.[5]

The authors agree with a growing body of craniofacial and neurosurgeons that posterior cranial distraction (PCD) is a minimally invasive way to slowly improve intracranial volume with potential to decrease mild to moderate elevations of ICP and help normalize the brachycephalic head shape by growing the skull in the anteroposterior axis. It is thus often ideal in syndromic craniosynostosis involving bicoronal or multisuture synostosis with brachycephaly and/or microcephaly.

CRANIOFACIAL TEAM

Syndromic craniosynostosis often involves multiple organ systems so an interdisciplinary team approach is now the standard of care for these complicated patients.[5] This team can include a plastic surgeon, pediatric otolaryngologist or facial plastic surgeon trained in craniofacial surgery, a pediatric neurosurgeon, an oral-maxillofacial surgeon, a pediatric anesthesiologist and intensivist, a pedodontist, orthodontist, a prosthodontist, a pediatric ophthalmologist, a psychologist, a geneticist, an audiologist, a speech pathologist, and pediatrician.[20]

DISTRACTION OSTEOGENESIS

Distraction osteogenesis (DO) can be used to advance the mandible, midface, orbits, and skull including lower level and higher level Le Fort osteotomies, PCD, or fronto-facial (Monobloc) advancements using either external or internal distractors (**Fig. 3**). Cranial distraction has been used to increase microcephalic skulls or provide added volume in the case of shunt-induced craniosynostosis. It has also been described for use across patent sutures and other more unconventional total cranial vault reconstruction in a recent paper describing 285 different cases of coronal, metopic, lambdoid, and sagittal synostosis, of which 33 were syndromic and 28 were secondary synostosis.[21] Typically an open bicoronal approach is used because eventual anterior cranial vault reconstruction (ACVR) with FOA and frontal cranioplasties are usually required months after distraction, although in cases of secondary synostosis, microcephaly, or persistent ICP elevation despite shunt, the approach can be accomplished through several small incisions and endoscopic assistance.

Table 1
Craniofacial anomalies with phenotype and known gene mutation

Condition	Craniofacial Phenotype	Gene[a]
Loeys-Dietz syndrome (aortic aneurysm, arterial tortuosity, hypertelorism, cleft palate/bifid uvula, craniosynostosis)	Craniosynostosis, cleft palate, hypertelorism	TGF β R1 TGF β R2
Apert syndrome	Craniosynostosis (brachycephaly); wide midline defect closes by coalescence of bony islands; midface malformations; dental crowding; cleft or narrow palate with swellings	FGFR2
Beare-Stevenson cutis gyrata syndrome	Craniosynostosis (kleeblattschädel) or cloverleaf skull	FGFR2
Boston-type craniosynostosis	Craniosynostosis (kleeblattschädel), forehead retrusion, frontal bossing	MSX2
Cleidocranial dysplasia	Delayed suture closure, frontal parietal bossing, wormian bones, hyperdontia, tooth eruption defects	RUNX2
Craniofrontonasal syndrome	Craniosynostosis (brachycephaly), central defect between frontal bones, hypertelorism, divergent orbits	EFNB1
Crouzon syndrome	Craniosynostosis (brachycephaly), pronounced digital impressions of skull, midface hypoplasia, shallow orbits	FGFR2
Crouzon syndrome with acanthosis nigricans	Craniosynostosis	FGFR3
Greig cephalopolysyndactyly	Craniosynostosis in small percentage of cases, frontal bossing, sagittal ridging, hypertelorism	GLI3
Muenke-type craniosynostosis (nonsyndromic)	Craniosynostosis (brachycephaly)	FGFR3
Parietal foramina	Symmetric parietal bone defects, cleft lip/palate	MSX2, ALX4
Parietal foramina with cleidocranial dysplasia	Symmetric parietal bone defects	MSX2
Pfeiffer syndrome	Craniosynostosis (brachycephaly)	FGFR1, FGFR2
Saethre-Chotzen syndrome	Craniosynostosis (especially brachycephaly), flat forehead, low hairline	FGFR2, TWIST1
Shprintzen-Goldberg (marfanoid) syndrome	Craniosynostosis (especially lambdoid and sagittal sutures), maxillary and mandibular hypoplasia, palatal abnormalities	SKI
Thanatophoric dysplasia II	Craniosynostosis (cloverleaf skull/kleeblattschädel deformity)	FGFR3

Abbreviations: EFNB1, Ephrin-B1; FBN, fibrillin; FGFR, fibroblast growth factor receptor; TGF-βR, tumor growth factor-β receptor.

[a] Gene abbreviations that have not been defined/spelled out are not acronyms or abbreviations.

Adapted from Rice DP. Craniofacial anomalies: from development to molecular pathogenesis. Curr Mol Med 2005;5:699, with updates from Online Mendelian Inheritance in Man (omim.org); and *From* Demke JC, Tatum SA. Craniofacial surgery for congenital and acquired deformities. In: Flint PW, Haughey BH, Lund V, et al, editors. Cummings otolaryngology. 6th edition. Philadelphia: Saunders; 2015. p. 2893. Chapter 186; with permission.

Following this approach, craniotomies are planned, marked, and performed either with a craniotome, Kerrison rongeurs, osteotomes, or peizosurgery device. Two to four single-vector cranial distractors are placed in the desired plane, typically anteroposterior for posterior vault distraction.

The incisions are closed and after a latency period (few days to a week), depending on the age of the patient, activation of the distraction commences at a typical rate of 0.5 mm twice daily. A commonly used internal device for PCD, made by KLS Martin (Jacksonville, FL), is 30 mm in length and has a

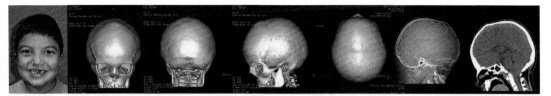

Fig. 2. A 6 year old with syndromic facies; no exorbitism; but mild midface hypoplasia, anterior open bite, and anterior crossbite with relative normocephaly (cephalic index 85%). 3D CT images reveal pansynostosis, lateral plain film shows thumb-printing (nonspecific for increased ICP), and sagittal CT shows Chiari malformation (asymptomatic). Genetic testing was negative for common fibroblast growth factor receptor and TWIST mutations.

switch that, once toggled, prevents parents from accidentally incorrectly turning the distractors in the wrong direction. Additionally, a ratcheting screw provides an audible and tactile click with each turn of the activating wrench/driver, giving parents additional feedback that they are correctly using the wrench and that the distraction is preceding appropriately. The desired volume is achieved after 3 to 5 weeks and a portion of the external distractor arms is thereafter removed in the office. After another 2 to 3 months of allowing the bony consolidate to calcify and mature, the patient is returned to the operating room for removal of distractors and at times concomitant ACVR. This approach is particularly useful in syndromic patients with brachycephaly in whom adequate advancement is difficult to achieve through conventional surgery.[22–25]

Transsutural DO (TSDO) has been described in which a simple suturectomy of the pathologic suture or even placement of distractors across patent sutures is used to distract the skull. TSDO potentially allows for greater cranial vault expansion compared with traditional posterior cranial vault reconstruction or ACVR, although it adds increased complexity and potential hardware complications by virtue of using greater number of distractors.

One TSDO study showed shorter mean operative time compared with most prior studies.[26–29] This results in decreased bleeding and transfusion volumes when compared with total cranial vault reconstruction with bone grafting.[29] TSDO has also been used with some success for total calvarial remodeling by removal of all sutures.[30] However, in this study approximately 50% developed Chiari malformations immediately after surgery and 50% with ocular abnormalities. The authors of this article have no experience with TSDO.

Theoretic advantages of distraction are that the soft tissue can be slowly stretched allowing for greater amounts of increased intracranial volume gained with lesser risk of relapse or tight scalp closures that are subject to dehiscence, scar widening, and exposure of hardware or bone grafts. In addition to improving the aesthetic appearance, there is functional benefit by giving the brain space (**Fig. 4**).

Risks of distraction include requiring secondary surgery to remove the distractors, infection, soft tissue ulceration around the distractors, dural injury, CSF leak, nonunion, and/or persistent

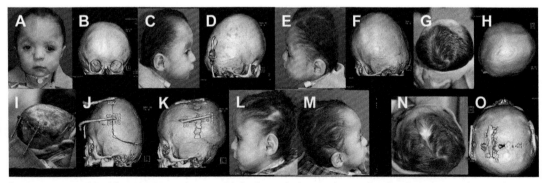

Fig. 3. A 2 year old with CHARGE syndrome with hydrocephalus s/p shunt who developed secondary multisuture craniosynostosis with resultant severe brachyturricephaly and underwent PCD. (*A–H*) Postshunt and predistraction photographs and 3D CT. (*I*) Intraoperative photograph demonstrating posterior craniotomies and distractor placement. (*J*) Immediately postoperative 3D CT scan. (*K, M*) Right, left, vertex 3D CT scan after consolidation phase. (*L, N, O*) Four weeks postdistractor removal, lateral and vertex photographs. s/p, status post.

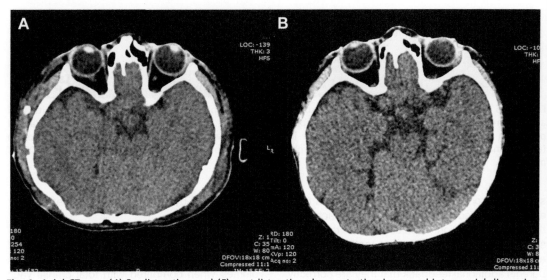

Fig. 4. Axial CT scan. (*A*) Predistraction and (*B*) postdistraction demonstrating improved intracranial dimensions and improvement in appearance of ventricles and gyri/sulci.

bony lacunae. With PCD, when the distractors are placed inferiorly along the coronal cuts, there is greater intracranial volume improvement but greater posterior occipital shelf/step-off deformity (**Fig. 5**).

The occipital shelf deformity (**Fig. 6**) is addressed by barrel staving, and reshaping or repositioning bone grafts of the posteroinferior occipital bone at the time of placement of the distractors or at time of their removal. Whenever possible we prefer to avoid this because it makes a minimally invasive operation more invasive and bloody. The occipital shelf is minimized by placing posterior vault distractors a little more cephalad on the cephalocaudal parietal craniotomy cuts. Doing this diminishes the potential for intracranial volume expansion but minimizes the posterior shelf/step-off deformity by allowing the bone to pivot posteriorly and open more like a clam shell rather

than slide like a drawer being pulled out. A certain amount of step-off is unavoidable unless addressed upfront or secondarily with either posterior camouflage bone cement cranioplasty or posterior cranial vault reconstruction with bone grafting/reshaping/respositioning with autologous bone.

When used for Le Fort advancements, distractions allows for the midface to advance in three directions: maxilla ± orbits advancing anteriorly, rotating clockwise or counterclockwise, with the mandible following suit.[31] CT data compared before and after distraction have demonstrated the amount of midface advancement to be significant.[31] Surgical correction with FOA is the gold standard to improve intracranial volume of the anterior cranial vault and improve orbital volume when supraorbital retrusion and bilateral coronal synostosis are present. Traditionally, a bifrontal craniotomy

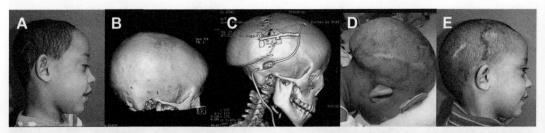

Fig. 5. A 5 year old with benign intracranial hypertension, increased ICP, and pansynostosis but relative normocephaly who underwent VP shunt but had persistent ICP elevation. (*A*) Right lateral photograph after VP shunt. (*B*) Right lateral 3D CT scan depicting pansynostosis before shunt. (*C*) Right lateral 3D CT scan after completion of PCD consolidation. (*D*) At time of distractor removal noted improvement in intracranial volume but severe occipital shelf deformity. (*E*) One week postoperative after removal of distractors and posterior cranial vault reconstruction with autologous bone graft repositioning to improve occipital shape. VP, ventriculoperitoneal.

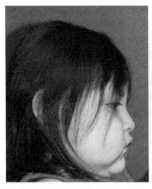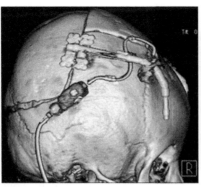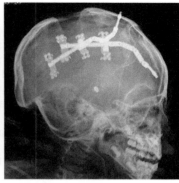

Fig. 6. A 2 year old with history of meningitis who developed hydrocephalus and Chiari, underwent VP shunting, developed shunt-induced craniosynostosis with brachyturricephaly status post-PCD and Chiari decompression. Moderate posterior occipital step-off deformity was addressed with bone-cement camouflage cranioplasty at time of distractor removal.

is performed and then a separate fronto-orbital bar or bandeau is osteotomized and when necessary reshaped, then advanced anteriorly and fixed in the midline near the glabella and bilaterally near the pterion. When pure advancement is required and there is no trigonocephaly or unilateral asymmetries, then FOA en bloc osteotomies have been alternatively reported.[32]

DO can be used to advance the face alone when coupled with Le Fort I, II, and III osteotomies or to advance the face and frontal skull as in Monobloc advancement (**Fig. 7**), which can be used as early as 4 years of age if deemed necessary because of neurosurgical, ophthalmologic, or airway issues or later in the teenage years to improve exorbitism, midface hypoplasia, and skeletal occlusal relationships that are poor. Distraction is considered by many to be less invasive, with greater potential to increase intracranial volume, often with decreased operative times, and in the case of Monobloc advancement decreased risk of CSF leak, and meningitis; however, until resorbable distractors become more reliable and available DO

still requires an additional surgery to remove the distractors.[32] In the case of syndromic craniosynostosis, it is reasonable to remove the distractors and do FOA in the same operation if both are determined to be expedient and necessary. For details regarding FOA, (see L Morris's article, "Non-Syndromic Craniosynostosis and Deformational Head Shape Disorders," in this issue) on isolated craniosynostosis elsewhere in this issue. FOA can be combined with Le Fort III if necessary and used with either external halotype distractors or internal distractors.

Another study stated four different movements were observed in DO: (1) anterior translation, (2) clockwise movement, (3) counterclockwise movement, and (4) anterocaudal translation.[33] With Le Fort III DO, a significant advancement is achievable, although the control of the vector of force may be difficult leading to unwanted counterclockwise movements.[33] Another study showed that frontofacial distraction produced long-term stable advancement in all cases and 88% achieved stable functional gains.[34]

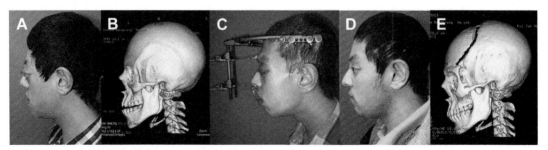

Fig. 7. A 13 year old with autosomal-dominant FGFR craniosynostosis. (*A*) Left lateral preoperative photograph demonstrating severe brachycephaly, midface hypoplasia, and exorbitism. (*B*) Preoperative left lateral 3D CT showing pansynostosis. (*C*) Two weeks postoperative with rigid external distractor in place for Monobloc distraction. (*D, E*) Left lateral photograph and 3D CT 2.5 years postoperative demonstrating improved midface and decreased proptosis despite some deficient cranial bone in region of frontal cranial distraction.

MOLECULAR GENETICS

A variety of mutations in transcription-derived growth factors, such as transmembrane fibroblast growth factor receptors (FGFR) 1, 2 and 3 and tumor growth factor-β receptors 1 and 2, are known to be involved in syndromic craniosynostosis (see **Table 1**).[35–38] In addition, connective tissue structural proteins, such as fibrillin-1 (FBN1) and TWIST, have also been implicated in association with syndromic craniosynostosis.

Defects in FGFR1 and FGFR2 have been linked to such syndromes as Pfeiffer syndrome and to conditions of which craniosynostosis is a feature.[39,40] Mutations in *FGFR2* have been reported to be responsible for Apert syndrome,[41,42] Beare-Stevenson cutis gyrata syndrome,[43] Crouzon syndrome,[44] and Jackson-Weiss syndrome.[45]

FGFR3 has recently been shown to play a role in regulation of skeletal growth with defective FGFR3 protein responsible for Crouzon syndrome with acanthosis nigricans.[46] Severe retardation of skeletal maturation has been seen in *Fgfr3* knockout mice.[42,47–49]

Transcription factor defects with TWIST and FBN1 are also involved in the pathogenesis of craniosynostosis. Most cases of Saethre-Chotzen syndrome are caused by haploinsufficiency of the *TWIST* gene, which seems to encode a transcription factor.[50] Mutations in *GLI3*, a transcription factor gene, are responsible for Greig cephalopolysyndactyly.[51,52] Defective *FBN1* results in Shprintzen-Goldberg syndrome with craniosynostosis and maxillary/mandibular hypoplasia.[53]

SYNDROMIC CRANIOSYNOSTOSIS ASSOCIATIONS
Hearing Loss

Literature review reveals a large range (4%–92%) in the incidence of hearing loss associated with FGFR in patients with syndromic craniosynostoses, such as Muenke, Apert, Pfeiffer, Crouzon, Jackson-Weiss, and Crouzon with acanthosis nigricans.[54] Most of the hearing loss is a conductive hearing loss, with the exception of Muenke syndrome, where most patients have a sensorineural hearing loss (SNHL), and Crouzon syndrome, where approximately 50% of patients have a pure or component of SNHL.[54]

Respiratory Difficulty

Syndromic craniosynostosis is associated with a high frequency of respiratory difficulty, with approximately 50% of patients with Apert, Crouzon, or Pfeiffer syndrome developing OSA.[55] Principally it

has been associated with midface hypoplasia, although relative adenotonsillar hypertrophy, pharyngeal collapse, nasopharyngeal stenosis, central neurologic factors, mandibular hypoplasia, and airway anomalies may play a role.[56] In addition, stenosis of the epipharynx caused by maxillary hypoplasia and that of the mesopharynx by mandibular hypoplasia,[57] and even normal-sized adenoids and tonsils, may contribute to airway obstruction.[58] Tracheotomy has traditionally been the standard method of airway protection in patients with craniosynostosis presenting with respiratory difficulty. Long-term nasopharyngeal airway use has been reported as a first-line intervention for airway obstruction and DO of the mandible and/or midface when appropriate may be options to avoid tracheotomy.[59,60] One study showed considerable numbers of cases with nasopharyngeal airway insertion were able to continue this form of treatment for more than 1 year without tracheotomy.[61] Other treatments, such as adenotonsillectomy and continuous positive airway pressure, although probably less effective, have lower morbidity, and are valuable adjuvant techniques that may control airway obstruction allowing craniofacial surgery to be delayed or avoided altogether.[56]

CRANIOFACIAL SYNDROMES

Craniofacial anomalies associated with syndromes vary distinctly in clinical presentation. Knowledge of the most common syndromes is important to focus the examination and understand when consultations are needed. The syndromes in the next sections are discussed from most common to least (**Fig. 8**).

Muenke Syndrome (1:30,000)

Muenke syndrome is AD and the most common syndromic craniosynostosis.[5,62] Muenke syndrome is caused by a proline-to-arginine substitution at amino acid 250 in the FGFR3 gene.[63] Patients commonly present with involvement of the coronal suture (bilateral > unilateral), carpal and/or tarsal bone coalition, developmental delay, and SNHL in addition to mild midfacial hypoplasia, high arched palate, and hypertelorism.[64] Muenke syndrome has considerable phenotypic variability from coronal synostosis to pan synostosis to no sutures. Tarsal coalition is a distinct feature of Muenke syndrome, as evidenced by its occasional description as "coronal craniosynostosis with brachydactyly and carpal/tarsal coalition."[65] Tarsal coalition also occurs as a part of several craniosynostosis syndromes caused by mutations in the FGFR genes,

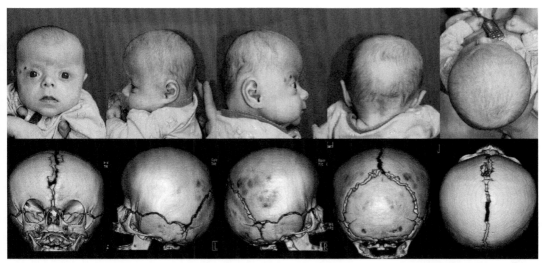

Fig. 8. A 2-month-old girl with brachyturricephaly and bicoronal synostosis, with midface hypoplasia.

including Apert, Crouzon, Jackson-Weiss, Muenke, and Pfeiffer syndromes.[66–70] Crouzon syndrome with acanthosis nigricans also involves the FGFR3 gene and has a similar phenotype; therefore, the only way to determine the difference between the two syndromes is through FGFR testing.

Saethre-Chotzen Syndrome (1:25,000–1:50,000)

Saethre-Chotzen syndrome is an AD disorder with full penetrance.[5,71] Patients have craniosynostosis, often with brachycephaly, brachydactyly, low hairline, ptosis, and a high arching palate with occasional palatal clefting.[71] Midface hypoplasia is not frequently seen.[71]

Crouzon Syndrome (1:62,500)

Crouzon syndrome is an AD condition with complete penetrance and variable expressivity.[5,71] It frequently involves the coronal sutures, resulting in brachycephaly, but multiple sutures may be affected.[71] Calvarial suture defects may occur before birth or throughout the first 5 years of life.[71] Although the mandible develops close to normal, hypoplasia of the midface leads to class III malocclusion.[71] Exorbitism occurs as a result of decreased bony orbital volume. Intelligence is generally normal if patients are managed properly (**Fig. 9**).[71]

Apert Syndrome (1:65,000–1:100,000)

Most cases of Apert syndrome arise sporadically through new mutations, although some familial cases with AD transmission have been reported.[5,72] Apert syndrome resembles Crouzon syndrome in several ways.[71] The disorder is characterized by brachycephaly (with resultant turricephaly) and midfacial hypoplasia (with associated orbital and dental issues).[71] Unlike Crouzon, Apert syndrome is associated with symmetric syndactyly of the hands and feet and other axial skeletal abnormalities.[71] Patients have high arching palates that may have clefting.[71] The defects in Apert syndrome are present at birth and intelligence may be affected.[71]

Pfeiffer Syndrome (1:100,000)

Pfeiffer syndrome is an AD disorder with features including craniosynostosis.[5,71] The coronal sutures are frequently involved, giving rise to brachycephaly, although the sagittal and lambdoid sutures may also be involved.[71] Affected patients may have midface hypoplasia with associated orbital and dental issues, and enlarged thumbs and big toes.[71]

Miscellaneous Syndromes

Jackson-Weiss syndrome is an AD disorder with high penetrance and variable expressivity with features similar to Pfeiffer syndrome.[71] Brachycephaly is common, the big toes are abnormally wide, but the thumbs are typically normal, unlike in Pfeiffer.[71] Midfacial hypoplasia is more common than in Pfeiffer syndrome.[71] Carpenter syndrome is a rare autosomal-recessive syndrome.[71] Craniosynostosis may involve the sagittal, lambdoid, and coronal sutures.[71] Midfacial hypoplasia, if present, is usually mild.[71] Other features include developmental delay, preaxial polysyndactyly of the feet, and other syndactyly.[71]

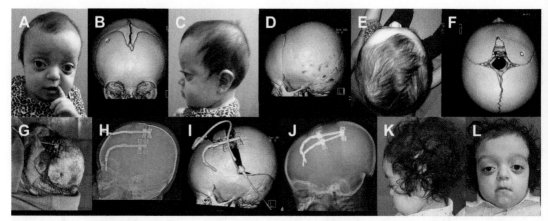

Fig. 9. A 9 month old with partial bicoronal synostosis, midface hypoplasia, and exorbitsim with underlying spontaneous FGFR2 mutation. (*A, C, E*) Preoperative frontal, left lateral, and vertex photographs at 9 months. (*B, D, F*) Frontal, left lateral, and vertex 3D CT after ICP pressure monitor performed. Results revealed a mild elevation of ICP. (*G*) Left lateral intraoperative photograph at time of PCD showing left internal posterior cranial distractor. (*H*) Left lateral skull radiograph after latency phase before beginning active distraction. (*I*) Left lateral 3D CT midway through active distraction when patient developed CSF leak, external ventricular drain placed, and endoscopic third ventriculostomy performed shortly thereafter. (*J*) Left lateral skull radiograph at conclusion of 30-mm active distraction. (*K, L*) One year after distractors removal and ACVR.

Secondary Craniosynostosis

Secondary synostosis can occur because of congenital, metabolic, iatrogenic, and infectious etiologies. Whatever the cause, the resultant underdeveloped brain fails to drive normal calvarial bone growth, cranial sutures fuse prematurely, and the head often remains microcephalic.[71] Blood disorders (eg, thalassemia, sickle cell anemia, polycythemia vera) can also cause cranial sutures to fuse prematurely.[73] Iatrogenic craniofacial anomalies can occur in patients receiving ventricular shunts in infancy and early childhood.[71] In children with patent cranial sutures overshunting of CSF leads to shunt-induced craniosynostosis and frequently microcephaly.[71] Trauma and neoplasms are rare causes of acquired craniofacial deformities.[71]

SUMMARY

Syndromic craniosynostosis is rare with characteristic craniofacial deformities, carpal-pedal anomalies, and cognitive impairment. Genetic mutations are associated with many forms of syndromic craniosynostosis. An interdisciplinary team approach and careful physical examination and history documentation is essential. DO is useful to increase intracranial volume often before the age of 1 year. FOA to gain additional cranial and orbital volume is still the mainstay of surgery around 9 to 12 months of age in most forms of syndromic craniosynostosis. Midface advancements can be done between 4 years of age and

adulthood to address skeletal hypoplasia and functional problems related to sleep-disordered breathing, OSA, malocclusion, and feeding.

REFERENCES

1. McLone DG. Pediatric neurosurgery. Surgery of the developing nervous system. 4th edition. Philadelphia: Saunders; 2001. Chapters 27 and 31.
2. Cinalli G, Renier D, Sebag G, et al. Chronic tonsillar herniation in Crouzon's and Apert's syndromes: the role of premature synostosis of the lambdoid suture. J Neurosurg 1995;83:575–82.
3. Agrawal D, Steinbok P, Cochrane D. Long term anthropometric outcomes following surgery for isolated cranial synostosis. J Neurosurg 2006;105(5 Suppl):357–60.
4. Addo NK, Javadpour S, Kandasamy J, et al. Central sleep apnea and associated Chiari malformation in children with syndromic craniosynostosis: treatment and outcome data from a supraregional national craniofacial center. J Neurosurg Pediatr 2013;11: 296–301.
5. Nagy L, Demke JC. Craniofacial anomalies. Facial Plast Surg Clin North Am 2014;22:523–48.
6. Del Bigio MR. Neuropathological changes caused by hydrocephalus. Acta Neuropathol 1993;85(6): 573–85.
7. Cinalli G, Sainte-Rose C, Kollar EM, et al. Hydrocephalus and craniosynostosis. J Neurosurg 1998; 88:209–14.
8. Driessen C, Joosten KF, Florisson JM, et al. Sleep apnea in syndromic craniosynostoses occurs

independent of hindbrain herniation. Childs Nerv Syst 2013;29(2):289–96.

9. Renier D, Arnaud E, Cinalli G, et al. Prognosis for mental function in Apert's syndrome. J Neurosurg 1996;85:66–72.

10. Van Der Meulen J, Van der Vlugt J, Okkerse J, et al. Early beaten-copper pattern: its long-term effect on intelligence quotients in 958 children with craniosynostosis. J Neurosurg Pediatr 2008;1:25–30.

11. Pollack IF, Losken HW, Biglan AW. Incidence of increased intracranial pressure after early surgical treatment of syndromic craniosynostosis. Pediatr Neurosurg 1996;24:202–9.

12. Thompson DN, Harkness W, Jones BM, et al. Aetiology of hindbrain herniation in craniosynostosis. An investigation incorporating intracranial pressure monitoring and magnetic resonance Imaging. Pediatr Neurosurg 1997;26:288–95.

13. Inagaki T, Kyotoku S, Seno T, et al. The intracranial pressure of the patients with mild form of craniosynostosis. Childs Nerv Syst 2007;23(12):1455–9.

14. Utria AF, Mundinger GS, Bellamy JL, et al. The importance of timing in optimizing cranial vault remodeling in syndromic craniosynostosis. Plast Reconstr Surg 2015;135:1077.

15. Hayward R, Gonsalez S. How low can you go? Intracranial pressure, cerebral perfusion pressure, and respiratory obstruction in children with complex craniosynostosis. J Neurosurg 2005;102:16–22.

16. Terner JS, Travieso R, Lee S, et al. Combined metopic and sagittal craniosynostosis: is it worse than sagittal synostosis alone? Neurosurg Focus 2011;31(2):E2.

17. Rollins N, Booth T, Shapiro K. MR venography in children with complex craniosynostosis. Pediatr Neurosurg 2000;32(6):308–15.

18. Seruya M, Boyajian MJ, Posnick JC, et al. Treatment for delayed presentation of sagittal synostosis: challenges pertaining to occult intracranial hypertension. J Neurosurg Pediatr 2011;8(1):40–8.

19. diRocco F, Juca CE, Arnaud E, et al. The role of endoscopic third ventriculostomy in the treatment of hydrocephalus associated with faciocraniosynostosis. J Neurosurg Pediatr 2010;6:17–22.

20. Mehta VA, Bettegowda C, Jallo GI, et al. The evolution of surgical management for craniosynostosis. Neurosurg Focus 2010;29(6):E5.

21. Park DH, Yoon SH. Transsutural distraction osteogenesis for 285 children with craniosynostosis: a single-institution experience. J Neurosurg Pediatr 2015;18:1–10.

22. Kobayashi S, Honda T, Saitoh A, et al. Unilateral coronal synostosis treated by internal forehead distraction. J Craniofac Surg 1999;10(6):467–71.

23. Alonso N, Goldenberg D, Fonseca AS, et al. Blindness as a complication of monobloc frontofacial advancement with distraction. J Craniofac Surg 2008;19(4):1170–3.

24. Akizuku T, Komuro Y, Ohmori K. Distraction osteogenesis for craniosynostosis. Neurosurg Focus 2000;9(3):E1.

25. Kazuaki Y, Keisuke I, Takuya F, et al. Cranial distraction osteogenesis for syndromic craniosynostosis: long-term follow-up and effect on postoperative cranial growth. J Plast Reconstr Aesthet Surg 2014;67:35–41.

26. Lauritzen CG, Davis C, Ivarsson A, et al. The evolving role of springs in craniofacial surgery: the first 100 clinical cases. Plast Reconstr Surg 2008;121:545–54.

27. Kim SW, Shim KW, Plesnila N, et al. Distraction vs remodeling surgery for craniosynostosis. Childs Nerv Syst 2007;23:201–6.

28. Park DH, Chung J, Yoon SH. Rotating distraction osteogenesis in 23 cases of craniosynostosis: comparison with the classical method of craniotomy and remodeling. Pediatr Neurosurg 2010;46:89–100.

29. Park DH, Yoon SH. The trans-sutural distraction osteogenesis for 22 cases of craniosynostosis: a new, easy, safe, and efficient method in craniosynostosis surgery. Pediatr Neurosurg 2011;47:167–75.

30. Park DH, Yoon SH. The total calvarial remodeling with transsutural distraction osteogenesis of 21 cases of craniosynostosis: new, efficient, safe and natural method in craniosynostosis surgery. Pediatr Neurosurg 2015;50:119–27.

31. Wery MF, Nada RM, van der Meulen JJ, et al. Three-dimensional computed tomographic evaluation of Le Fort III distraction osteogenesis with an external device in syndromic craniosynostosis. Br J Oral Maxillofac Surg 2015;53:285.

32. Satoh K, Mitsukawa N, Kubota Y, et al. Appropriate indication of fronto-orbital advancement by distraction osteogenesis in syndromic craniosynostosis: beyond the conventional technique. J Craniomaxillofac Surg 2015;43:2079–84.

33. Bouw FP, Nout E, van Bezooijen JS, et al. Three-dimensional position changes of the midface following Le Fort III advancement in syndromic craniosynostosis. J Craniomaxillofac Surg 2015;43:820.

34. Gwanmesia I, Jeelani O, Hayward R, et al. Frontofacial advancement by distraction osteogenesis: a long-term review. Plast Reconstr Surg 2015;135:553.

35. Albright AL, Pollack IF, Adelson PF. Principles and practice of pediatric neurosurgery. 2nd edition. New York: Thieme; 2007. p. 265. Chapter 17.

36. Britto JA, Moore RL, Evans RD, et al. Negative autoregulation of fibroblast growth factor receptor 2 expression characterizing cranial development in cases of Apert (P253R mutation) and Pfeiffer (C278F mutation) syndromes and suggesting a basis for differences in their cranial phenotypes. J Neurosurg 2001;95:660–73.

37. Chumas PD, Cinalli G, Arnaud E, et al. Classification of previously unclassified cases of craniosynostosis. J Neurosurg 1997;86:177–81.

38. Lajeunie E, Le Merrer M, Arnaud E, et al. Trigonocephaly: isolated, associated and syndromic forms. Genetic study in a series of 278 patients. Arch Pediatr 1988;5(8):873–9.

39. Rutland P, Pulleyn LJ, Reardon W, et al. Identical mutations in the FGFR2 gene cause both Pfeiffer and Crouzon syndrome phenotypes. Nat Genet 1995;9:173.

40. Robin NH, Feldman GJ, Mitchell HF, et al. Linkage of Pfeiffer syndrome to chromosome 8 centromere and evidence for genetic heterogeneity. Hum Mol Genet 1994;3:2153.

41. Wilkie AO, Slaney SF, Oldridge M, et al. Apert syndrome results from localized mutations of FGFR2 and is allelic with Crouzon syndrome. Nat Genet 1995;9:165.

42. Wilkie AO. Craniosynostosis: genes and mechanisms. Hum Mol Genet 1997;6:1647.

43. Bratanic B, Praprotnik M, Novosel-Sever M. Congenital craniofacial dysostosis and cutis gyratum: the Beare-Stevenson syndrome. Eur J Pediatr 1994; 153:184.

44. Reardon W, Winter RM, Rutland P, et al. Mutations in the fibroblast growth factor receptor 2 gene cause Crouzon syndrome. Nat Genet 1994;8:98.

45. Jabs EW, Li X, Scott AF, et al. Jackson-Weiss and Crouzon syndromes are allelic with mutations in fibroblast growth factor receptor 2. Nat Genet 1994;8:275.

46. Meyers GA, Orlow SJ, Munro IR, et al. Fibroblast growth factor receptor 3 (FGFR3) transmembrane mutation in Crouzon syndrome with acanthosis nigricans. Nat Genet 1995;11:462.

47. Deng C, Wynshaw-Boris A, Zhou F, et al. Fibroblast growth factor receptor 3 is a negative regulator of bone growth. Cell 1996;84:911.

48. Colvin JS, Bohne BA, Harding GW, et al. Skeletal overgrowth and deafness in mice lacking fibroblast growth factor receptor 3. Nat Genet 1996;12:390.

49. Robin NH. Molecular genetic advances in understanding craniosynostosis. Plast Reconstr Surg 1999;103:1060.

50. Howard TD, Paznekas WA, Green ED, et al. Mutations in TWIST, a basic helix-loop-helix transcription factor, in Saethre-Chotzen syndrome. Nat Genet 1997;15:36.

51. Vortkamp A, Gessler M, Grzeschik KH. GLI3 zinc-finger gene interrupted by translocations in Greig syndrome families. Nature 1991;352:539.

52. Brueton L, Huson SM, Winter RM, et al. Chromosomal localisation of a developmental gene in man; direct DNA analysis demonstrates that Greig cephalopolysyndactyly maps to 7p13. Am J Med Genet 1988;31:799.

53. Sood S, Eldadah ZA, Krause WL, et al. Mutation in fibrillin-1 and the Marfanoid-craniosynostosis (Shprintzen-Goldberg) syndrome. Nat Genet 1996; 12:209.

54. Agochukwu NB, Solomon BD, Muenke M. Hearing loss in syndromic craniosynostoses: otologic manifestations and clinical findings. Int J Pediatr Otorhinolaryngol 2014;78:2037.

55. Banninl E, Nout E, Wolvius B, et al. Obstructive sleep apnea in children with syndromic craniosynostosis: long-term respiratory outcome of midface advancement. Int J Oral Maxillofac Surg 2010;39: 115–21.

56. Nash R, Possamai V, Manjaly J, et al. The management of obstructive sleep apnea in syndromic craniosynostosis. J Craniofac Surg 2015;26:1914.

57. Kakitsubata N, Sadaoka T, Motoyama S, et al. Sleep apnea and sleep-related breathing disorders in patients with craniofacial synostosis. Acta Otolaryngol 1994;517:6–10.

58. Adam JW, James DR. Adenotonsillectomy for the management of obstructive sleep apnea in children with congenital craniosynostosis syndromes. J Craniofac Surg 2012;23:1020–2.

59. Jahangir A, Damian M, Leslie C, et al. The role of the nasopharyngeal airway for obstructive sleep apnea in syndromic craniosynostosis. J Craniofac Surg 2008;19:659–63.

60. Randhawa RS, Ahmed J, Nouraei SR, et al. Impact of long-term nasopharyngeal airway on health-related quality of life of children with obstructive sleep apnea caused by syndromic craniosynostosis. J Craniofac Surg 2011;22:125–8.

61. Kouga T, Tanoue K, Matsui K. Airway statuses and nasopharyngeal airway use for airway obstruction in syndromic craniosynostosis. J Craniofac Surg 2014;25:762.

62. Boulet SL, Rasmussen SA, Honein MA. A population-based study of craniosynostosis in metropolitan Atlanta, 1989–2003. Am J Med Genet A 2008;146A:984–91.

63. Bellus G, McIntosh I, Smith EA, et al. A recurrent mutation in the tyrosine kinase domain of fibroblast growth factor receptor3 causes hypochondroplasia. Nat Genet 1995;10:357–9.

64. Agochukwu NB, Solomon BD, Benson LJ, et al. Talocalcaneal coalition in Muenke syndrome: report of a patient, review of the literature in FGFR-related craniosynostoses, and consideration of mechanism. Am J Med Genet A 2013;161(3): 453–60.

65. Graham JM Jr, Braddock SR, Mortier GR, et al. Syndrome of coronal craniosynostosis with brachydactyly and carpal/tarsal coalition due to Pro250Arg mutation in FGFR3 gene. Am J Med Genet 1998; 77:322–9.

66. Anderson PJ, Hall CM, Evans RD, et al. The feet in Crouzon syndrome. J Craniofac Genet Dev Biol 1997;17:43–7.

67. Anderson PJ, Hall CM, Evans RD, et al. The feet in Pfeiffer syndrome. J Craniofac Surg 1998;9:98–102.

68. Anderson PJ, Hall CM, Evans RD, et al. The feet in Apert's syndrome. J Pediatr Orthop 1999;19:504–7.

69. Jackson CE, Weiss L, Reynolds WA, et al. Craniosynostosis midface hypoplasia, and foot abnormalities: an autosomal dominant phenotype in a large Amish kindred. J Pediatr 1976;88:963–8.

70. Muenke M, Gripp KW, McDonald-McGinn DM, et al. A unique point mutation in the fibroblast growth factor receptor 3 gene (FGFR3) defines a new craniosynostosis syndrome. Am J Hum Genet 1997;60:555–64.

71. Flint PW. Cummings otolaryngology – head and neck surgery. 6th edition. Philadelphia: Saunders; 2015. Chapter 186.

72. Katzen JT, McCarthy JG. Syndromes involving craniosynostosis and midface hypoplasia. Otolaryngol Clin North Am 2000;33:1257, vi.

73. Reimann F, Gokmen M, Inceman S. On the behavior of the cranial sutures in thalassemias. IV. Further studies on changes in the skeletal system in severe blood diseases. Blut 1968;17:214 [in German].

Tessier Clefts and Hypertelorism

Ryan Winters, MD

KEYWORDS

- Tessier cleft • Hypertelorism • Craniofacial surgery • Congenital

KEY POINTS

- Tessier's classification of craniofacial clefts denotes their position on the skull and face relative to the orbit.
- It provides no information regarding the severity of the cleft, only the location.
- Orbital hypertelorism refers to true increased distance between the bony orbits.
- Surgical repair must be tailored to the individual cleft based on severity and structures involved.

The rarity, complexity, and great variety of craniofacial clefts have all contributed to the difficulty in establishing a concise yet comprehensive classification system for these anomalies. In 1887, Morian proposed a basic schema with the infraorbital foramen as the reference.[1,2] Morian type I clefts existed in the space between the infraorbital foramen and the facial midline, and type II existed lateral to the infraorbital foramen. Clearly significant ambiguity exists within each of these 2 categories regarding structures involved in the clefting process, and a more precise classification system was needed. Boo-Chai subdivided the oro–ocular clefts described by Morian in an attempt at further refinement, and Karfik was the first to attempt classification by embryologic origin in 1966.[2,3]

In 1976, Tessier proposed a classification system based on his personal experience with 336 patients,[4,5] and the resultant ordered numbering system has greatly facilitated communication between reconstructive surgeons. Tessier's system has gained widespread acceptance and is now the most consistently used method of describing craniofacial clefts in the literature. It is centered on the orbit, with clefts assigned a number in a counterclockwise rotation. Facial clefts are numbered from 0 to 7, with 0 a midline facial cleft, and the cranial clefts are numbered 8 to 14, with 14 being a midline cranial cleft. Midline mandibular cleft is assigned number 30 (**Fig. 1**). Each of these clefts may involve both soft tissue and bone, and the number does not provide information regarding severity of tissue involvement, merely the location on the face and/or skull.

The remainder of this article explores the various Tessier clefts in more detail, followed by a discussion of orbital hypertelorism (an abnormally widened distance between the bony orbits), which may be present in association with some craniofacial clefts.

CLEFT DESCRIPTIONS

What follows is a description of each cleft type, with the bony and soft tissue manifestations discussed in further detail. Within each cleft type there is a spectrum of severity, both of soft tissue and bony involvement.

TESSIER 0

Tessier 0 cleft is a true midline facial cleft, which may be accompanied by a Tessier 14 cleft (extension of the midline cleft to the cranium), with a

Disclosure: The author has no conflicts to disclose.
Surgery Service Line, Sunrise Health System and Sunrise Children's Hospital, 3201 South Maryland Parkway, Suite 300, Las Vegas, NV 89109, USA
E-mail address: ryan.winters@gmail.com

Facial Plast Surg Clin N Am 24 (2016) 545–558
http://dx.doi.org/10.1016/j.fsc.2016.06.013

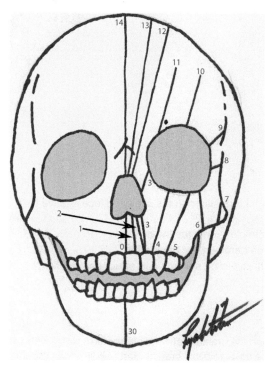

Fig. 1. Clefts numbered according to Tessier.

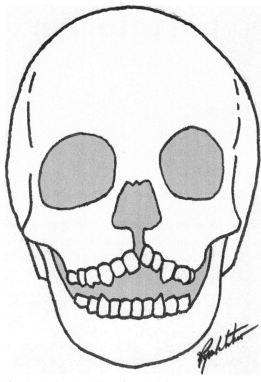

Fig. 2. Tessier 0 midline facial cleft.

resultant variable degree of hypertelorism. This is among the more common of the "atypical facial clefts," although it is still very rare, with a incidence reported as 1 in 1 million live births.[6]

Soft Tissue

The subtlest manifestation is a broadening of the philtrum, with a typical bifid nasal tip and columella, which are widened with a central concavity. In more complete cases, a true midline cleft lip may be present.[4,6] The nose will thus appear shortened, and the nasal ala laterally displaced and the alar base widened.

Bone

The midline cleft alveolus appears between the central incisors (**Fig. 2**), producing a characteristic sloping alveolar ridges toward the cleft bilaterally, described as keel shaped.[2] This will typically create an anterior open bite deformity from vertical deficiency of the maxilla in the region of the midline cleft. Involvement of the nasal septum is variable, and ranges from mild thickening of the septal cartilage and thickening and flattening of the maxillary crest, to lateral displacement of the nasal processes of the maxilla, to true duplication of the septal structures and significant lateral displacement of the nasal bones.[7]

In severe cases, where the cleft extends superiorly or exists in conjunction with a Tessier 14 cleft, the ethmoid sinuses are volumetrically enlarged and prolapsed inferiorly and laterally. There may be widening of the floor of the anterior cranial fossa and hypertelorism. The sphenoid sinus may prolapse anteroinferiorly, although the body of the sphenoid bone is characteristically normal.[2,8] The pterygoids may be displaced somewhat laterally.

TESSIER 1

A Tessier 1 cleft is similar to a "typical" cleft lip. This is a paramedian cleft in the Cupid's bow, extending superiorly to the dome of the alar cartilage or even to the medial aspect of the brow. Extension beyond the medial orbit/brow denotes a Tessier 13 cleft, which may exist simultaneously.[2,9,10]

Soft Tissue

A paramedian cleft lip is present, extending above the lip into the dome of the alar cartilage. The lower lateral cartilage and alar dome are cleft, with a short, wide columella.[2,10] The lateral remnant of the ala and lower lateral cartilage may be atrophic, curled, and deviated away from the cleft margin. Extension of the cleft into the upper lateral cartilage and nasal sidewall or paramedian nasal dorsum ranges from subtle furrow in the soft tissue to frank cleft toward the medial brow and orbit. Severe manifestations of the Tessier 1 cleft result in severe telecanthus and a variable degree of true hypertelorism, depending on bony involvement.[9]

Bone

As in "typical" cleft lip and palate, Tessier 1 may extend posteriorly into the maxilla, resulting in a paramedian cleft alveolus or complete cleft palate. There is frequently a partial anterior open bite on the cleft side (**Fig. 3**), and the maxilla is hypoplastic ipsilaterally, with severe maxillary hypoplasia potentially creating paradoxic choanal atresia.[11] The medial maxillary wall is preserved, although distortion of the nasal septum may flatten the nasal dorsum. There is distortion of the anterior cranial fossa, with relative hypoplasia of the ipsilateral pterygoids and sphenoid wings.[2,10]

TESSIER 2

Tessier 2 cleft is also a paramedian cleft lip with concomitant underdevelopment of the nasal ala on the cleft side. There is no true notching of the ala nasi, helping to distinguish Tessier 2 from Tessier 1. The base of the nose is widened, and the lateral crus of the cleft side lower lateral cartilage is flattened. The root of the nose is also widened and flattened, and bony notching of the nasal bone is present, with resultant hypertelorism. Cranial

extension corresponds with Tessier 12. The cleft alveolus is present at the lateral incisor and extends into the pyriform aperture. It does not disrupt the medial wall of the maxillary sinus[2,11,12] (**Fig. 4**).

Soft Tissue

The cleft lip extends into the nostril as a wide cleft, with a flattened and laterally displaced lower lateral cartilage. There is no notching of the cartilage itself. There is a flattening of the nasal dorsum and sidewall, and a soft tissue groove may be present extending to the root of the nose. The eyebrows are intact.[12,13]

Bone

The alveolar cleft is present in the area of the lateral incisor and extends as a unilateral complete cleft palate. The nasal septum is deviated to the noncleft side and is intact. The cleft side maxilla is hypoplastic, and cases of paradoxic choanal atresia (cleft side and bilateral) have been described. The ethmoid is broadened with resultant orbital hypertelorism, and notching of the nasal bones is present. The ipsilateral frontal sinus is not pneumatized, and the orbit is narrowed.[2,13]

TESSIER 3

As seen in Tessier clefts 1 and 2, there is a paramedian cleft lip. Unlike Tessier 1 and 2, the cleft

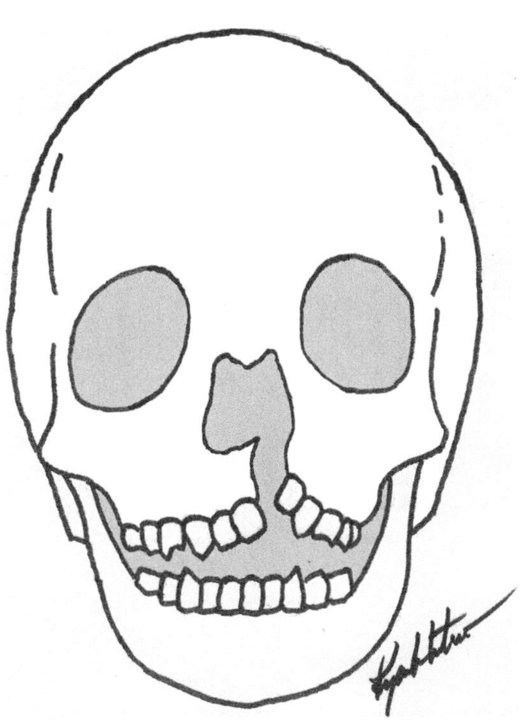

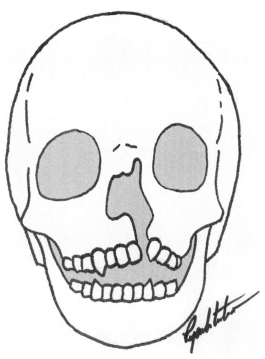

Fig. 3. Tessier 1 paramedian facial cleft.

Fig. 4. Tessier 2 paramedian facial cleft with widening of pyriform aperture.

does not involve the nasal base or lower lateral cartilage. The cleft extends superiorly involving the lower eyelid medial to the punctum (**Fig. 5**). The medial canthi are disrupted, as is the nasolacrimal system. Concurrent microphthalmia or anophthalmia may be present. The cleft alveolus is more lateral than in the typical cleft palate, coursing between the lateral incisor and canine. The medial wall of the maxillary sinus is absent, and the medial and inferior orbital walls are disrupted, leading to direct communication between the oral cavity, nasal cavity, and orbit. Cranial extension results in Tessier cleft 11.[2,14,15]

Soft Tissue

There is extreme vertical soft tissue deficiency of both margins of the cleft, resulting in superior displacement of the alar base and minimal soft tissue present between the alar base and the lower eyelid. The inferior lacrimal punctum is visible at the margin of the cleft eyelid, and the lacrimal sac opens directly onto the cheek and does not communicate with the nasal cavity.[15]

Bone

The alveolar cleft is present between the lateral incisor and canine, and the medial maxillary wall is absent. The maxilla is hypoplastic on the cleft side, and the nasal septum deviates away from the cleft. The cleft may extend superiorly to the medial and inferior orbital walls and onto the inferior orbital rim. This results in communication between the orbit, nasal, and oral cavity. The cleft side pterygoid is displaced medially, and the orbit and floor of the anterior cranial fossa are displaced inferiorly.[2,14]

TESSIER 4

Tessier 4 cleft involves the lip at the midpoint between the commissure and philtral column. It extends onto the cheek, lateral to the alar base and pyriform aperture, and can involve the lower eyelid lateral to the punctum, sparing the nasolacrimal system. The alveolar cleft occurs between the lateral incisor and canine, courses through the maxillary sinus medial to the infraorbital foramen and may involve the medial aspect of the inferior orbital rim[4] (**Fig. 6**).

Soft Tissue

Similar to the Tessier 3 cleft, there is significant vertical soft tissue deficiency along the margins of the cleft, with the medial margin of the cleft lip extending onto the medial margin of the cleft lower eyelid. The nasal ala is displaced superiorly, and the nose is shortened. Muscle may be congenitally absent in the medial aspect of the cleft lip. Significant vertical dystopia and hypoglobus may be present owing to skeletal deficiencies of the orbital rim and medial orbital wall, although both globes are otherwise normal.[2,16]

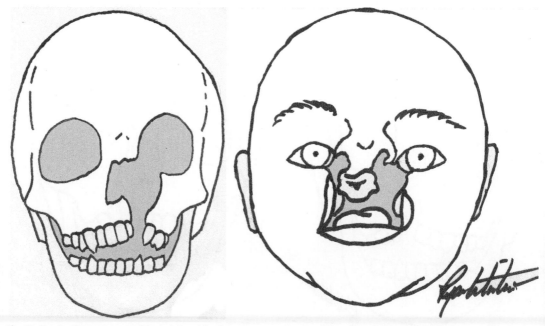

Fig. 5. Tessier 3 oro–naso–orbital cleft with direct communication between all 3 cavities. Bilateral cleft shown in soft tissue illustration.

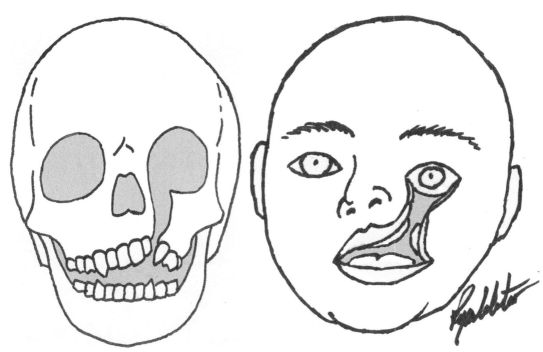

Fig. 6. Tessier 4 medial orbito–maxillary–oral cleft.

Bone

The alveolar cleft passes between the lateral incisor and canine, extending as a unilateral complete cleft palate. The cleft involves the maxillary sinus, which is hypoplastic, although the medial wall remains intact and extends to involve the inferior orbital rim and floor. Direct communication between the orbit, maxillary sinus, and oral cavity exists, but the nasal cavity is separate.[2] There is severe midfacial hypoplasia, and asymmetry of the sphenoid is present. The cleft does not extend to the skull base.[16–18]

TESSIER 5

The cleft lip originates just medial to the oral commissure, though the commissure itself is uninvolved (distinguishing Tessier 5 from Tessier 7). The cleft extends across the cheek and terminates at the lateral one-third of the lower eyelid. Eye malformations are common, particularly microphthalmia. The alveolar cleft is in the premolar area and extends superiorly to involve the orbital floor and lateral inferior orbital rim[2,4,19] (**Fig. 7**).

Soft Tissue

There is vertical soft tissue deficiency along both margins of the cleft, although it is more severe between the lip and lower eyelid. There is mild shortening of the nose on the cleft side with some superior displacement of the alar base.[19] There is

no involvement of the upper eyelid, brow, or hairline and the globes are normal. Vertical dystopia and facial asymmetry are present as a result of underlying bony abnormalities.

Bone

Bony involvement is variable. In mild cases, a simple bony depression exists along the face of the maxilla, whereas in more severe cases, a wide bony cleft is present coursing lateral to the infraorbital foramen and hypoplastic maxillary sinus. This cleft can extend to the lateral inferior orbital rim, although it does not communicate with the inferior orbital fissure. There is a shortening of the lateral orbital wall and greater wing of the sphenoid. The cleft side pterygoid plates are medialized and underdeveloped.[2,19,20]

TESSIER 6

Tessier 6 is a rare zygomaticomaxillary cleft typically manifest as a furrow in soft tissue extending from the oral commissure to the lateral one-third of the eyelid where coloboma exists. On occasion, this furrow originates at the angle of the mandible rather than the oral commissure. If bony involvement is present, the cleft occurs between the zygoma and maxilla, passing through the lateral inferior orbital rim to enter the inferior orbital fissure with an intact zygomatic arch (**Fig. 8**). This cleft is clinically similar to clefts observed in Treacher–Collins syndrome.[2,21]

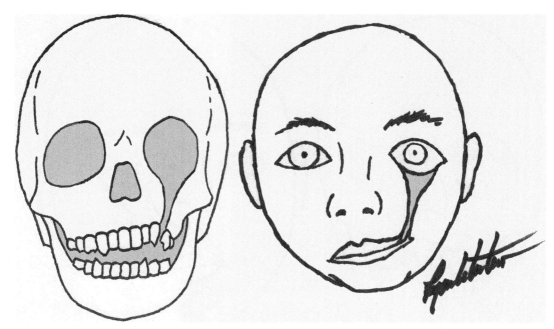

Fig. 7. Tessier 5 lateral orbito–maxillary–oral cleft.

Soft Tissue

The previously described soft tissue furrow is associated with a laterally displaced lower eyelid coloboma and antimongoloid palpebral slant. There may be a mild degree of brow ptosis and

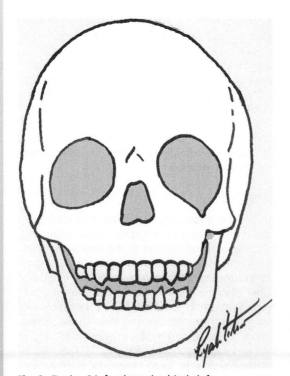

Fig. 8. Tessier 6 inferolateral orbital cleft.

associated anophthalmia has been described, although this is rare.[2]

Bone

When bony involvement is present, it is characterized by a cleft at the zygomaticomaxillary suture. The zygomatic arch is intact and relatively normal in shape. There is no alveolar or palatal defect. The orbits may be hypoplastic, and there is an inferior slant to the lateral orbital floor.[2]

TESSIER 7

This is the most common of the Tessier clefts, and occurs in both Treacher–Collins syndrome and craniofacial microsomia. The cleft originates at the oral commissure with resultant macrostomia, and extends laterally as a transverse facial cleft. There can be associated malformations of the facial nerve, external and middle ear, temporalis muscle, and preauricular hair (especially in Treacher–Collins syndrome). The bony defect is at the pterygomaxillary junction with resultant vertical hypoplasia of the maxilla and potential absence of the zygomatic arch. There can be associated abnormalities of the mandibular condyle, coronoid, and ramus as well.[2,22]

Soft Tissue

The cleft originates at the oral commissure and courses toward the preauricular region (**Fig. 9**). Mild forms present as a soft tissue furrow owing

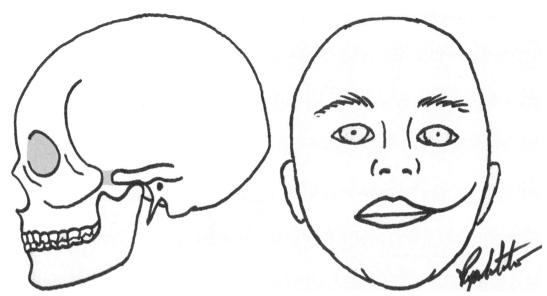

Fig. 9. Tessier 7 soft tissue cleft at oral commissure (*right*) with underlying bony cleft of zygomatic arch (*left*).

to underlying muscular diastasis, and more severe cases see a true cleft of all facial layers resulting in significant macrostomia. The parotid gland may be hypoplastic and congenital facial palsy is possible, as is associated microtia. Underlying skeletal anomalies can lead to lateral canthal dystopia, although the eyelids are uninvolved.[22,23]

Bone

Typical bony clefting is at the pterygomaxillary junction in the molar area, leading to posterior open bite. The maxilla is vertically hypoplastic, leading to an occlusal cant, and partial duplication of the maxilla has been reported.[22,23] The mandibular ramus, condyle, and coronoid are hypoplastic and may be absent. There is significant skull base asymmetry with asymmetric location of the glenoid fossae, and the pterygoids are hypoplastic or absent on the cleft side.[2]

TESSIER 8

Tessier 8 is a frontozygomatic cleft that is also found in Treacher–Collins and Goldenhar syndromes, with skeletal defects common in Treacher–Collins syndrome and soft tissue clefts more commonly seen in Goldenhar syndrome.[2,3] The Tessier 8 cleft is a lateral eyelid coloboma with absence of the lateral canthus, and may have associated globe anomalies, such as epibulbar cysts. There is absence of the lateral orbital rim and wall, together with a hypoplastic greater wing of the sphenoid.[24] These skeleton defects produce the classic findings of lateral canthal

dystopia (a widening of the distance between the medial canthi) and antimongoloid slanting of the palpebrae.

Soft Tissue

The soft tissue findings of Treacher–Collins and Goldenhar syndromes are well-described. Specific to the Tessier 8 cleft, soft tissue involvement can be as subtle as a furrow or shadow at the level of the lateral canthus, or more severe, as a true coloboma with absence of the lateral canthus altogether.[25]

Bone

The bony defect in Tessier 8 cleft is absence of the lateral orbital wall and rim (**Fig. 10**). The lateral border of the orbit is formed by the greater wing of the sphenoid, and rudimentary bony buds may be present in lieu of the zygoma. There is soft tissue communication between the orbit, and temporal and infratemporal fossa owing to these defects.[2,24]

TESSIER 9

Tessier 9 is a superolateral orbital cleft (**Fig. 11**). It originates in the lateral one-third of the upper eyelid and orbital rim and extends through the superior lateral orbital angle into the cranium.[4,5]

Soft Tissue

The lateral one-third of the upper eyelid is involved as a true coloboma and the lateral canthus may be distorted, preventing normal apposition of the

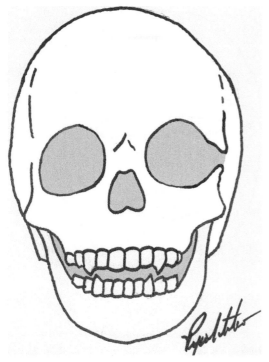

Fig. 10. Tessier 8 lateral orbital cleft.

eyelid and globe. Superior extension of the cleft may present as a soft tissue furrow owing to diastasis of the orbicularis oculi, or may appear as a frank cleft if bony involvement is present.[2,26]

Bone

Bony involvement may be a simple superolateral bony notch, or the cleft may involve the roof of the orbit, superolateral orbital rim, and extend into the temporal fossa. Intracranial extension is rare. There is often some degree of anteroposterior volume reduction of the anterior cranial fossa, and some authors postulate this represents cranial extension of Tessier 5 cleft, although this combination of clefts is very rare.[26]

TESSIER 10

Tessier 10 cleft is a cleft of the superomedial eyelid and orbital rim (**Fig. 12**). A coloboma of the medial or central one-third of the upper eyelid exists, in severe cases total ablepharia is present. Associated colobomata of the iris or other ocular abnormalities may be present. The brow is disrupted, often absent medially, and the cleft may extend as a soft tissue furrow or true cleft superomedially, with diastasis of the orbicularis oculi, procerus, and frontalis muscles. In severe cases, paramedian encephalocele is present. The bony cleft

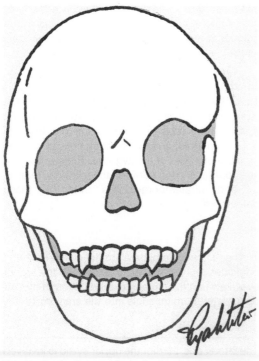

Fig. 11. Tessier 9 superolateral orbital cleft extending to temporal fossa.

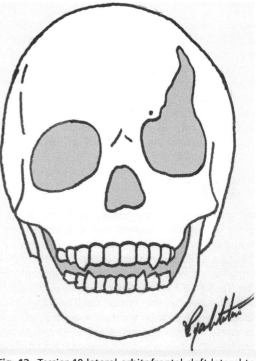

Fig. 12. Tessier 10 lateral orbitofrontal cleft lateral to supraorbital foramen with hypertelorism.

originates in the middle region of the superior orbital rim and can involve the medial roof of the orbit and frontal bone lateral to the supraorbital nerve. In cases with encephalocele, lateral displacement of the cleft-side orbit will yield hypertelorism.[2,26,27]

Soft Tissue

As a result of the medial or total ablepharia, the palpebral fissure on the cleft side is elongated horizontally. The brow is deficient medially or absent, and thins laterally possibly connecting with an anterior projection of the frontotemporal hairline (this can also be seen in Tessier clefts 9 and 11).[28,29] If an encephalocele is present, it is typically broad and located in the middle one-third of the forehead, and the supraorbital ridge and orbital rim will be involved.

Bone

The existence of a true bony cleft heralds the presence of a frontal encephalocele, involving the anterior one-half of the medial orbital roof, the supraorbital rim, and a variable amount of the frontal bone lateral to the supraorbital nerve. The orbit is displaced inferiorly, and the anterior cranial fossa is distorted.[2]

TESSIER 11

Tessier 11 cleft is a true superomedial orbital cleft, involving the medial one-third of the upper eyelid, medial one-third of the superior orbit medial to the supraorbital nerve, and extending through the brow to the frontal hairline. This cleft often presents as an extension of Tessier 3. The cleft will either pass lateral to the ethmoid or directly through the ethmoid cells and through the supraorbital rim, resulting in hypertelorism[2,30] (**Fig. 13**).

Soft Tissue

The soft tissue cleft originates at the medial one-third of the eyelid, lateral to the superior punctum, with variable disruption of the lacrimal system. The medial brow demonstrates irregularity in the direction of hair growth, and the lateral brow is thinned, and may connect with an anterior projection of the frontotemporal hairline, as seen in Tessier 9 and 10.[2,30]

Bone

Bony involvement originates at the medial supraorbital rim and extends into the frontal bone. With complete bony clefting, a frontal encephalocele is present in the mid forehead. The cleft side ethmoid and frontal sinuses are pneumatized and

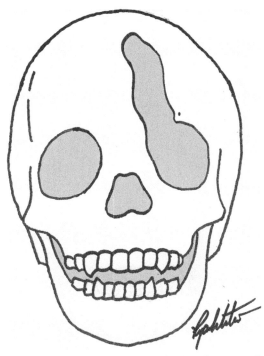

Fig. 13. Tessier 11 superomedial orbitofrontal cleft medial to supraorbital foramen with hypertelorism.

enlarged, and a variable degree of hypertelorism may be present.[30] The sphenoid and remainder of the skull base are characteristically normal.

TESSIER 12

Tessier 12 is a medial cranial cleft originating from the root of the eyebrow, medial to the medial canthus (**Fig. 14**). There is a resultant lateral expansion of the ethmoid with hypertelorism, although the cribriform is of normal size. The frontal sinuses are enlarged, though the frontal bone is flattened. Encephalocele is rare.[2,31]

Soft Tissue

The cleft originates medial to the medial canthus, with resultant telecanthus and true hypertelorism, the latter owing to underlying skeletal anomalies. There is extension into the root of the brow, with thinning of the skin and hair. There is often a short, asymmetric, downward paramedian projection of the frontal hairline on the cleft side.[2]

Bone

There is an increase in the transverse dimension of the ethmoid cavity, creating hypertelorism. There is minor flattening of the frontal bone in the region of the cleft. The frontal and ethmoid sinuses are well-pneumatized, and the anterior and middle

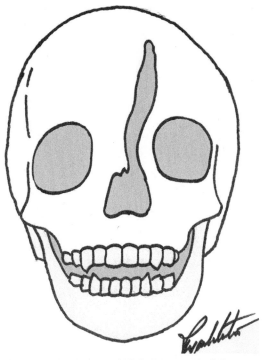

Fig. 14. Tessier 12 medial frontocranial cleft originating at medial superior orbital rim.

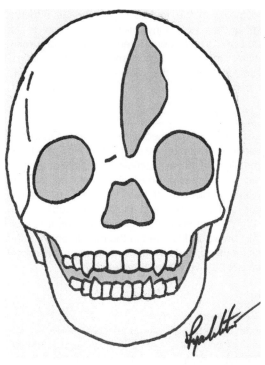

Fig. 15. Tessier 13 paramedian nasofrontal cleft with hypertelorism.

cranial fossae are broadened on the cleft side, though encephalocele is rare as the bony defect is typically limited to the anterior table of the frontal bone.[2] This is thought to be a cranial extension of Tessier 2.

TESSIER 13

This is a frontal paramedian cleft frequently associated with encephalocele. The soft tissue cleft passes medial to an otherwise normal medial brow. The cribriform, olfactory groove, and ethmoid are all widened in a transverse dimension, with resultant hypertelorism[2,4] (**Fig. 15**).

Soft Tissue

Tessier 13 is a cranial extension of Tessier 1, with broadening of the nasal dorsum, root of the nose, and marked hypertelorism. There is asymmetric widening of the root of the nose and forehead, and encephalocele may be present in a medial, although still paramedian, location.[2,32]

Bone

Tessier 13 originates in a paramedian location at the nasal bone and extends through the full height of the frontal bone. In these severe cases,

paramedian encephalocele is the norm. The cleft extends posteriorly through the cribriform and ethmoid sinuses to the lesser wing of the sphenoid, leading to orbital hypertelorism.[2]

TESSIER 14

This is a true midline cranial cleft, representing a cranial extension of Tessier 0 (**Fig. 16**). The nasal root is broad, and the nose bifid. There is marked orbital hypertelorism and there may be associated median frontal encephalocele, although there is a range of frontal bony involvement. There is an increased transverse distance between the olfactory grooves and the crista galli is widened (although it can be duplicated completely, or can be absent). There is significant inferior displacement of the ethmoid bone.[33,34]

Soft Tissue

There is a broad flattening of the glabella corresponding with the midline bony defect through which the frontal encephalocele herniates, with extreme telecanthus. The eyelids, orbits, and periorbita are otherwise normal. There is often a long midline projection of the frontal hairline, denoting the superior extent of the midline cleft.[33–35]

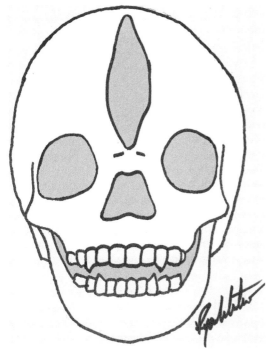

Fig. 16. Tessier 14 median nasofrontal cleft with hypertelorism.

Bone

The midline frontal bone defect provides the path of egress for the frontal encephalocele. In isolated Tessier 14, it begins at the glabella and extends cephalad. Both frontal sinuses are typically absent and the cribriform plate, crista galli, and perpendicular plate of the ethmoid are bifid. The sphenoid sinus is widened but fully pneumatized, and the greater and lesser wings of the sphenoid are rotated symmetrically laterally.[2]

TESSIER 30

The Tessier 30 cleft is a median cleft of the mandibular symphysis. Adherence of the tongue to the midline floor of mouth may exist, and there can be a median cleft of the lower lip. Soft tissue involvement of the midline neck may be present as a continuation of the oromandibular cleft, or may exist as an isolated soft tissue cleft of the midline neck without mandibular bony involvement.[36,37]

Soft Tissue

In the mildest form, the soft tissue involvement may be confined to the skin and subcutaneous tissues of the neck, often referred to as a congenital midline cervical cleft[38,39] **(Fig. 17)**. More complete clefting may involve the lower lip and anterior floor of

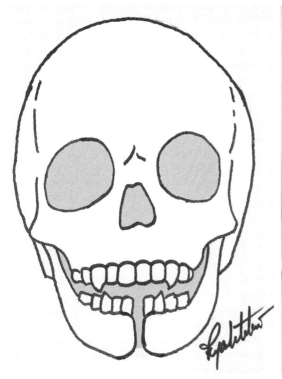
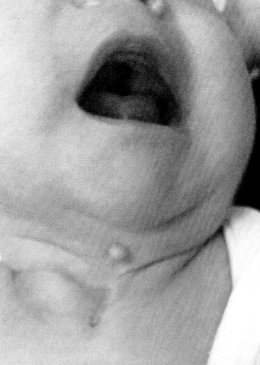

Fig. 17. Median mandibular cleft (*left*) and isolated soft tissue cervical cleft (*right*).

mouth, with vertical shortening of the lip along both cleft borders and functional ankyloglossia owing to severe shortening or agenesis of the lingual frenulum. Rarely, the tongue may be bifid.[38,40]

Bone

When bony involvement is present, it occurs as a midline nonunion at the mandibular symphysis between the medial mandibular incisors. The hyoid bone is characteristically intact and normal in appearance. There have been reports of paramedian mandibular clefts not corresponding with the Tessier system, and ongoing research will elucidate their relationship to known congenital phenomena.[41]

HYPERTELORISM

Orbital hypertelorism denotes an abnormally widened distance between the bony orbits. This must be distinguished from telecanthus (abnormally widened distance between the medial canthi, but with normal bony orbital position), because both the causes and treatments are radically different. Hypertelorism is owing to failure of the orbits to rotate into their normal position during embryogenesis, and found in a number of congenital anomalies and genetic syndromes. Trauma may produce telecanthus, but will not produce true hypertelorism. For the sake of brevity in this article, we focus on hypertelorism owing to facial clefting.

The true expansion of midline or paramedian facial structures as a result of a cleft can result in widening of the interorbital distance. This can be owing to cleft expansion of the median or paramedian bony structures, or can be owing to such clefts leading to local encephalocele, which lateralizes the orbits without creating excess bone between them. Depending on the causative cleft, there will be a variable degree of vertical dystopia, enophthalmos, and associated ocular abnormalities.[42] Correction of these anomalies is an integral part of repairing the underlying Tessier clefts, although such procedures carry an additional risk to the orbital structures and optic nerve as the orbits and globes are repositioned.[43]

In Tessier's original description of hypertelorism repair, he proposed a grading system from 1 to 3 based on the interorbital distance measured at the skull.[44] First-degree hypertelorism is euryopia or possible telecanthus, second-degree (interorbital distance >34 mm) finds the orbits of normal or near-normal shape but farther apart than usual, and in third-degree hypertelorism (interorbital distance ≥40 mm), the cribriform is prolapsed and the orbits themselves may be morphologically abnormal.[44] The degree of severity can help to guide goals of surgery, and with increasing grade of hypertelorism, the potential for multiple operations increases. In correcting hypertelorism, excess bony tissue between the orbits is reduced via paramedian wedge osteotomies to allow corrective rotation of the orbit, and box osteotomies are combined with circular osteotomies to free the orbits individually from the remainder of the craniofacial skeleton. These units are rotated and medialized into the desired position and secured with absorbable plates.

Mild degrees of hypertelorism may be corrected with extracranial/subcranial techniques, but more severe malformations will require combined intracranial/subcranial approaches to sufficiently reposition the orbits and other tissues involved with any concurrent facial cleft.

SUMMARY

Rare craniofacial clefts can present challenging and humbling scenarios for the reconstructive surgeon. The classification system proposed by Tessier can assist the craniofacial surgeon in understanding structures involved in the cleft process, thereby facilitating the surgical plan.

REFERENCES

1. Morian R. Ueber die schrege Gesichtsspalte. Arch Klin Chir 1887;35:245.
2. David DJ, Moore MH, Cooter RD. Tessier clefts revisited with a third dimension. Cleft Palate J 1989;26(3): 163–85.
3. Butow K, Botha A. A classification and construction of congenital lateral facial clefts. J Craniomaxillofac Surg 2010;38:477–84.
4. Tessier P. Anatomical classification of facial, craniofacial and laterofacial clefts. J Maxillofac Surg 1976;4:69–92.
5. Kawamoto HK. The kaleidoscopic world of rare craniofacial clefts: order out of chaos (Tessier classification). Clin Plast Surg 1976;3:529–72.
6. Mishra S, Sabhlok S, Panda PK, et al. Management of midline facial clefts. J Maxillofac Oral Surg 2015; 14(4):883–90.
7. Kolker AR, Sailon AM, Meara JG, et al. Midline cleft lip and bifid nose deformity: description, classification, and treatment. J Craniofac Surg 2015;26(8):2034–8.
8. Tada M, Nakamura N. Sphenoethmoidal encephalomeningocele and midline anomalies of face and brain. Hokkaido Igaku Zasshi 1985;60(1):48–56.
9. Savastano CP, Bernardi P, Seuanez HN, et al. Rare nasal cleft in a patient with holoprosencephaly due

to a mutation in the Z1C2 gene. Birth Defects Res A Clin Mol Teratol 2014;100(4):300–6.

10. Addona T, Friedman A, Post A, et al. Complete calvarial agenesis in conjunction with a Tessier 1-13 facial cleft. Cleft Palate Craniofac J 2012;49(4):484–7.

11. Garabedian EN, Ducroz V, Roger G, et al. Nasal fossa malformations and paramedian facial cleft: new perspectives. J Craniofac Genet Dev Biol 1999;19(1):12–9.

12. Altuntas A, Yilmaz MD, Khaveci OK, et al. Coexistance of choanal atresia and Tessier's facial cleft number 2. Int J Pediatr Otorhinolaryngol 2004;68(8):1081–5.

13. Ozek C, Gundogan H, Bilkay U, et al. Rare craniofacial anomaly: Tessier no. 2 cleft. J Craniofac Surg 2001;12(4):355–61.

14. Allam KA, Lim AA, Elsherbiny A, et al. The Tessier number 3 cleft: a report of 10 cases and review of literature. J Plast Reconstr Aesthet Surg 2014; 67(8):1055–62.

15. Da Silva Freitas R, Alonso N, Busato L, et al. Oral-nasal-ocular cleft: the greatest challenge among the rare clefts. J Craniofac Surg 2010;21(2):390–5.

16. Alonso N, Freitas Reda S, de Oliviera e Cruz GA, et al. Tessier no. 4 facial cleft: evolution of surgical treatment in a large series of patients. Plast Reconstr Surg 2008;122(5):1505–13.

17. Longaker MT, Lipshutz GS, Kawamoto HK Jr. Reconstruction of Tessier no. 4 clefts revisited. Plast Reconstr Surg 1997;99(6):1501–7.

18. Resnick JI, Kawamoto HK Jr. Rare craniofacial clefts: Tessier no. 4 clefts. Plast Reconstr Surg 1990;85(6): 843–9.

19. Abdollahifakhim S, Shahidi N, Bayazian G. A bilateral Tessier number 4 and 5 facial cleft and surgical strategy: a case report. Iran J Otorhinolaryngol 2013;25(73):259–62.

20. Da Silva Freitas R, Alonso N, Shin JH, et al. The Tessier number 5 facial cleft: surgical strategies and outcomes in six patients. Cleft Palate Craniofac J 2009;46(2):179–86.

21. Bilkay U, Gundogan H, Ozek C, et al. A rare craniofacial cleft: bilateral Tessier no. 5 accompanied by no. 1 and no. 6 clefts. Ann Plast Surg 2000;45(6): 654–7.

22. Woods RH, Varma S, David DJ. Tessier no.7 cleft: a new subclassification and management protocol. Plast Reconstr Surg 2008;122(3):898–905.

23. Borzabadi-Farahani A, Yen SL, Francis C, et al. A rare case of accessory maxilla and bilateral Tessier no. 7 clefts, a 10-year follow-up. J Craniomaxillofac Surg 2013;41(6):527–31.

24. Raulo Y, Tessier P. Mandibulo-facial dysostosis analysis: principles of surgery. Scand J Plast Reconstr Surg 1981;15:251–6.

25. Fuente-del-Campo A. Surgical correction of Tessier number 8 cleft. Plast Reconstr Surg 1990;86(4):658–61.

26. Pereira FJ, Milbratz GH, Cruz AA, et al. Ophthalmic considerations in the management of Tessier cleft 5/9. Ophthal Plast Reconstr Surg 2010;26(6):450–3.

27. Ortube MC, Dipple K, Setoguchi Y, et al. Ocular manifestations of oblique facial clefts. J Craniofac Surg 2010;21(5):1630–1.

28. Toriyama K, Hatano H, Yagi S, et al. Long follow-up of craniofacial cleft treated by the folded vascularized calvarial bone. J Craniofac Surg 2013;24(3): e202–3.

29. Lee HM, Noh TK, Yoo HW, et al. A wedge-shaped anterior hairline extension associated with a Tessier number 10 cleft. Ann Dermatol 2012;24(4): 464–7.

30. Bodin F, Salazard B, Bardot J, et al. Craniofacial cleft: a case of Tessier No. 3, 7 and 11 cleft. J Plast Reconstr Aesthet Surg 2006;59(12): 1388–90.

31. Moon SY, Kim SG, Park YJ, et al. Correction of bilateral Tessier no. 2, 3, and 12 facial cleft with anophthalmia. J Korean Assoc Maxillofac Plast Reconstr Surg 2013;35(4):243–7.

32. Gargano F, Szymanski K, Bosman M, et al. Tessier 1-13 atypical craniofacial cleft. Eplasty 2015;15: ic32.

33. Nam SM, Kim YB. The Tessier number 14 facial cleft: a 20 year follow-up. J Craniomaxillofac Surg 2014; 42(7):1397–401.

34. Pidgeon TE, Flapper WJ, David DJ, et al. From birth to maturity: midline Tessier 0-14 craniofacial cleft patients who have completed protocol management at a single craniofacial unit. Cleft Palate Craniofac J 2014;51(4):e70–9.

35. Sleg P, Hakim SG, Jacobsen HC, et al. Rare facial clefts: treatment during charity missions in developing countries. Plast Reconstr Surg 2004;114(3): 640–7.

36. Ladan P, Sailer HF, Sabnis R. Tessier 30 symphyseal mandibular cleft: early simultaneous soft and hard tissue correction: a case report. J Craniomaxillofac Surg 2012;41(8):735–9.

37. Rao AY. Complete midline cleft of lower lip, mandible, tongue, floor of mouth, with neck contracture: a case report and review of literature. Craniomaxillofac Trauma Reconstr 2015;8(4):363–9.

38. Surendran N, Varghese B. Midline cleft of lower lip with cleft of the mandible and midline dermoid in the neck. J Pediatr Surg 1991;26(12):1387–8.

39. Sinopidis X, Kourea HP, Panagidis A, et al. Congenital midline cervical cleft: diagnosis, pathologic findings, and early stage treatment. Case Rep Pediatr 2012;2012:951040.

40. Halli R, Kini Y, Kharkar V, et al. Treatment of midline cleft of the mandible – a 2-stage approach. J Craniofac Surg 2011;22(1):220–2.

41. Tanna N, Wan DC, Perry AD, et al. Paramedian mandibular cleft: revisiting the Tessier classification. J Craniofac Surg 2012;23(1):e38–40.

42. Marchac D, Sati S, Renier D, et al. Hypertelorism correction: what happens with growth? evaluation of a series of 95 surgical cases. Plast Reconstr Surg 2012;129(3):713–27.

43. Pagnoni M, Fadda MT, Spalice A, et al. Surgical timing of craniosynostosis: what to do and when. J Craniomaxillofac Surg 2014;42(5):513–9.

44. Tessier P. Orbital hypertelorism: 1. Successive surgical attempts. material and methods. causes and mechanisms. Scand J Plast Reconstr Surg 1972;6(2):135–55.

Vascular Lesions

 CrossMark

Keimun A. Slaughter, MD[a,b,c,d,e], Tiffany Chen, MD[a,d,e],
Edwin Williams III, MD[a,b,c,d],*

KEYWORDS

- Vascular lesions • Vascular malformations • Hemangiomas • Port wine stains
- Lymphovascular malformations • Capillary malformations • Vascular defects

KEY POINTS

- Classification of vascular lesions based of off the biological behavior has greatly facilitated more accurate diagnoses, optimally defined treatment plans, and better outcomes.
- Treatment of vascular lesions has taken a more conservative surgical approach with reliance on select medical treatment options, which has greatly reduced morbidity and mortality resulting from extensive surgery.
- A multidisciplinary approach involving multiple surgical and pediatric subspecialties has led to advancement in both understanding and ideal treatment strategies of these lesions.

INTRODUCTION

The study of vascular lesions has spanned many medical and surgical subspecialties within academia over the last several decades. Much of the understanding regarding the nonsurgical management of these lesions has been predicated by pediatric subspecialties and complemented by advances in surgical management of these lesions and vice versa. Furthermore, because many of these lesions have involved the craniofacial region, this area has been thoroughly investigated by surgical subspecialties, including facial plastic surgery along with oral maxillofacial and craniofacial surgery.

Since the advent of the current classification system approved by the International Society for the Study of Vascular Anomalies in 1996 (and updated in 2014), relatively few advances in treatment of these lesions have occurred.[1] This classification system was derived from Mulliken and Glowacki's system,[2] which was published in 1982 and based on the biological behavior of the lesions. In general, the overlying theme has been toward more conservative surgical approaches and a greater reliance on the advances in medical management, which in turn has led to more effective treatment with a greatly reduced morbidity.

Specifically, the lesions can be divided into vascular tumors, including the more common infantile hemangiomas, rapidly and noninvoluting congenital hemangiomas, and kaposiform hemangioendotheliomas, among others; and vascular malformations, including low-flow venous, lymphatic, and capillary/port-wine stain subtypes, high-flow arteriovenous malformations (AVM), and combined complex capillary-venous, capillary-arteriovenous, and lymphaticovenous subtypes. In this article, the more common lesions, and specifically the classification, diagnosis, and management, are focused on, with an emphasis on an aesthetic approach regarding surgical technique when indicated (**Box 1**).

VASCULAR TUMORS: HEMANGIOMA

Considered the most common tumor of infancy and childhood, hemangiomas have an estimated

[a] Albany Medical Center, 43 New Scotland Avenue, Albany, NY 12208, USA; [b] New England Laser and Cosmetic Surgery Center, 1072 Troy Schenectady Road #101, Latham, NY 12110, USA; [c] Williams Center Plastic Surgery Specialists, 1072 Troy Schenectady Road #201, Latham, NY 12110, USA; [d] St Peters Hospital, 315 S Manning Boulevard, Albany, NY 12208, USA; [e] Stratton VA, 113 Holland Avenue, Albany, NY 12208, USA
* Corresponding author. Williams Center Plastic Surgery Specialists, 1072 Troy Schenectady Road #201, Latham, NY 12110.
E-mail address: edwilliamsmd@gmail.com

Facial Plast Surg Clin N Am 24 (2016) 559–571
http://dx.doi.org/10.1016/j.fsc.2016.06.009

advocated for aggressive management with surgical excision, cauterization, carbon dioxide snow, surface radium, radioactive implants, external beam radiation, interstitial gamma radiation, and sclerosing agents. However, serious complications arose, such as malignant transformation after radiation therapy and poor cosmetic results due to significant scar formation secondary to resection and other ablative procedures. Conversely, proponents of more conservative benign neglect strategies argued that the natural course of most hemangiomas included involution with no residual deformity. The stark polarity in treatment algorithms was centered around the fact that vascular tumors and malformations were often categorized as similar or related entities—for example, the term capillary hemangioma was used to describe port-wine stains, which are capillary malformations, whereas strawberry nevi and cavernous hemangiomas were used to describe true hemangiomas. [5] This early misclassification of vascular lesions is what led to a lack of consensus in regards to management, which again was addressed by Mulliken and Glowacki's delineation of vascular tumors (hemangiomas) and malformations based on biological behavior, resulting in the current classification.[1]

CLINICAL PRESENTATION AND DIAGNOSIS

Infantile hemangiomas are usually visible within the first few weeks of life, whereas congenital hemangiomas are fully formed at birth and grow with variable intensity. Superficial hemangiomas are contained within the papillary dermis and are characterized by bright red, macular, or papular lesions with well-defined borders. The macular variety can be confused with port-wine malformations; however, over time the hemangioma will change in size, whereas the port-wine malformation remains relatively stable. Deep hemangiomas are contained in the reticular dermis or subcutaneous tissue and present as a blue, subcutaneous mass with bluish or colorless overlying skin depending on the depth. These hemangiomas may appear similar to lymphatic malformations on examination. Compound hemangiomas have features of both superficial and deep lesions **(Fig. 1)**.[3,5]

Hemangiomas exhibit 2 distinct clinical stages, including proliferation and involution. Proliferation occurs during the first 12 months of life and occasionally as late as 18 months. An initial growth phase during the first few months of life followed by a subsequent growth phase at 4 to 6 months establishes a bimodal pattern of growth. Cosmetic deformity or functional obstruction of the eye,

prevalence of 10% by age 1, with 30% evident at birth, and a female predilection of 4:1.[3] Ninety percent of all vascular tumors are infantile hemangiomas.[4] Although 40% to 60% involve the head and neck, 80% of these lesions tend to be solitary.[3] There are various syndromes that can be associated with hemangiomas, including PHACES (*p*osterior fossa malformations, *h*emangiomas, *a*rterial anomalies, *c*oarctation of the aorta and cardiac defects, *e*ye abnormalities, and *s*ternal defects), and other symptoms such as stridor in a patient with cutaneous hemangiomas should be further investigated along with the potential for visceral hemangiomas and hemangiomas overlying the lumbosacral spine due to the increased association with spinal cord and genitourinary anomalies.[3] Imaging studies, such as screening ultrasounds and confirmatory MRIs, should be strongly considered in these patients.[5]

Historically, treatment of these lesions involved the use of various modalities. Many investigators

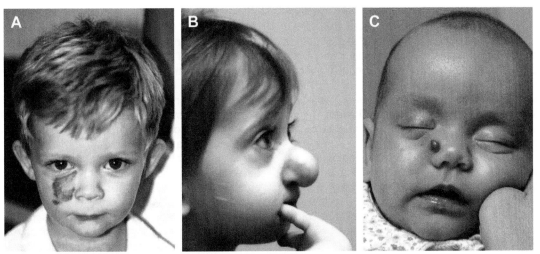

Fig. 1. (*A*) Superficial hemangiomas are bright red macular or papular lesions. (*B*) Deep hemangiomas present as bluish, subcutaneous masses. (*C*) Compound hemangiomas exhibit features of both superficial and deep hemangiomas.

nose, or airway typically arises during the first growth phase (**Fig. 2**).[3] Histologic features during the proliferative phase include plump proliferating endothelial cells and pericytes with barely perceptible vascular channels.[5] Involution, occurring over the first several years of life, is characterized by a decrease and then cessation in growth of the lesion. The lesion changes from bright red to dark maroon and eventually patches of ashen gray, evolving from a firm, tense consistency to a lobular, soft, compressible mass on palpation. Histologically, there is a gradual flattening of endothelial cells with progressive deposition of fibrous tissue and vessel ectasia, resulting in superficial telangiectasia and subcutaneous fibrofatty residuum (**Fig. 3**).[3]

Although imaging is not required for diagnosis, it can be useful to evaluate the extent of involvement in deeper lesions as well as rule out other vascular tumors. Ultrasound findings demonstrate a solid

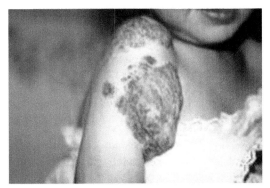

Fig. 2. Rapidly proliferating hemangioma in the same infant in **Fig. 1C**, 5 months later, unresponsive to intralesional steroids or PDL, now with astigmatism, partial visual obstruction, and impending amblyopia.

Fig. 3. Late involuting hemangioma demonstrating darkening skin color and patches of ashen gray. Significant subcutaneous fibrofatty residuum will require surgical excision.

mass with increased/high color flow within it; Doppler ultrasound can demonstrate the arterial feeder and venous drainage. MRI characteristics include lesions that exhibit enhancement on T2-weighted images, which are relatively isointense on T1-weighted images with homogenous contrast enhancement; internal serpiginous flow voids within the lesion in T2-weighted images represent the arterial feeder, which can be an important diagnostic clue.[4]

The diagnosis of infantile hemangiomas can also be assisted with the use of immunohistochemical markers because endothelial cells in these lesions stain strongly for the glucose transporter protein isoform 1, whereas most other vascular tumors, such as congenital hemangiomas, do not.[4]

The psychology of children with these lesions has also been studied. It is known that children begin to develop self-awareness at 18 to 24 months of age with a significant body image well under development by 3 years of age.[6] Individual studies by Williams and colleagues[6] and Dieterich-Miller and colleagues[7] comparing children 3 to 5 years of age with hemangiomas of the head and neck with unaffected children found that children with hemangiomas perceived that others valued them significantly lower compared with the unaffected group. Furthermore, parental interviews revealed reports of strangers questioning child abuse, children burying their faces or hiding lesions with their hair, and family and friends commenting openly on intervention.[6,7] Preventing the aforementioned scenarios makes diagnosis, classification, and effective treatment of these lesions extremely important in the pediatric population with respect to psychosocial affects.

TREATMENT: HEMANGIOMAS

Treatment of hemangiomas historically has involved various approaches, including surgical excision, steroids, and benign neglect; current therapy has evolved to include interventions such as laser therapy and propranolol. Review of the literature on pediatric facial hemangiomas revealed 25% to 40% will result in an unacceptable aesthetic outcome when no intervention is performed.[5] Finn and colleagues[3] found that of 50% of lesions that involuted early (before age 5), 19% resulted in a substantial aesthetic deformity, including residual scar, redundant skin, or telangiectasia, whereas of the 50% that involuted late (after age 5), 60% were cosmetically unacceptable.

The treatment algorithm is dependent on the classification of the lesion, and deciding when to observe or intervene is the most important decision (Fig. 4).[3] If observation is determined to be the approach, then unlike the practice of benign neglect, it must be an active process with routine monitoring every 3 months. This frequency of evaluation must be increased to every 2 to 4 weeks with demonstrated interval change or for a lesion in a cosmetically sensitive area. The decision to treat proliferating lesions should be based on the rate of proliferation, presence of or pending ulcerating, and aesthetic result in the setting of possible involution with no resulting deformity. Goals for therapy include reduction in size and induction of involution. The mainstay of interventions for these lesions includes intralesional or systemic steroids, pulsed dye laser (PDL), and surgical excision.

Hemangiomas that are involuting require monitoring for 8 to 12 months. Serial photography and questioning on history during early involution will reveal regression or provide information on the degree of stabilization of the lesion. Early involuters show regression by age 2, whereas later involuters do not have evidence of regression by this time. Hemangiomas that have not somewhat regressed in size by 8 to 12 months are most likely late involuters.[5] Early involuters are monitored every 6 months until 4 to 4.5 years of age, at which time surgical treatment for atrophic skin or fibrofatty residuum or PDL treatment for telangiectasia can be pursued. Approximately 20% of early involuters require additional intervention for an aesthetic deformity, whereas 60% of later involuters leave a cosmetically imperfect result.[5] The mainstay interventions for these lesions include observation, PDL, and surgical excision.

PDL therapy is indicated for more superficial hemangiomas that rapidly proliferate, ulcerate, or demonstrate pending ulceration, lead to nasal airway obstruction, or are located in more cosmetically sensitive areas (Fig. 5). Treatment of proliferating ulcerative hemangiomas is efficacious because of their inhibitory effect on the growth rate of the hemangioma, which allows re-epithelialization to occur.[3,5] Treatment is delivered at 4- to 6-week intervals until resolution of ulceration or cessation of proliferation. A wavelength of 595 nm is selected to allow deeper penetration into the thickened aspects of the hemangioma, and selective photothermolysis at this wavelength corresponds to the second and third absorption peak for hemoglobin and oxyhemoglobin, respectively.[3] Starting with a fluence around 9 J/cm^2 with a 5-mm hand piece or 8 J/cm^2 for a 7-mm hand

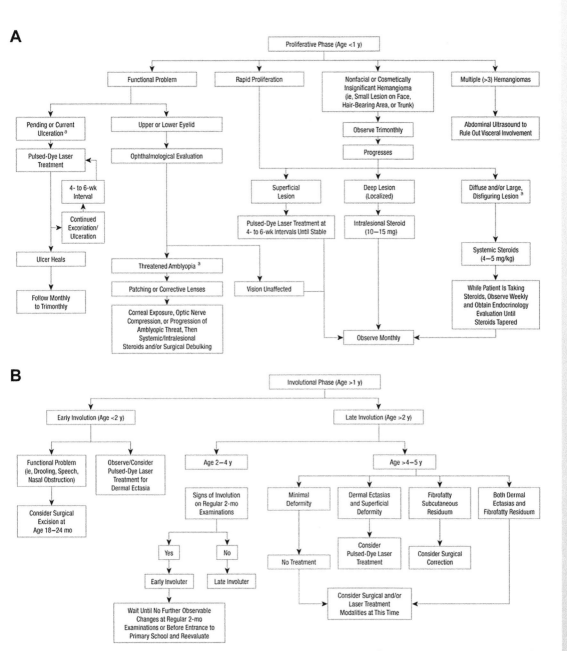

Fig. 4. Algorithm developed by the senior author (E.F.W.) for management of hemangiomas during the proliferative (*A*) and involutional phase (*B*). [a] Consider initiation of propranolol in infantile hemangioma. (*Adapted from* Batniji RK, Buckingham ED, Williams EF. An aesthetic approach to facial hemangiomas. Arch Facial Plast Surg 2005;7:301–6; with permission.)

piece, this should be increased until the desired degree of purpura is achieved. The addition of a cryogen spray via a dynamic cooling device (DCD) attached to the hand piece allows cooling of the superficial epidermis with continued penetration of laser energy to the lesion, theoretically resulting in less superficial thermal injury, scarring, and discomfort. It has been the authors'

experience and observation that use of the DCD can diminish the effect of the laser on the lesion, and for select lesions, they do see better treatment response with deactivation of the DCD. One should be extremely mindful of fluence levels and tissue response if the DCD is deactivated because the potential for thermal injury is greatly increased. Of note, first-generation lasers have a pulse time of

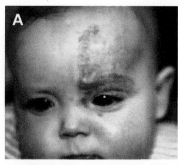
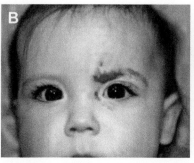
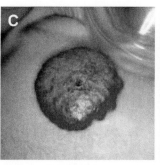

Fig. 5. Indications for PDL during the proliferative phase. (*A, B*) Prelaser and postlaser ablation of a superficial hemangioma in a potentially cosmetically disfiguring area. (*C*) Presence of ulceration or impending ulceration. Can also consider initiation of propranolol therapy if not medically contraindicated.

450 to 500 microseconds, which is significantly shorter than the thermal relaxation time of skin of 700 to 900 microseconds, thus increasing the safety profile for these lasers, but second-generation lasers have an increased pulse time of 1500 microseconds to increase efficacy for larger vessels.[3] As the PDL is relatively ineffective for deeper lesions due to the inability to penetrate tissue to the necessary depth, intralesional potassium titanyl phosphate or Nd:YAG lasers have been suggested; however, the concern for scarring and damage to underlying structures is greatly increased.

For deeper or more compound lesions, systemic or intralesional steroids can be used, especially for rapidly proliferating and aesthetically or functionally debilitating lesions. These medications were used historically but have been replaced by safer, more effective alternatives. Kenalog is used primarily for intralesional injection and is delivered to the bulk of the tumor. Ten milligrams per milliliter in a 1-mL syringe with a 27′ or 30′ needle is used to deliver a total of 10 to 15 mg depending on the size of the lesion, or roughly 2 to 3 mg/kg. The treatment is repeated every 4 to 6 weeks until the lesion stabilizes, decreases, or requires additional intervention. In order to prevent increased bleeding with the injection, ensure that the needle is passed through normal skin, avoiding the thinned epidermis involved with the lesion. If you opt for dual therapy with use of the laser, laser treatment should be performed first in order to avoid interference of injection-associated bleeding with accuracy of laser pulses. Systemic steroids can also be considered for proliferating hemangiomas. The optimal dosing regimen has not been completely delineated; however, increased responsiveness has been noted with higher dosing but at the expense of greater adverse effects. Side effects such as Cushingoid features, hypertension, hyperglycemia, immune suppression, behavioral

disturbances, and growth retardation are observed and increased in likelihood with higher and prolonged steroid dosing. The authors propose an effective and safe regimen consisting of prednisone 4 mg/kg as a single starting dose. This dose is maintained for 3 weeks if stabilization or shrinkage of the lesion is observed or can be increased to 5 mg/kg daily, if tolerated, for a week if no response is noted. At around the 3-week follow-up, the steroid is tapered over 4 to 8 weeks. If rebound proliferation occurs during tapering, the dosage should be increased to the next highest level for an additional week, and then tapering can be reattempted. Ideally, this should be done in collaboration with the primary care physician or pediatrician and endocrinologist. Antireflux prophylaxis should be initiated and live vaccines avoided. The patient should be followed monthly, and the lesion re-evaluated after completion of the taper. A dose of 4 mg/kg daily can be resumed for 1 week if there is continued proliferation but should be tapered over 4 weeks if improvement is noted.[3,5] Although there are indications for steroid use, treatment has fallen out of favor because of the adverse side effects and has been replaced largely by the use of propranolol.

Propranolol, which is traditionally used by cardiologists in infants with tachyarrhythmias, has been shown to be an effective treatment for select hemangiomas.[8] Propranolol has been found to be rapidly effective for infantile hemangiomas and well tolerated, with the most frequently reported serious complications including hypotension, bronchial hyperreactivity due to inhibition of adrenergic broncodilation, hypoglycemia or hypoglycemic seizure, asymptomatic bradycardia, and hyperkalemia.[8] Commonly reported adverse effects include sleep disturbances, diarrhea, and gastroesophageal reflux disease.[8] The mechanism of action has not been clearly elucidated with various proposed hypotheses, including vasoconstriction, decreased renin production, inhibition of angiogenesis, and stimulation of apoptosis proposed.[8] Consensus recommendations from 2011 encourage treatment of ulceration, ocular compromise, airway obstruction, and risk of permanent disfigurement and should be initiated and managed by a medical team familiar with hemangiomas and the medication in pediatric populations.[8] The dose is started low with escalation to a target dose of 1 to 3 mg/kg daily in 3 divided doses.[8] Initiation should be considered with inpatient hospitalization in infants less than 8 weeks of age or any infant with inadequate social support or comorbid conditions.[8] Peak effect on blood pressure and heart rate occurs 1 to 3 hours after administration.[8]

Surgical excision has also been an effective treatment option for carefully selected lesions. Planning is paramount when considering surgical intervention and should be considered during involution in order to minimize blood loss. Incisions should be placed in the junction of facial subunits or relaxed skin tension lines to conceal scars. Atrophic scar tissue and ulceration should be incorporated into the skin excision, and careful identification and management of feeding vessels with bipolar cautery will result in less blood loss and avoidance of blood products. Use of M-plasty technique can shorten incision lines (**Fig. 6**).[3,5] Ten percent of the lesion should be left behind if full excision will result in violation of aesthetic lines or an unsightly incision. The remaining lesion can be observed or treated with PDL (**Figs. 7** and **8**).[3,5] When considering treatment of hemangiomas in the periorbital region, management should include consultation with an ophthalmologist. Treatment is indicated with amblyopia or

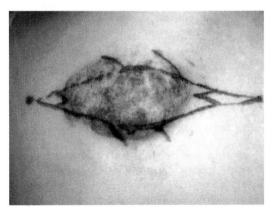

Fig. 6. Z-plasty is used for scar camouflage and M-plasty is used to shorten the length of the incision line.

rapid proliferation (**Fig. 9**). Surgical management is reserved for functional concerns and nonresponders to steroid or laser therapy. If orbital structures are compromised, then a portion of the lesion is left behind and treated with intralesional steroid injections or PDL therapy.[5] Special consideration should also be given to nasal and lip hemangiomas with respect to placement of incisions within aesthetic subunits and avoidance of aggressive resection (**Fig. 10**).

VASCULAR TUMORS: KAPOSIFORM HEMANGIOENDOTHELIOMA

Kaposiform hemangioendothelioma is a rare vascular tumor that is present at birth or within the first few months of life, but may also present later in childhood.[4] It presents as an ill-defined, purpuric solid mass that is often painful and destructive—infiltrative growth differentiates this lesion from a hemangioma.[4] Histology reveals cells that form a slitlike lumina containing erythrocytes resembling Kaposi sarcoma.[4] It is associated with Kasabach-Merritt phenomenon in up to 50% of patients with a high mortality due to coagulopathy or complications from local tumor infiltration.[4] Imaging reveals a solid mass with ill-defined borders and variable echogenicity on ultrasound, whereas MRI usually demonstrates a lesion involving multiple soft tissue planes with skin, subcutaneous fat, muscle, and bony cortex infiltration.[4] Treatment is primarily medical because the tumor is usually too extensive for surgical resection.[9]

VASCULAR MALFORMATIONS

Vascular malformations are vascular lesions that are present at birth with a growth rate that is dependent on the principal type of vessel and proportional to the individual without spontaneous regression.[8] These lesions can experience rapid expansion when triggered by hormonal factors, trauma, or infection, but can also remain dormant with a presentation later in childhood or adulthood.[4] Histology reveals vascular spaces lined with flat, mature, mitotically quiescent epithelium with the subtype classified by the constituent vessel, presence or absence of arteriovenous shunting, and flow dynamics—specifically low flow versus high flow.[4]

Venous, lymphatic, and capillary malformations comprise low-flow lesions. Venous malformations present as soft, compressible, bluish lesions that infiltrate multiple tissue planes (**Fig. 11**). They may enlarge with Valsalva maneuvers and exhibit skin involvement. Spontaneous thrombosis and

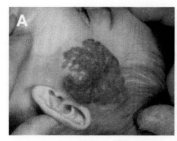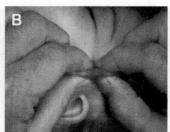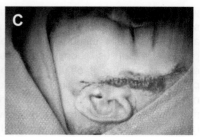

Fig. 7. (A, B) Significant tissue expansion effect of lesion. (C) Residual hemangioma after closure allows for postoperative involution and tissue creation with PDL.

thrombolysis can occur resulting in elevated D-dimer levels.[4] MRI is the best imaging modality and reveals hyperintense serpiginous lesions with phleboliths on T2-weighted images and possible fat or muscle interspersed between venous channels.[4] Easily compressible, spongelike networks of tubular structures with low velocity or no venous flow are demonstrated on ultrasound.[4] Lymphatic malformations present as soft, compressible cystic lesions filled with chylous material. They are classified as microcystic, macrocystic, or mixed. MRI varies depending on internal hemorrhage and inflammation, with high-signal T2-weighted images with gadolinium demonstrating mild peripheral enhancement without internal enhancement; ultrasound reveals no flow within major spaces.[4] Capillary vascular malformations (port-wine stains) present as flat lesions with a red to pink hue that may lighten during the first year of life, but eventually darken into a deeper red or blue lesion with thickening and nodularity.[10] These lesions are the most common type of

malformations noted in 3/1000 births with an equal sex distribution and head and neck involvement in 80% of cases.[10] These lesions do not resolve spontaneously, grow proportionally with the patient, and are associated with syndromes such as Sturge-Weber (malformation distributed in the first trigeminal division, with possible V2 or V3 involvement, glaucoma, and central nervous system abnormalities) and Klippel-Trenaunay syndrome (malformation involving a unilateral lower extremity with associated hypertrophy, varicose veins, lymphedema and phleboliths).[10]

AVM comprise rare high-flow lesions with an unpredictable course, making treatment aesthetically challenging.[11] These lesions enlarge more readily because of higher inflowing pressures (absence of capillary transition between arterial and venous systems) and recruitment and collateralization, and as such, usually present as a pulsatile lesion with an associated bruit or murmur.[4] These lesions can lead to high-output cardiac failure in some cases.[4] The diagnosis should be made with MRI or computed tomographic angiography, and biopsy should be avoided due to the high risk of bleeding. MRI reveals prominent flow-related signal voids and allows for visualization of feeding and draining vessels, whereas Doppler ultrasound shows arterial flow within prominent high-flow draining vessels.[4] Histology exhibits beds of venules and arterioles intermixed with large-caliber arteries and veins.[4] The Schobinger scale can be used to classify the severity **(Table 1)**.[4]

TREATMENT: VASCULAR MALFORMATIONS

Treatment varies depending on the type of lesion. Low-flow lesions can be treated effectively with sclerotherapy, PDL, and surgery in select lesions, whereas high-flow lesions are usually managed with a multimodality approach.

Percutaneous sclerotherapy can be used as a first-line agent for small low-flow vascular

Fig. 8. Avoid overdeveloping the plane between skin and hemangioma to maintain a safe skin flap thickness. Residual hemangioma is left behind to ensure flap survival.

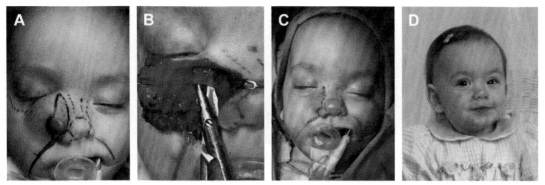

Fig. 9. (*A*) Preoperative photograph of the infant from **Figs. 1C** and **2** before surgical debulking during proliferation. (*B*) Surgical plane deep to the hemangioma is easily defined; rarely are deeper structures involved. (*C, D*) Immediate and delayed postoperative result.

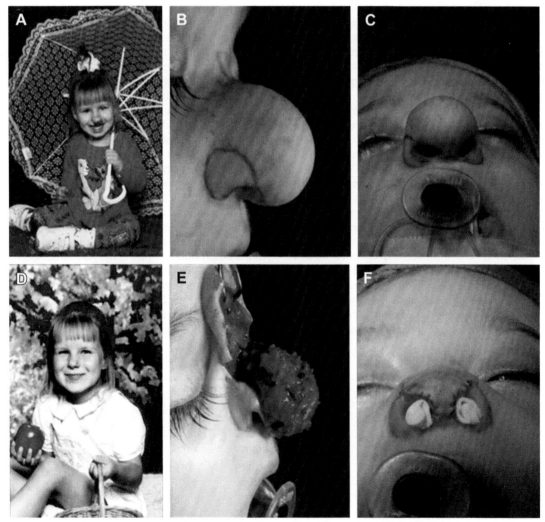

Fig. 10. External rhinoplasty approach to a deep hemangioma of the nose. (*A–C*) Preoperative views. (*D, F*) Postoperative views. (*E*) Intraoperative view with cutaneous flap elevated to demonstrate superolateral cutaneous extensions of marginal incision at the subunit junction.

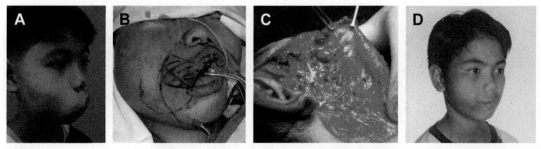

Fig. 11. Venous malformation resection. (*A*) Preoperative view. (*B, C*) Intraoperative views. (*D*) Postoperative view.

malformations or as a preoperative modality in an attempt to induce lesion regression before resection.[12–14] These treatments have been proposed to avoid significant morbidity and suboptimal cosmetic outcomes associated with surgical excision after failed conservative management. Sclerosants include ethanol, OK-432 (penicillin-killed *Streptococcus pyogenes*), sodium tetradecyl sulfate/sodium dodecyl sulfate (anionic surfactant), doxycycline, bleomycin, and gelatin adhesive, to name a few. They are injected in the malformation to induce endothelial damage, inflammation, thrombosis, and fibrosis and cause eventual destruction of the lesion.[12,13] Advantages include reduced risk of damage to nearby structures, such as nerves, absence of an incision, low risk of infections, and rapid recovery. Disadvantages include need for multiple treatments, limited application if lesions surround important structures, or ill effects from sclerosants that enter the systemic circulation.[12,13]

PDL treatment is particularly effective for low-flow capillary malformations or port-wine stains (**Fig. 12**). Before this, cosmetic camouflage and the argon laser were used to treat these lesions; however, the argon laser caused significant scarring. PDL has been established as the gold

standard for treatment because it selectively targets the vascular chromophore, minimizing lesion-induced deformity with little morbidity.[10] Complications are rare but can include scarring, uneven pigment distribution, transient alopecia, cutaneous infections, and ocular injuries. It remains the authors' practice to treat no earlier than 6 months of age because this reduces the anesthesia risk with a plan for 3 to 5 treatment sessions approximately 6 weeks apart. The authors favor earlier laser therapy because mature lesions may be recalcitrant to laser intervention. It is important to educate the patient and family about the progressive, natural course of the disease, the need for repeated treatments, and the concept that port-wine stains cannot be completely eradicated, only lightened and flattened with the laser.[10] In fact, 50% of these lesions return to the initial appearance before treatment over time.[10] Preoperatively, outline the extent of the lesion before induction of anesthesia to ensure treatment of the lesion without treating the normal surrounding skin, because this can become more difficult to discern after anesthesia is administered. Ensure standard laser protocols for the patient (corneal shields or eye patches, surgical lubricant over hair-bearing structures to avoid damage) and staff

Table 1
Schobinger scale of severity of arteriovenous malformations

Stage	Stage Name	Description
I	Quiescence	Pink-bluish stain and warmth
II	Expansion	Enlarged swelling with pulsation, thrill, and bruit. Tense and tortuous veins
III	Destruction	Stage II with ulceration, bleeding, pain, and tissue necrosis
IV	Decompensation	Stage III with cardiac failure

Adapted from Tekes A, Koshy J, Kalayci TO, et al. S.E. Mitchell Vascular Anomalies Flow Chart (SEMVAFC): a visual pathway combining clinical and imaging findings for classification of soft-tissue vascular anomalies. Clin Radiol 2014;69:443–57; with permission.

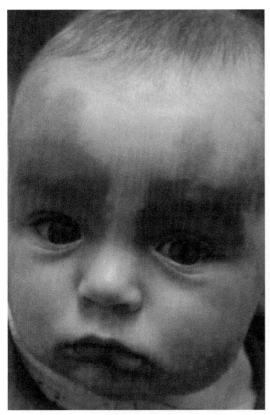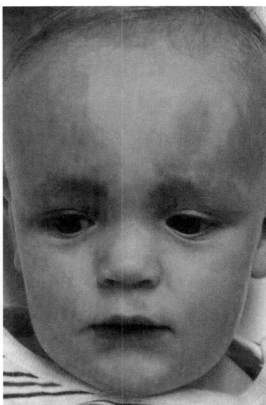

Fig. 12. Preoperative (6 months) and postoperative (1 year old) views of a child with bilateral V1 port-wine stains. There is noticeable lightening of the lesions after completing 3 laser treatments.

(safety glasses). By using a 5-mm hand piece with higher fluences (5–7 J/cm^2 for infants and patients with more sensitive skin, 8–12 J/cm^2 for patients >2 years of age), precise control can be attained at the periphery, whereas a 7-mm hand piece allows for a wider arc of coverage with lower fluences in the central areas. Target the perimeter of the lesion initially to disrupt the border of demarcation between normal and abnormal skin. Apply bacitracin as a dressing at the conclusion of treatment (**Fig. 13**).[10]

Treatment of high-flow lesions such as AVMs requires a multimodality therapeutic approach. Surgical resection is often the end result of management and is most effective with judicious resection and reconstruction using local and expanded tissue rearrangement. Preoperative embolization is highly recommended for complicated and extensive lesions that would otherwise be unsafe or surgically inoperable. The timing of surgical intervention is paramount as earlier intervention may minimize psychological distress and prevent growth of the lesion; however, older children are typically more tolerant of a potentially large operation. The focus surgically should be

minimization of intraoperative hemorrhage via meticulous surgical principles with respect to vessel ligation and dissection. Once resected, the defect should be immediately reconstructed or allowed to heal by secondary intention if indicated (see **Fig. 13**).

SUMMARY

The ideal management strategy of vascular lesions rests on establishing the appropriate diagnosis, which historically was difficult until the advent of an effective classification system. Once the diagnosis has been secured, treatment of the lesion can follow a clear and usually successful algorithm. A multidisciplinary approach is paramount to successful management, and extensive surgical planning should be performed preoperatively if resection is anticipated. A conservative approach for the appropriate lesion has certainly reduced morbidity and optimized aesthetic outcomes. It is the surgeon's responsibility to exhaust all treatment strategies before considering operative management, unless early surgical intervention for established indications is necessary. With early

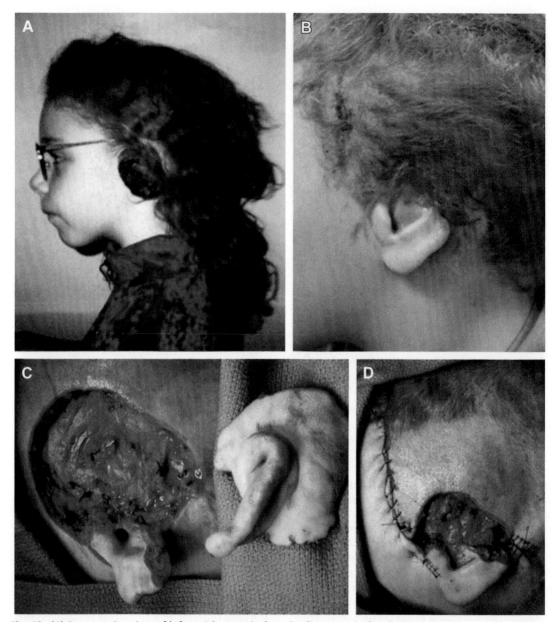

Fig. 13. (*A*) Preoperative view of left auricle AVM before the first round of embolization and surgical resection. (*B*) Postoperative view at 3 months after repeat surgical resection; complete closure of the wound by secondary intention occurred over a 3-week period. (*C*) Resected AVM lying adjacent to the surgical defect. (*D*) Surgical defect after rotation-advancement flap.

involvement of other specialists and the development of a comprehensive plan, safe and effective results can consistently be achieved.

REFERENCES

1. Wassef M, Blei F, Adams D. Vascular anomalies classification: recommendations from the International Society for the Study of Vascular Anomalies. Pediatrics 2015;136:e203–14.

2. Mulliken JB, Glowacki J. Hemangiomas and vascular malformations in infants and children: a classification based on endothelial characteristics. Plast Reconstr Surg 1982;69:412–20.

3. Finn MC, Glowacki J, Mulliken JB. Congenital vascular lesions: clinical application of a new

classification. Journal of Pediatric Surgery 1983;
18(6):894–900.

4. Tekes A, Koshy J, Kalayci TO, et al. S.E. Mitchell
Vascular Anomalies Flow Chart (SEMVAFC): a visual
pathway combining clinical and imaging findings for
classification of soft-tissue vascular anomalies. Clin
Radiol 2014;69:443–57.

5. Batniji RK, Buckingham ED, Williams EF. An
aesthetic approach to facial hemangiomas. Arch
Facial Plast Surg 2005;7:301–6.

6. Williams EF, Hochman M, Rodgers BJ, et al.
A psychological profile of children with hemangiomas and their families. Arch Facial Plast Surg
2003;5:229–34.

7. Dieterich-Miller CA, Cohen BA, Liggett J. Behavioral
adjustment and self-concept of young children with
hemangiomas. Pediatr Dermatol 1992;9:241–5.

8. Drolet BA, Frommelt PC, Chamlin SL, et al. Initiation
and use of propranolol for infantile hemangioma:
report of a consensus conference. Pediatrics 2013;
131:128–40.

9. Foley LS, Kulungowski AM. Vascular anomalies in
pediatrics. Adv Pediatr 2015;62:227–55.

10. Lam SM, Williams EF. Practical considerations in the
treatment of capillary vascular malformations, or
port wine stains. Facial Plast Surg 2004;20:71–6.

11. Lam SM, Dahiya R, Williams EF. Management of an
arteriovenous malformation. Arch Facial Plast Surg
2003;5:334–7.

12. Gurgacz S, Zamora L, Scott NA. Percutaneous
sclerotherapy for vascular malformations: a systemic review. Ann Vasc Surg 2014;28:1335–49.

13. Colletti G, Valassina D, Bertossi D, et al. Contemporary management of vascular malformations. J Oral
Maxillofac Surg 2014;72:510–28.

14. Smith MC, Zimmerman MB, Burke DK, et al. Efficacy
and safety of OK-432 immunotherapy of lymphatic
malformations. Laryngoscope 2009;119:107–15.

Facial Nerve Rehabilitation

Lisa E. Ishii, MD, MHS

KEYWORDS

- Facial palsy • Facial paralysis • Free tissue transfer • Synkinesis

KEY POINTS

- Facial nerve paralysis occurs in the pediatric population from several causes.
- Management goals include eye protection, treatment for nasal obstruction, smile restoration, and treatment of synkinesis.
- Free tissue transfer is the preferred method of smile restoration, with results equivalent to or superior to results of similar methods in adults with facial nerve disorders.

INTRODUCTION

Our face is our window to the world, serving not only as the primary method of identification, but also as our portal for expression of emotion. Disorders of the face, and specifically those impacting facial movement such as facial nerve disorders, can have substantial negative psychosocial impact. In addition to the psychosocial impact, the functional deficits resulting from facial nerve disorders may also be significant, manifesting with incomplete eye closure, drooling, and difficulty eating, to name a few. Consideration for facial nerve rehabilitation specifically in children is of utmost importance as a growing body of literature documents the specific negative impact of facial nerve paralysis on perception by others.[1–3] This is of particular importance for children actively developing their self-esteem, self-confidence, and perceptions of self. Although facial nerve rehabilitation in adults has been extensively described, a considerable body of literature exists to guide in the management of children with facial nerve disorders as well.

Facial nerve disorders are fortunately rare in infants and children, with a calculated incidence of 21.1 in 100,000 described in children younger than age 15 in one prospective study of 106 patients.[4]

Another study in a pediatric population estimated the incidence to be 2.7 per 100,000 under age 10 years, and 10.1 per 100,000 between ages 10 and 20 years.[5] Similar to adults, even in the pediatric population, the most common cause of unilateral facial paralysis remains idiopathic or Bell palsy, accounting for ranges of 40% to 75% of cases.[5]

CAUSES (NOT EXHAUSTIVE)

Congenital
1. Syringobulbia—fluid-filled cavities, or syrinxes, that affect the brainstem. Typically congenital but may be caused by tumor
2. Mobius syndrome—bilateral or unilateral facial paralysis, prevalence reported at 1 in 150,000 live births, affecting cranial nerves (CN) VI and CN VII with other CN variably involved, leads to "blank" faces of affected children
3. Goldenhar-Gorlin syndrome (several craniofacial abnormalities, including hemifacial microsomia, epibulbar dermoid, and microtia)
4. Hemifacial microsomia

Acquired
1. Trauma—surgical or nonsurgical (temporal bone trauma)

The author has nothing to disclose.
Facial Plastic & Reconstructive Surgery, Department of Otolaryngology-Head & Neck Surgery, Johns Hopkins School of Medicine, 601 North Caroline Street, Suite 6231, Baltimore, MD 21287, USA
E-mail address: Learnes2@jhmi.edu

facialplastic.theclinics.com

2. Infection—Ramsey Hunt syndrome, Epstein-Barr virus, Lyme disease, human immunodeficiency virus, cytomegalovirus, adenovirus idiopathic, Bell palsy
3. Neoplasm—schwannomas of CN VII, hemangiomas, parotid tumors

REHABILITATION

Facial nerve rehabilitation is conceptually more challenging in children for unique concerns, including growing anatomy, and requirement for parental consent on behalf of the children. Although facial reanimation procedures are generally deferred until children are at least 5 or 6 years of age, with methods of eye protection incorporated earlier as appropriate, the literature does not support any untoward effects of the procedures on facial growth. Facial rehabilitation aims to restore both resting facial symmetry and symmetry with motion for aesthetic and functional purposes, including emotion, articulation, and eating, to name a few.

EYE PROTECTION

The first issue of paramount concern for special consideration, regardless of age, is eye protection. Methods to achieve corneal coverage in patients with upper division nerve involvement and any possibility of corneal exposure should be used first. This is of even greater significance if the area is not sensate due to other CN involvement (ie, the patient cannot feel irritation). Protection methods for children, similar to adults, include the following:

- Copious lubrication with saline eye drops
- Moisture chamber (possibly as simple as taping a small square of Saran Wrap over the affected eye)
- Eyelid weighting with platinum chain[6]
- Tarsal strip procedures (however, generally speaking, children do not have the laxity that is an issue for many adults)

Of note, Terzis and Karypidis[7] described dynamic blink rehabilitation in pediatric patients and recommended consideration of this technique in patients with severe eye involvement. Improved blink scores were reported. These methods included the following:

- Nerve transfers: cross-face nerve grafting to the affected nerve, minihypoglossal nerve transfers
- Eye sphincter substitution: pedicled frontalis and temporalis muscles, and free platysma and pectoralis minor free flaps

Direct orbicularis oculi muscle neurotization was the superior method, and the indicated method in cases of partial innervation.

Nasal Deviation

- Indicated in cases of severe deviation of the nasal base away from the paralyzed side and external nasal valve collapse
- A fascia lata sling from the lateral thigh is placed in a subcutaneous tunnel on the paralyzed side running from a preauricular incision to an incision in the alar crease.
- The sling is adjusted until appropriate position is achieved and the lateral sling is secured to the temporalis.
- Lindsay and colleagues[8] demonstrated improvement in disease-specific quality of life in a series of adults who underwent this procedure. It is reasonable to expect similar improvements would be demonstrated in the pediatric population.

Smile Restoration

As noted, the psychosocial ramifications of facial nerve disorders are substantial, and of particular significance as related to the asymmetric smile.[1–3] For pediatric patients, particular attention and optimal methods should be used for smile restoration. Both static and dynamic methods have been described as achieving good results, but dynamic methods, despite the additional challenges of execution, are clearly preferred. Multiple studies demonstrated the success of free muscle transfer in children and found it to be superior to that in adults with regards to smile excursion and flap failure, without any morbidity related to active growth.[9–11]

Temporalis regional dynamic flaps

- Leboulanger and colleagues[12] evaluated a series of temporalis flaps for children with congenital facial paralysis and reported 80% achieved adequate smile excursion.
- Advantages include single-stage, low-morbidity procedure with immediate results.
- Disadvantages include lack of spontaneous smile, muscle bulk in midface, and depression in temporal fossa.

Free muscle transfer dynamic flaps

- The first-line treatment for pediatric patients with facial palsy
- Described with gracilis, pectoralis minor, and latissimus dorsi muscles

- Goal is spontaneous smile with a procedure with low morbidity and high reliability
- Two-stage procedure ideal in patients with an intact contralateral facial nerve. The first stage is coaptation of cross-face nerve (typically sural nerve) tunneled through upper lip to intact facial nerve branches on uninvolved side; after 6 to 12 months, the second stage is performed with muscle harvest (in children, gracilis is ideal) and placement on the paralyzed side.
- Single-stage procedure described for patients who failed the 2-stage procedure, or those without an intact facial nerve or an at-risk facial nerve (neurofibromatosis). The transferred muscle is powered by the masseteric nerve. Advantage to single stage is single neurorrhaphy, quicker results. Disadvantage is lack of spontaneous smile.
- In their series of 48 patients with Möbius and Möbius-like syndromes, of the 20 patients for whom gracilis-free transfer was performed, there was no flap loss, and symmetry with facial smiling was noted in 87% of patients.[13]
- Free tissue transfer for facial reanimation in the pediatric population is generally a low-morbidity procedure, with the most common complication being hematoma; bedside evacuation is the standard treatment for hematoma. Flap failure from vascular insufficiency is uncommon.

Synkinesis

- Involuntary muscle movements that accompany voluntary muscle contraction and occur as a result of aberrant axonal regeneration
- Nonsurgical treatments include botulinum toxin injections to paralyze the muscles contracting involuntarily and physical therapy also to decrease involuntary activity
- Terzis and Karypidis[14] described surgical methods to break the synkinesis cycle; cross-face nerve grafting to the affected facial nerve branches was performed to overcome the inappropriate neural firing; this surgical method combined with biofeedback and botulinum toxin injections was effective for restoring facial function and symmetry.

REFERENCES

1. Ishii L, Dey J, Boahene KD, et al. The social distraction of facial paralysis: objective measurement of social attention using eye-tracking. Laryngoscope 2016;126(2):334–9.
2. Ishii L, Godoy A, Encarnacion CO, et al. Not just another face in the crowd: society's perceptions of facial paralysis. Laryngoscope 2012;122(3):533–8.
3. Ishii LE, Godoy A, Encarnacion CO, et al. What faces reveal: impaired affect display in facial paralysis. Laryngoscope 2011;121(6):1138–43.
4. Jenke AC, Stoek LM, Zilbauer M, et al. Facial palsy: etiology, outcome and management in children. Eur J Paediatr Neurol 2011;15(3):209–13.
5. Katusic SK, Beard CM, Wiederholt WC, et al. Incidence, clinical features, and prognosis in Bell's palsy, Rochester, Minnesota, 1968-1982. Ann Neurol 1986;20(5):622–7.
6. Silver AL, Lindsay RW, Cheney ML, et al. Thin-profile platinum eyelid weighting: a superior option in the paralyzed eye. Plast Reconstr Surg 2009;123(6):1697–703.
7. Terzis JK, Karypidis D. The outcomes of dynamic procedures for blink restoration in pediatric facial paralysis. Plast Reconstr Surg 2010;125(2):629–44.
8. Lindsay RW, Bhama P, Hohman M, et al. Prospective evaluation of quality-of-life improvement after correction of the alar base in the flaccidly paralyzed face. JAMA Facial Plast Surg 2015;17(2):108–12.
9. Hadlock TA, Malo JS, Cheney ML, et al. Free gracilis transfer for smile in children: the Massachusetts Eye and Ear Infirmary Experience in excursion and quality-of-life changes. Arch Facial Plast Surg 2011;13(3):190–4.
10. Terzis JK, Konofaos P. Reanimation of facial palsy following tumor extirpation in pediatric patients: our experience with 16 patients. J Plast Reconstr Aesthet Surg 2013;66(9):1219–29.
11. Terzis JK, Olivares FS. Long-term outcomes of free-muscle transfer for smile restoration in adults. Plast Reconstr Surg 2009;123(3):877–88.
12. Leboulanger N, Maldent JB, Glynn F, et al. Rehabilitation of congenital facial palsy with temporalis flap–case series and literature review. Int J Pediatr Otorhinolaryngol 2012;76(8):1205–10.
13. Bianchi B, Copelli C, Ferrari S, et al. Facial animation in patients with Moebius and Moebius-like syndromes. Int J Oral Maxillofac Surg 2010;39(11):1066–73.
14. Terzis JK, Karypidis D. Therapeutic strategies in post-facial paralysis synkinesis in pediatric patients. J Plast Reconstr Aesthet Surg 2012;65(8):1009–18.

Microtia Reconstruction

Randall A. Bly, MD[a], Amit D. Bhrany, MD[b], Craig S. Murakami, MD[c],
Kathleen C.Y. Sie, MD[d],*

KEYWORDS

- Microtia • Auricular reconstruction • Cartilage graft • Autologous reconstruction
- Alloplastic reconstruction • Microtia management

KEY POINTS

- Children with outer ear anomalies should have diagnostic audiological assessment.
- Management of hearing should be considered when developing a plan for auricular reconstruction because it may impact the timing and order of procedure(s) because atresia is present in 75% of microtia.
- Options for management of microtia include observation, prosthetic management, and reconstruction.
- Reconstruction options include staged autologous costal cartilage reconstruction and single-stage reconstruction with alloplastic framework.
- Families should be educated on all treatment options in terms of both hearing rehabilitation and reconstruction options.

INTRODUCTION

Microtia, or small or malformed ear, occurs with an incidence of 1 to 10 per 10,000 births.[1–3] Although associated with many syndromes, it occurs in isolation and unilaterally in most cases. The right side is more commonly affected, and boys have a 30% higher affected rate than girls. Ethnic groups with the highest incidence include Andeans, Native Americans, Asians, and Hispanics.[4,5] Aural atresia is found with microtia in 75% of cases.[6]

Embryologically, the external ear begins to form at 6 weeks from tissue derived from first and second branchial arches. The 6 hillocks of His become the tragus, helix, concha cymba, antihelix, and antitragus. A meatal plug expands and forms the tympanic membrane by 13 weeks. At 18 weeks, the meatus is fully formed, as are all parts of the external ear.

In addition to ethnicity and male sex, risk factors for microtia include low birth weight and acute maternal illness.[7] In utero exposure to teratogens such has thalidomide and retinoids are strongly associated with microtia.[8] Higher levels of folate ingestion during pregnancy have been found to reduce the incidence of microtia. The precise mechanism for the development of microtia is a topic of ongoing research.

The microtia phenotype appears in a spectrum of disorders of which the most common include craniofacial microsomia, Goldenhar, and Treacher Collins.[9] Multiple other syndromes or genetic causes have been identified and are associated with microtia in less than 50% of cases (**Box 1**). Although the contralateral ear appears normal

Disclosure Statement: The authors have nothing to disclose.

[a] Pediatric Otolaryngology, Seattle Children's Hospital, University of Washington, 4800 Sand Point Way NE, Seattle, WA 98105, USA; [b] Department of Otolaryngology-Head and Neck Surgery, University of Washington, 1959 Pacific Avenue NE, Seattle, WA 98195, USA; [c] Division of Otolaryngology Head and Neck Surgery, Virginia Mason Medical Center, University of Washington, 1201 Terry Avenue, Seattle, WA 98101, USA; [d] Childhood Communication Center, Richard and Francine Loeb Endowed Chair in Childhood Communication Research, Seattle Children's Hospital, University of Washington, 4800 Sand Point Way NE, Seattle, WA 98105, USA
* Corresponding author. Seattle Children's Hospital, OA.9.220, 4800 Sand Point Way Northeast, Seattle, WA 98105.
E-mail address: kathleen.sie@seattlechildrens.org

Box 1
Syndromes or disorders associated with microtia

Auriculo-condylar

Bixler (hypertelorism-microtia-clefting)

Bosley-Salih-Alorainy

Branchio-oculo-facial

Branchio-oto-renal/branchio-otic

CHARGE

Fraser

Kabuki

Klippel-Feil

Labyrinthine aplasia

Meier-Gorlin

Miller

Nager

Oculo-auricular

Pallister-Hall

Townes-Brocks

Treacher Collins

Wildervanck (cervico-oculo-acoustic)

Data from Luquetti DV, Heike CL, Hing AV, et al. Microtia: epidemiology and genetics. Am J Med Genet A 2012;158A:124–39; and Bartel-Friedrich S. Congenital auricular malformations: description of anomalies and syndromes. Facial Plast Surg 2015;31(6):567–80.

---

size in most cases, detailed measurement reveals that it is actually smaller than a normal control group.[10] There may be other abnormalities that have not fully been evaluated or discovered in their association with microtia. For example, a recent study found high correlations with chest wall deformities when detailed analysis of thoracic imaging was performed.[11]

DIAGNOSIS AND EVALUATION

Patients with microtia and malformed ears are diagnosed at birth and should undergo audiological testing. Microtic ears should be carefully examined for the presence of an ear canal. Newborn hearing screen should be performed in all ears with a patent ear canal. Over the long term, even if unilateral microtia is present, an otolaryngologist and audiologist should maintain regular clinical encounters because the contralateral ear is at higher risk for abnormalities than the general population.[12,13]

If bilateral atresia is present, diagnostic brainstem auditory-evoked responses should be performed. Amplification and enrollment in early

intervention should be initiated, ideally within the first few months of life. On examination, it is important to accurately describe the malformed ear. **Fig. 1** shows normal external auricle anatomy.

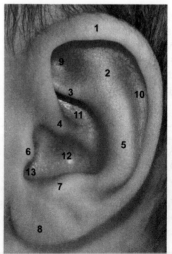

1- Helix
2- Superior Crus
3- Inferior Crus
4- Helical Root
5- Antihelix
6- Tragus
7- Antitragus
8- Lobile
9- Triangular Fossa
10- Scaphoid Fossa
11- Concha Cymba
12- Concha Cavum
13- Intertragal Notch

Fig. 1. Normal anatomic landmarks of external auricle.

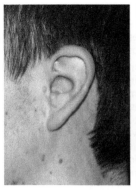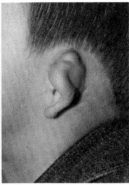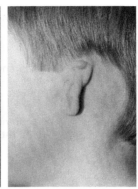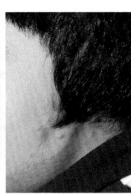

Fig. 2. Class I, II, III, IV microtia.

Table 1
HEAR MAPS classification incorporating multiple grading scales

Hear	Air-bone gap (dB HL)
Ear	Microtia grade 1–4
Atresia	Jahrsdoerfer CT scale (1–10)
Remnant earlobe	Grade 1–4
Mandible asymmetry	Grade 1–4
Asymmetry soft tissue	Grade 1–4
Paresis of the facial nerve	House-Brackmann scale (1–6)
Syndrome	(Yes/No)

Table 2
Hearing rehabilitation options in unilateral aural atresia

Approach	Advantages	Disadvantages
Observation	Minimize risk	Unilateral hearing loss
Band-retained bone conduction sound processor	No surgery	Cosmesis Device required Comfort
Osseointegrated implant-retained bone conduction sound processor	Simple surgery Predictable Excellent hearing result Magnetic option available	Cosmesis Device required Must be at least 5 years old Soft tissue issues (nonmagnetic)
Atresiaplasty	Cosmesis Accommodation of ear level hearing aid if necessary No device	Complex surgery Less predictable result Modest hearing benefit Ongoing care required

Table 3
Microtia management options

Type	Details	Advantages	Disadvantages
Observation		No risk	Cosmesis Psychosocial issues
Prosthetic	Adhesive retained	Appearance	Insecure Ongoing prosthetic care Daily maintenance Use restrictions
	Implant retained	Appearance Secure retention	Multiple procedures Removal of remnant and soft tissue Ongoing prosthetic care Daily maintenance Use restrictions
Reconstruction	Costal cartilage (autologous)	Autologous tissue Minimal maintenance Becomes sensate Atresia repair	Appearance Donor sites Multiple surgeries
	Alloplastic	Less donor site morbidity Less variability in carving Appearance Single surgery	Foreign body More challenging to do atresia repair

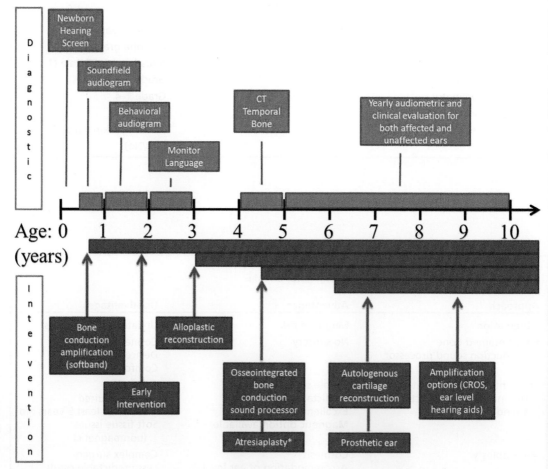

Fig. 3. Timeline of diagnostic and treatment interventions for microtia and atresia. Diagnostic studies are shown in blue and interventions in red. CROS, contralateral routing of signal. * Atresiaplasty is considered if patient has favorable findings on high resolution computed tomography of the temporal bones.

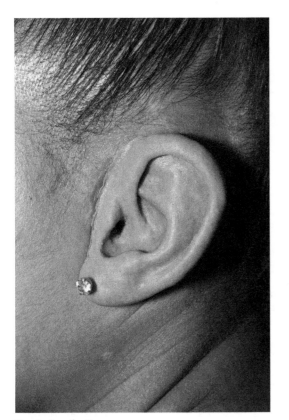

Fig. 4. Prosthetic ear.

Multiple classification schemes are used to describe the degree of microtia.[14–19] **Fig. 2** displays 4 classes of microtia as proposed by Marx and modified by Rogers. In grade I, the ear is small or abnormal, but all landmarks are discernible. In grade II, some of the landmarks are identifiable. Grade III has very small external auricle components, often only a skin tag. Grade IV is anotia. Nagata[20] proposed a classification scheme of

descriptive terms, including lobule-type, concha-type, and small concha-type. In lobule type, there is a remnant of the lobule and auricle with no canal, concha, nor tragus. Concha-type has variable presence of the lobule and tragus. Small concha-type has a small indentation of the concha and remnant of lobule and auricle. He also used anotia and atypical in the scheme, in which the ear did not fit into the above types.

Other classification schemes to summarize the craniofacial anomalies associated with microtia have been described. OMENS is a classification system for hemifacial microsomia proposed by Mulliken that examines variables of orbital, mandibular, ear, neural, and soft tissue phenotypes.[21] Research using OMENS has found that 67% of patients with hemifacial microsomia have extracraniofacial anomalies and 26% have cardiac anomalies, which has modified the classification scheme to OMENS-Plus if an extracraniofacial anomaly is present.[22] Recently, a classification scheme called HEAR MAPS that incorporates multiple other staging systems was proposed to improve communication among the multiple disciplines of providers (**Table 1**).[23]

INDICATIONS AND COUNSELING

Indications for microtia management should be based on a discussion with the patient and patient's family. There is an overall increased rate of depression and anxiety in microtia patients compared with a control cohort.[24,25] Studies have shown reduced psychological stressors after undergoing microtia reconstruction and overall patient satisfaction.[26–28] Furthermore, a reconstructed auricle will permit retention of a hearing aid or glasses.

Most microtia patients also have aural atresia, and the management of the conductive hearing loss has implications on microtia reconstruction. All options, both for hearing rehabilitation and

Table 4 Microtia reconstruction technique summary using autologous cartilage		
	3 Stage (Brent)	**2 Stage (Nagata)**
Surgical stages	1. Framework 2. Lobule transposition 3. Elevation	1. Framework/lobule transfer 2. Elevation
Advantages	Possibly better for lobule-type microtia	2 Stages Better for conchal bowl-type microtia Stacked framework
Disadvantages	3 stages	First stage more complex Stacked framework

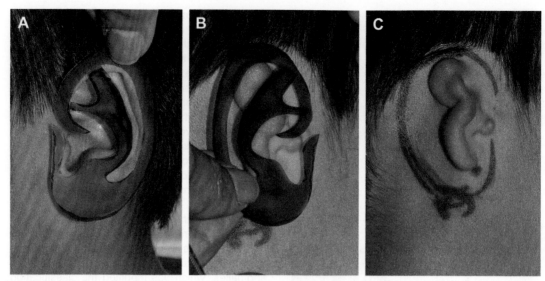

Fig. 5. (*A*) Template of normal left ear made from radiograph film. (*B*) Template placed over right microtic ear and (*C*) used to help position incisions for graft placement.

for auricular reconstruction, should be thoroughly discussed with the patient and family. It is important for the surgeon and the family to generate a cohesive plan that includes management of the ear and hearing. The hearing management options are summarized in **Table 2**, and the microtia management options are summarized in **Table 3**.

From a surgical planning perspective, one of the main decision points is atresiaplasty candidacy, which is based on high-resolution computed tomography (CT) of the temporal bones typically done around age 4 years. Obtaining the CT scan at about 4 years of age obviates sedation, allows for mastoid growth, and may mitigate the potential effects of radiation on the developing brain. This timing also allows for the

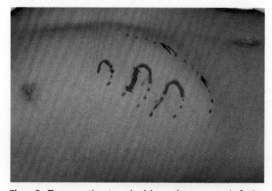

Fig. 6. Two-centimeter incision drawn at inferior aspect of superior limb of synchondrosis to be harvested.

CT scan to screen for occult congenital cholesteatoma. Traditionally, autologous costochondral microtia reconstruction was performed before atresiaplasty. More recently, multiple surgeons have reported atresiaplasty before or simultaneous with microtia reconstruction with good outcomes.[29]

The only surgical reconstruction option for many years used autologous costochondral cartilage, and surgeons preferred to wait until the patient was at least 6 years of age for multiple reasons: (1) the contralateral ear is near full size, (2) the costochondral cartilage is of adequate size, and (3) the patient is able to understand the reconstructive options.[30] The last point could be considered a disadvantage in that families may prefer to undergo the reconstruction as soon as possible and before school begins. The introduction of alloplastic reconstruction options has modified the timeline for decisions with the patient's families because reconstruction as young as age 3 is now possible (**Fig. 3**).

In addition to the alloplastic reconstruction technique, other technologies are also changing options available to families. Prosthetic ears are now more affordable and potentially easier to fabricate with the aid of 3-dimensional printing. In the past, molding and creating the prosthesis required significant cooperation from the patient and typically was not done until after age 6 (**Fig. 4**). The technology for bone conduction amplification is rapidly advancing, and the magnetic sound processor (eg, BahaAttract; Cochlear, Sydney, Australia) does not require an abutment to protrude through the skin, reducing the risk of skin and soft tissue issues. It is important for family counseling to understand all options and stay current as new devices become available. Patients are encouraged to review photographs of patients who have undergone various reconstruction techniques to aid in their decision; this also serves to set appropriate expectations.

SURGICAL TECHNIQUE
Autologous Cartilage Reconstruction

The surgical technique described is a modification of the 2-stage technique described by Nagata (**Table 4**). The authors have also incorporated techniques described by Siegert and colleagues[31] and Firmin and Marchac.[32]

Stage I
The procedure is done under general anesthesia and with the table rotated 180°. Two surgical teams increase efficiency as one team can harvest the cartilage while the other team prepares the recipient site. A template of the unaffected ear is created on radiographic film or face shield plastic (**Fig. 5**). A horizontal 2-cm incision is designed over the contralateral costochondral synchondrosis of ribs 6, 7, and 8 (**Fig. 6**). Local anesthetic is infiltrated. The face and both ears are included in the operative field.

A 2-cm incision is made over the anterior aspect of rudimentary ear lobe, and the existing cartilage is removed. A skin flap of approximately 6 × 6 cm is created and thinned to accommodate the cartilage framework. The lobule is transferred using a

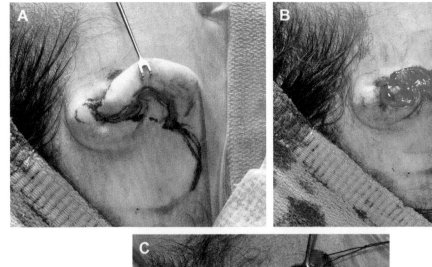
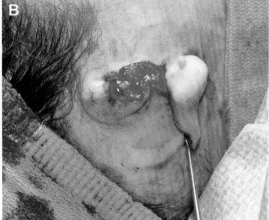
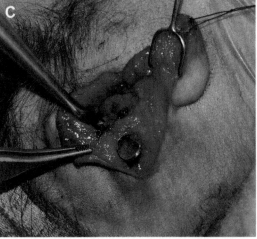

Fig. 7. (*A*) Incision made along microtic ear lobule and then onto postauricular scalp to permit microtic remnant removal and lobule transposition. (*B*) Lobule transposed into desired position. (*C*) Mastoid pocket elevated with maintenance of subcutaneous pedicle to superior flap (superficial to retractor).

z-plasty technique. With the Nagata technique, a 1-cm vascularized pedicle is also maintained (**Fig. 7**).

Rib harvest After incision, the rectus muscle is divided widely (with extension past the skin incision medially and laterally) with needle tip cautery. The medial aspect of the free floating rib is identified and grasped with an Allis clamp (**Fig. 8**A). A Cottle elevator is used to dissect and isolate the cartilage, which is divided in a beveled fashion (avoiding sharp or protuberant edges) near the bone-cartilaginous junction. The perichondrium overlying the synchondrosis of ribs 6, 7, and 8 is sharply divided. The deep perichondrium is preserved to minimize risk of pleural violation. The limbs of the synchondrosis are divided at the bony cartilaginous junctions in a beveled fashion, and they are elevated from lateral to medial with perichondrial elevators (see **Fig. 8**). The body of

the synchondrosis is dissected and divided as superiorly as possible to maximize the size of the synchondrosis removed. The wound is irrigated and observed with Valsalva maneuvers up to a pressure of 40 cm of water to check for air leak. The rectus muscle is closed with horizontal mattress sutures. The superficial chest wound is closed after framework carving so that excess cartilage can be banked for use at the second stage. The excess cartilage is placed superficial to the rectus muscle. Then, Scarpa fascia, deep dermal, and skin layers are closed without drain placement.

Framework carving A number 15 blade and 2- and 4-mm skin biopsy punches are used for carving. The inferior and superior crura of the triangular fossa and the antihelical fold are accentuated by a y-shaped cartilage placed on the lateral surface of the framework. The scaphoid fossa is defined

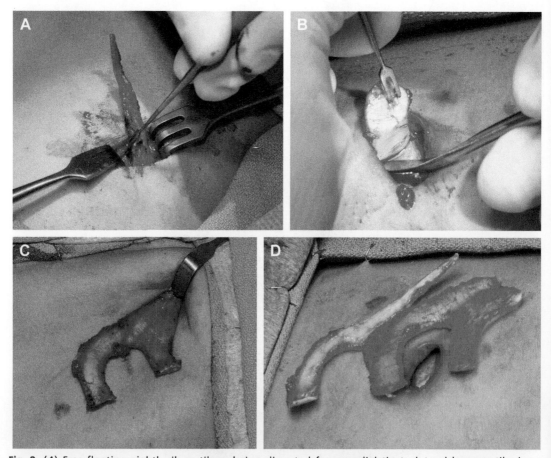

Fig. 8. (*A*) Free-floating eighth rib cartilage being dissected from medial tip to lateral bony-cartilaginous junction. (*B*) Inferior limb being dissected from lateral to medial using hook for retraction. (*C*) Entire synchondrosis harvested before final superior limb cut. (*D*) Eighth free floating ribs and synchondrosis completely harvested.

by deepening the groove, and 2-mm holes are placed to allow for a single drain to be placed deep to the framework. Another piece of cartilage is used to create the antitragus, incisura, and tragus. The free floater segment is thinned and formed into the helical rim. The 4 pieces of cartilage are sutured using horizontal mattress clear nylon sutures to create the framework (**Fig. 9**).

The framework is inserted into the soft tissue envelope, ensuring adequate position based on symmetry. The wound is closed over a single suction drain (**Fig. 10**). A xeroform bolster is carefully sutured over the skin and into the concavities of the reconstructed ear (**Fig. 11**). Postoperatively, the drain remains to continuous wall suction for 2 days. The patient wears a Glasscock dressing until seen in clinic in 1 to 2 weeks when the bolster is removed.

Stage II

The second-stage operation is typically done as an outpatient. An incision is made around the framework, and the ear is elevated (**Fig. 12**). The position of the lobule and any irregularities of soft tissue overlying the framework can be adjusted as needed during this stage. The banked cartilage from the chest is retrieved to create a wedge. The wedge is secured to the posterior aspect of the elevated framework and covered with an anteriorly based soft tissue flap. A postauricular scalp flap is advanced to cover most of the mastoid cortex. Advancement of the scalp will result in a standing cone in the hairline. The position of the standing cone will determine the angle of the ear. A towel clip is placed to define the standing cone (see **Fig. 12**). A deep 3-0 polydioxanone suture is placed, as a double horizontal mattress to remove

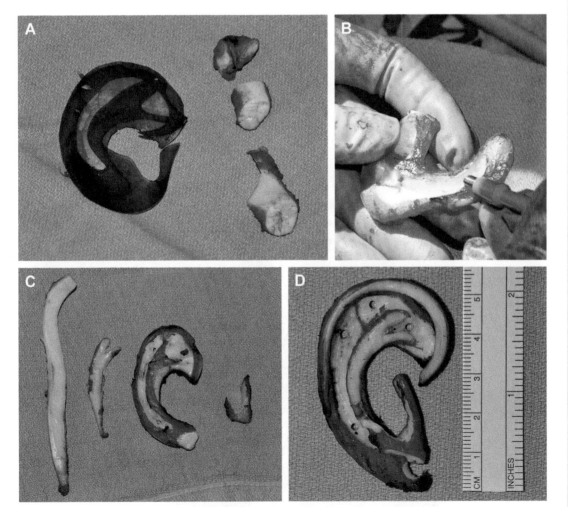

Fig. 9. (*A*) Template used to guide carving of auricular framework from rib synchondrosis with excess pieces removed. (*B*) Framework carved with 15 blade and skin biopsy punches. (*C*) Rib cartilage pieces shown separately: helical rim, antihelix projection, base framework, and antitragus-tragus complex. (*D*) Framework constructed.

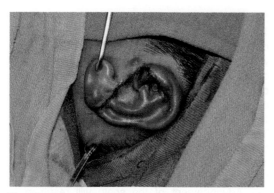

Fig. 10. Completion of stage 1 autologous reconstruction (note that the tragus is native).

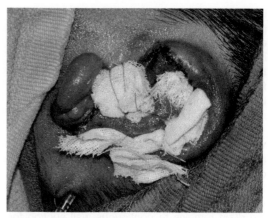

Fig. 11. Bolster in place after completion of stage 1 autologous reconstruction.

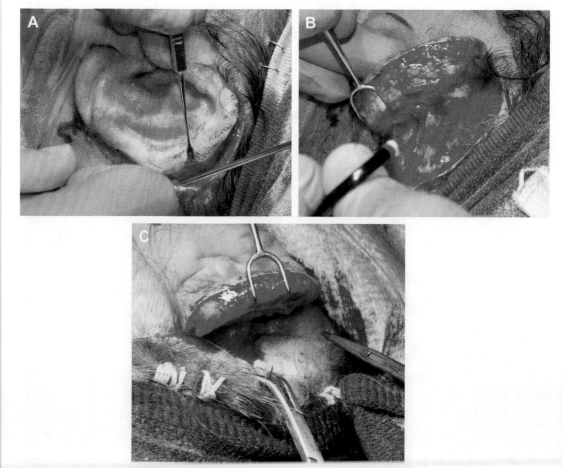

Fig. 12. (*A*) Incision made around framework. (*B*) Auricular framework elevated exposing postauricular surface of framework to be grafted and mastoid cortex. (*C*) Postauricular scalp flap advanced with towel clip in place.

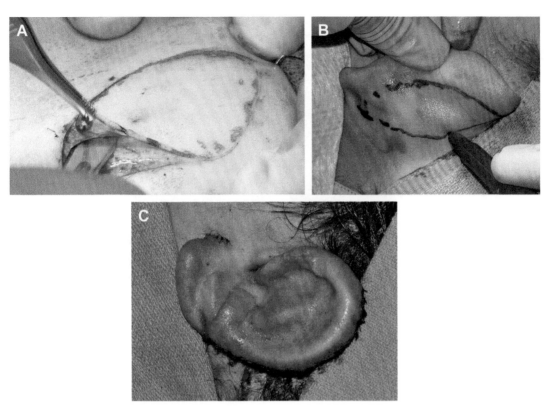

Fig. 13. (*A*) Elliptical skin graft designed on upper thigh and harvested with number 20 blade. (*B*) Additional postauricular skin graft harvested from contralateral ear. (*C*) Ear elevated after scalp flap advancement and placement of skin grafts.

any tension, and the towel clip is removed. The standing cone is excised, and the triangle of skin is thinned to create a small hair-free skin graft that will be used to cover the mastoid aspect of the neosulcus. The incision created by excision of the standing cone is closed with deep interrupted 4-0 polydiaxanone sutures. The skin edges are approximated with a running locked 5-0 chromic gut suture.

A full-thickness skin graft (typically 9 cm × 4 cm) is harvested as an ellipse from the groin to serve as the postauricular sulcus skin (**Fig. 13**A). If contralateral otoplasty is indicated, then full-thickness skin graft can also be harvested from the

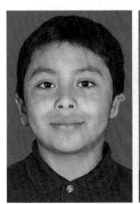
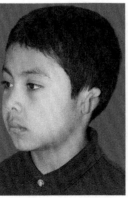
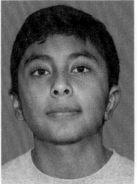
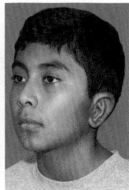

Fig. 14. Preoperative and postoperative photographs of left microtia and autologous cartilage reconstruction.

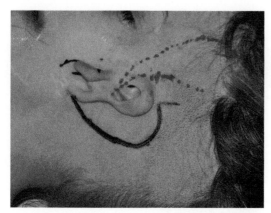

Fig. 15. Preoperative marking for superficial temporal artery in preparation for harvest of TPF flap (*red*) and "c"-shaped incision (*black*).

contralateral postauricular area (**Fig. 13**B). The skin graft is sutured in place; a bolster is applied, and a Glasscock dressing is used in the postoperative period. The donor sites are closed primarily, and the bolster is removed after 1 to 2 weeks.

Fig. 14 shows preoperative and postoperative photographs of left microtia and autologous cartilage reconstruction after stage I and II are completed.

Alloplastic Reconstruction

Reinisch[33] has pioneered alloplastic microtia reconstruction using a temporoparietal fascial (TPF) flap, which significantly reduced the rate of implant exposure.[34,35] The procedure is done as a single stage under general anesthesia. Surgical planning includes radiograph

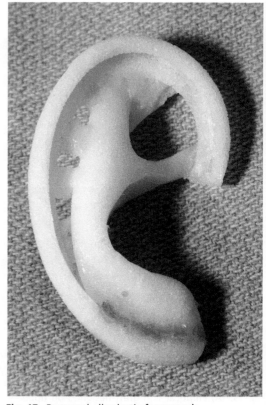

Fig. 17. Prepared alloplastic framework.

film tracing of the contralateral ear for template purposes, positioning of ear, and measuring TPF flap dimensions (13 cm in height and approximately 10 cm wide). A "c"-shaped 6-cm incision is made posterior to planned position of alloplastic implant (**Fig. 15**). The lobule is preserved. Rudimentary cartilage is removed,

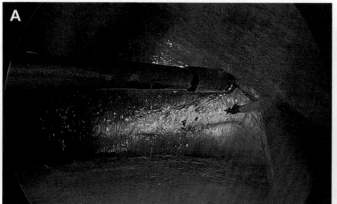

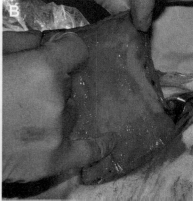

Fig. 16. (*A*) Endoscopic view of TPF harvest, distal TPF flap dissected away from subcutaneous tissue using extended length needle tip cautery. (*B*) TPF flap elevated.

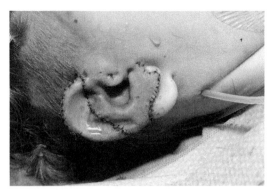

Fig. 18. Alloplastic framework in place with skin graft.

and overlying skin is thinned. A TPF flap is elevated using needle tip cautery. A headlight, lighted retractors, endoscopes, and extended length cautery tips can be used to facilitate distal flap dissection through a relatively small incision (**Fig. 16**). The superficial temporal artery pedicle is identified and preserved. The deep layer of the flap is defined, and it is divided superiorly, anteriorly, and posteriorly. The temporal branch of the facial nerve (often termed "frontal branch") is identified and preserved deep to the TPF at Pitanguy line (0.5 cm inferior from tragus to 1.5 cm superolateral from lateral eyebrow).[36] The high-density porous polyethylene implant is assembled and adjusted to achieve symmetry with the contralateral ear (**Fig. 17**). This is done using a battery-operated handheld high temperature cautery unit that works to apply heat and melt the components of the implant together. A smoke evacuator

should be used. Ear projection is defined by removing material on the medial portion of the implant. The TPF flap is draped over the implant. The position and rotation of the ear are defined. Two temporary suction drains are placed in the scalp and deep to the TPF flap. Skin grafts are obtained from groin or contralateral postauricular sites for skin coverage over the TPF flap (**Fig. 18**). A silicone mold is applied over the implant to maintain soft tissue contour, and the suction drains are removed in the operative room. A soft dressing is applied.

Fig. 19 shows preoperative and postoperative photographs of alloplastic (Medpor; Stryker, Kalamazoo, MI, USA) reconstruction.

COMPLICATIONS

In cartilage reconstruction, the most common complications include cartilage exposure and associated local infection. This can often be treated with topical wound care and antibiotics. A local flap may be needed for coverage. There is also malposition, low-lying hair, cartilage resorption, delayed framework fractures, and framework disarticulations.

Alloplastic reconstruction has seen a dramatic reduction in complications in recent years. Comparing newer techniques with initial attempts, Reinisch reports reductions in implant fracture (28% to <9%) and implant exposure (44% to <5%).

SUMMARY

Surgeons should consider management of hearing and counsel families about reconstructive options. Techniques for microtia reconstruction

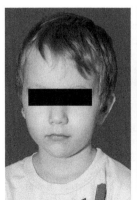
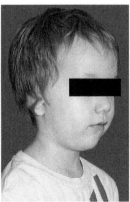
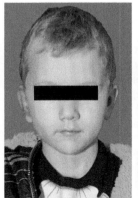
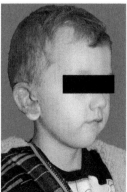

Fig. 19. Preoperative and postoperative photographs of right microtia with alloplastic reconstruction.

using both autologous costochondral frameworks and alloplastic implants have improved over the past 20 years. Surgeons undertaking the challenge of microtia reconstruction must constantly work on improving outcomes for these patients.

ACKNOWLEDGMENTS

The authors thank Eden Palmer for her contribution in figure preparation.

REFERENCES

1. Luquetti DV, Leoncini E, Mastroiacovo P. Microtia-anotia: a global review of prevalence rates. Birth Defects Res A Clin Mol Teratol 2011;91(9):813–22.
2. Luquetti DV, Heike CL, Hing AV, et al. Microtia: epidemiology and genetics. Am J Med Genet A 2012;158A(1):124–39.
3. Mastroiacovo P, Corchia C, Botto LD, et al. Epidemiology and genetics of microtia-anotia: a registry based study on over one million births. J Med Genet 1995;32(6):453–7.
4. Harris J, Källén B, Robert E. The epidemiology of anotia and microtia. J Med Genet 1996;33(10):809–13.
5. Castilla EE, Orioli IM. Prevalence rates of microtia in South America. Int J Epidemiol 1986;15:364–8.
6. van Nunen DP, Kolodzynski MN, van den Boogaard MJ, et al. Microtia in the Netherlands: clinical characteristics and associated anomalies. Int J Pediatr Otorhinolaryngol 2014;78(6):954–9.
7. Orioli IM, Castilla EE. Epidemiological assessment of misoprostol teratogenicity. BJOG 2000;107:519–23.
8. Anderka MT, Lin AE, Abuelo DN, et al. Reviewing the evidence for mycophenolate mofetil as a new teratogen: case report and review of the literature. Am J Med Genet A 2009;149A:1241–8.
9. Shaw GM, Carmichael SL, Kaidarova Z, et al. Epidemiologic characteristics of anotia and microtia in California 1989–1997. Birth Defects Res A Clin Mol Teratol 2004;70:472–5.
10. Matsuka K, Hata Y, Yano K, et al. Comparative study of auricular dimensions for the normal auricles of microtia patients, their parents, and normal individuals. Ann Plast Surg 1994;32(2):135–40.
11. Wu R, Jiang H, Chen W, et al. Three-dimensional chest computed tomography analysis of thoracic deformities in patients with microtia. J Plast Reconstr Aesthet Surg 2015;68(4):498–504.
12. Billings KR, Qureshi H, Gouveia C, et al. Management of hearing loss and the normal ear in cases of unilateral microtia with aural atresia. Laryngoscope 2015;126(6):1470–4.
13. Lipan MJ, Eshraghi AA. Otologic and audiology aspects of microtia repair. Semin Plast Surg 2011;25(4):273–8.
14. Hunter A, Frias JL, Gillessen-Kaesbach G, et al. Elements of morphology: standard terminology for the ear. Am J Med Genet A 2009;149A(1):40–60.
15. Tanzer RC. Microtia. Clin Plast Surg 1978;5(3):317–36.
16. Weerda H. Classification of congenital deformities of the auricle. Facial Plast Surg 1988;5(5):385–8.
17. Microtia NS. Auricular reconstruction. In: Achauer B, Erikkson E, editors. Plastic surgery: indications, operations, outcomes, vol. 2. St Louis (MO): Mosby; 2000. p. 1023–55.
18. Anatomy RB. Embryology, and classification of auricular deformities. In: Tanzer R, Edgerton M, editors. Symposium on reconstruction of the auricle, vol. 10. St Louis (MO): CV Mosby; 1974. p. 3–11.
19. Marx H. Die Missbildungen des ohres. In: Denker A, Kahler O, editors. Handbuch der spez path anatomie histologie. Berlin: Springer; 1926. p. 131.
20. Nagata S. Total auricular reconstruction with a three-dimensional costal cartilage framework Annales de Chirugerie Plastique et Esthetique 1995;40(3):371–99.
21. Vento AR, LaBrie RA, Mulliken JB. The OMENS classification of hemifacial microsomia. Cleft Palate Craniofac J 1991;28:68–77.
22. Horgan JE, Padwa BL, LaBrie RA, et al. OMENS-Plus: analysis of craniofacial and extracraniofacial anomalies in hemifacial microsomia. Cleft Palate Craniofac J 1995;32(5):405–12.
23. Roberson JB Jr, Goldsztein H, Balaker A, et al. HEAR MAPS a classification for congenital microtia/atresia based on the evaluation of 742 patients. Int J Pediatr Otorhinolaryngol 2013;77(9):1551–4.
24. Li D, Chin W, Wu J, et al. Psychosocial outcomes among microtia patients of different ages and genders before ear reconstruction. Aesthetic Plast Surg 2010;34(5):570–6.
25. Jiamei D, Jiake C, Hongxing Z, et al. An investigation of psychological profiles and risk factors in congenital microtia patients. J Plast Reconstr Aesthet Surg 2008;61(Suppl 1):S37–43.
26. Johns AL, Lucash RE, Im DD, et al. Pre and postoperative psychological functioning in younger and older children with microtia. J Plast Reconstr Aesthet Surg 2015;68(4):492–7.
27. Steffen A, Wollenberg B, König IR, et al. A prospective evaluation of psychosocial outcomes following ear reconstruction with rib cartilage in microtia. J Plast Reconstr Aesthet Surg 2010;63(9):1466–73.
28. Brent B. Auricular repair with autogenous rib cartilage grafts: two decades of experience with 600 cases. Plast Reconstr Surg 1992;90(3):355–74 [discussion: 375–6].

29. Roberson JB Jr, Reinisch J, Colen TY, et al. Atresia repair before microtia reconstruction: comparison of early with standard surgical timing. Otol Neurotol 2009;30(6):771–6.

30. Im DD, Paskhover B, Staffenberg DA, et al. Current management of microtia: a national survey. Aesthetic Plast Surg 2013;37(2):402–8.

31. Siegert R, Weerda H, Magritz R. Basic techniques in autogenous microtia repair. Facial Plast Surg 2009; 25(3):149–57.

32. Firmin F, Marchac A. A novel algorithm for autologous ear reconstruction. Semin Plast Surg 2011; 25(4):257–64.

33. Reinisch J. Ear reconstruction in young children. Facial Plast Surg 2015;31(6):600–3.

34. Reinisch JF, Lewin S. Ear reconstruction using a porous polyethylene framework and temporoparietal fascia flap. Facial Plast Surg 2009;25(3): 181–9.

35. Baluch N, Nagata S, Park C, et al. Auricular reconstruction for microtia: a review of available methods. Plast Surg (Oakv) 2014;22(1):39–43.

36. Pitanguy I, Ramos AS. The frontal branch of the facial nerve: the importance of its variations in face lifting. Plast Reconstr Surg 1966;38(4): 352–6.

The Evolution of Complex Microsurgical Midface Reconstruction

A Classification Scheme and Reconstructive Algorithm

Daniel Alam, MD[a],*, Yaseen Ali, MD[b],
Christopher Klem, MD[a], Daniel Coventry, BSc[c]

KEYWORDS

- Midface • Microvascular • Free flap • Reconstruction • Orbit • Malar • Maxilla

KEY POINTS

- Complex midface reconstruction has evolved from prosthesis-based rehabilitation to surgical reconstruction.
- The authors present a new surgically based classification scheme for complex midface ablative surgical defects.
- Three-dimensional modeling of both bony and soft tissue elements is critical to achieving good outcomes.

INTRODUCTION

The orbito-malar framework is one of the most difficult regions to reconstruct if there is significant tissue loss. The complexity of the 3-dimensional (3D) interplay of bone, soft tissue, vital neuromuscular structures, and skin makes this area such a challenge. Beyond the anatomy, the region is a critical part of the face where aesthetic outcomes become paramount. Observers can identify a few millimeters of malposition of anatomic landmarks (eg, the lower lid margin) because of the robustness of our facial recognition systems. This ability places a unique reconstructive burden on the surgeon. The combination of anatomic complexity and the psychological and functional importance of the region have made its reconstruction a high-stakes affair.

HISTORICAL CLASSIFICATION SCHEMES

As the first step in approaching any reconstructive procedure is developing an understanding of the missing normal anatomy, the initial efforts to establish a management scheme were aimed at defining the anatomic aspects of the region. In an attempt to achieve a unified classification system of the midface after maxillectomy, at least 15 individual classification systems have been proposed in the past half-century. However, there remains no surgical or prosthodontic consensus on which one to use. Concurrent with the advent of numerous classification schemes has been the evolution of the surgical techniques to manage them. As we progressed from purely prosthetic-based approaches to fully surgically based reconstructions, the schemes were constantly revised to

Disclosure Statement: No disclosures for any of the authors.

[a] University of Hawaii, John A Burns School of Medicine, Honolulu, HI, USA; [b] Facial Plastic and Reconstructive Surgery, Queens Medical Center, Honolulu, HI, USA; [c] Oxford University School of Medicine, Oxford, UK

* Corresponding author. University of Hawaii, John A Burns School of Medicine, 1380 Lusitana Street, Honolulu, HI 96813.

E-mail address: dalam@queens.org

Facial Plast Surg Clin N Am 24 (2016) 593–603
http://dx.doi.org/10.1016/j.fsc.2016.06.012

account for the ever-changing playing field of maxillary reconstruction. As each new classification has emerged, new parameters have been included. Aramany[1] designed a system from a purely prosthodontic angle, discussing mainly the palate and maxillary alveolar ridge. McGregor and McGregor[2] chose to use a simple 3-class system, based on interruption (or not) of the orbital floor. Others then extended their systems to include midfacial skin.[3–5] Spiro and colleagues[6] defined maxillectomy defects based on the removal of specific antral walls: limited maxillectomy as removal of only one (unspecified) antral wall, subtotal maxillectomy as removal of 2 (unspecified) antral walls, and total maxillectomy as removal of the entirety of the maxilla. Davison and colleagues[7] discuss maxillectomy defects and advocate their "filling," if obturator use is impossible or intolerable.

In this era of classification schemes, the defects were characterized simply on anatomic characteristics and landmarks with little focus given to reconstructive options. Surgical reconstruction remained a last resort for volumetric reduction of defects as maxillary prosthodontics remained the mainstay for rehabilitation.

SURGICAL RECONSTRUCTION OF COMPLEX MIDFACE DEFECTS

Although microsurgical reconstruction became commonplace after its initial introduction in the early 1980s, it is important here to note that microvascular reconstructions of the midface were not attempted until the 1990s and complex osseocutaneous free flaps did not make an appearance until the twenty-first century. Better understanding of flap anatomy, increasing comfort level with flap modification and inset geometry, and improved flap survival rates all contributed to this evolving clinical path. As the mode of reconstruction has changed, the classifications before this have limited value in directing the complex microvascular free flap reconstructions performed today.

At the turn of the century, the paradigm began to shift as the free flaps used for midface reconstruction began to increase in complexity and provide better functional outcomes. Comparative studies measuring quality-of-life metrics offered evidence of better self-esteem and psychosocial outcomes in patients who had surgical reconstruction when compared with their prosthesis-based rehabilitation counterparts.[8,9] As the pendulum shifted to surgery, the surgical approaches continued to improve. Instead of using solely large soft tissue flaps to obliterate defects, the goals changed to

better osseous reconstructive methods to improve functional outcomes.

Techniques to rebuild midface buttresses and provide a framework of alveolus for dental implantation began to become more commonplace in the literature with investigators advocating specific reconstructive constructs (C shaped, Omega shaped, stacked, and so forth) and different donor flaps (fibula, iliac crest, scapula). Umino and colleagues,[10] Davison and colleagues,[7] Brown and colleagues,[11] Triana and colleagues,[12] Cordiero and Santamaria,[13] Okay and colleagues,[14] Yamamoto and colleagues,[15] Futran and Mendez,[16] and Rodriguez and colleagues[17–19] have all entered their individual classification schemes and surgical algorithms into the reconstructive arena.

The Evolution of the Classification Systems

If the classification schemes of old were lacking in appropriate algorithms for reconstruction, the newer literature became focused on individual techniques for specific defects. In doing so, the individual reports became less universal as guidelines for management. Also, most, if not all, of the work has been directed at bony reconstruction with little technical guidance as to how to establish an appropriate volumetric reconstruction. There is often discussion of what bone is missing but little emphasis on which specific structures need replacing and to what end. For example, the widely accepted schema of Cordiero and Santamaria's[13] classification system describes 4 groups, depending on the lost maxillary bony borders. The classification is used to guide the choice of osseocutaneous free flap. Bone is the tissue to be addressed first; the soft tissues are mentioned, though not with regard to restoring normal architecture.

A commonly used classification system comes from Brown and Shaw.[20] They describe the defect by its vertical and horizontal extensions, in terms of numbers and letters, respectively. Their intentions are (1) to provide a framework for nonsurgical health care workers to plan their input (eg, the prosthodontist), (2) to predict future outcomes (eg, midfacial collapse following resection of the orbital floor), and (3) to guide reconstruction of the defect. In 2010, this system was revised to include orbito-maxillary and nasomaxillary defects. New recommendations are made with regard to reconstructive approach, depending on the descriptor given to a defect. (There is no mention of volume replacement to counteract enophthalmos in class III or replacing the inferior orbital rim with bone/implant. They also advocate 3 distinct bone flaps for the same defect, each with a different morphologic outcome, ie, not like-for-like).

The intellectual gap between detailed classification schemes lacking surgical guidance and surgically based schemes but with a narrow bone-centric approach remains a problem. This problem has led to articles in recent years[21,22] to argue that not one system has succeeded to include all relevant factors. In fact, they think the myriad published classifications serve to muddy the waters and that most reconstructive dentists refer back to Aramany's[1] 1978 system still.

The authors see 2 overriding needs within a classification system for the midface. The first is a surgically based approach to anatomically categorize the region into discrete operative procedures. In this perspective, the authors do not advocate any single technique or approach for orbito-malar reconstruction but instead recommend a series of procedures based on the nature of the defect. The second important concept that the authors hope to convey within the schema is adherence to the Gillies principle, which lies at the core of all reconstructive procedures. It is critical to replace like with like. In the midface, this is not only bony reconstruction but also soft tissue and critical volumes such as that of the orbit. Within the framework of the classification, directed approaches to 3D analysis of bone, the osseous framework, and the soft tissue are discussed. Although a few reports have addressed this issue, such as Costa and colleagues,[23] the integrated combination of a surgically derived scheme based on discrete volumetric modeling is novel.

The ultimate goal of reconstruction is to reestablish normalcy for patients. Although this is almost never a realizable outcome, precision and proper planning can help us come closer to this asymptote.

SURGICAL APPROACH–BASED CLASSIFICATION SCHEME

The authors' current reconstructive algorithm is presented in **Fig. 1**. Each of the anatomic defects represents a specific surgical approach based on the overarching goal of like-to-like reconstruction. Within each group, the individual 3D framework goals vary. In some regions, bone buttress reconstitution and geometry are the primary metrics and in others the role of volumetric soft tissue is the critical element. The authors think that achieving the optimal reconstructive outcome specifically in the maxilla depends on the principle of restoring the structures as close to their normal original tissue makeup as possible, rather than just

obliterating a defect. In order to effectively approximate normality, it is critical to provide the soft tissue volumes needed at the different areas of reconstruction to bring patients back to precancer status. The use of computer-aided design–based technology in the form of state-of-the-art 3D stereotactic models provides a great tool and guide in these cases, especially if the cancer causes significant destruction and distortion of the tissues. A model is often created as a mirror image of the anatomy on the normal side of the face, which can then form the template for the reconstruction to achieve the desired outcome.

With the Gillies principle in mind, the authors have devised an algorithm to try and simplify the maxillary reconstruction by categorizing the defects into simpler general reconstructive categories and describe, what is in their opinion, the best reconstructive method for the given defect category.

CATEGORIES OF DEFECTS
Category 1

This category denotes inferior maxillectomy involving a limited hard palate (up to one-third of the maxillary alveolus) and any amount of soft tissue.

- In this category, facial support mechanisms and structures are not affected by the defect.

Category 2

This category denotes anterior or extensive inferior maxillectomy involving the anterior support buttresses but sparing the infraorbital rim (orbito-malar).

- The facial support is affected in this category in the premaxillary region and along the alveolus.

Category 3

This category denotes superior maxillectomy whereby the inferior portion of the maxilla is spared and the defect could involve the cheek, orbital rim, and lateral part of the maxilla.

Category 4

This category denotes a combined total defect that involves both superior and inferior components of the maxilla, including the infraorbital rim and floor, anterior buttresses, and hard palate.

These individual defect types are not delineated based on exact anatomic landmarks but are intended to serve as the clinical map for specific

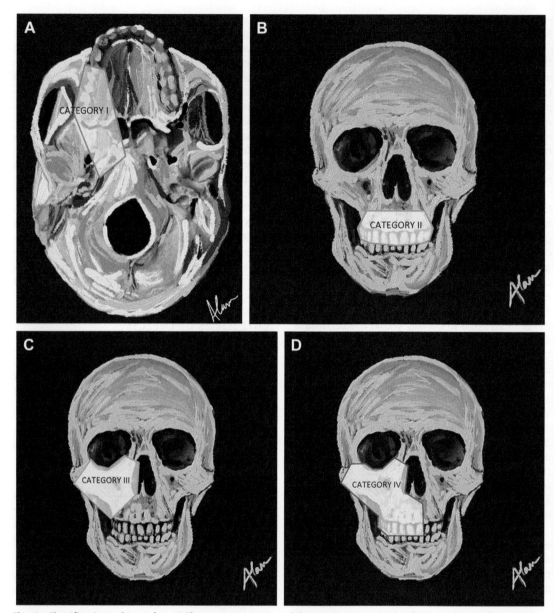

Fig. 1. Classification scheme for midface reconstruction. (*A*) Category I: partial inferior palate defect without anterior buttress involvement; (*B*) category II: inferior maxillectomy up to complete LeFort I defect (*C*); category III: orbito-malar defect with an intact palate; (*D*) category IV: total maxillectomy with simultaneous orbital and palate involvements.

reconstructions. This scheme is more inspired and influenced by the most optimal reconstructive method for each defect type rather than the defect type itself, as is evident in the next section of this article.

CATEGORY-BASED MANAGEMENT ALGORITHM

The classification and management algorithm are summarized in **Table 1**.

Category 1

This category includes posterior palatal defects that do not disrupt the anterior alveolus. The oncological resection of these tumors will often have extension to the buccal space, and the pedicle geometry will require passage of the vessels through the ipsilateral cheek into the neck. For defects that only involve the posterior hard palate, bony flaps are often too bulky and create obvious deformities in patients requiring subsequent

Table 1
Summary of the classification and management algorithm

Category	Anatomical Boundaries	Management Algorithm	Virtual Surgical Planning
Category 1	Limited inferior maxillectomy Up to one-third of maxillary alveolus Any amount of soft tissue	Radial forearm free flap	Assess soft tissue Volume lost and needed for reconstruction
Category 2	Anterior or extensive inferior maxillectomy Vertical buttress Any amount of soft tissue	Composite fibula free flap	Surgical planning for bony support design and placement Assess volume lost and needed for reconstruction
Category 3	Superior maxillectomy Infraorbital rim Vertical buttress Lateral maxilla Any amount of soft tissue	Composite fibula free flap or Anterolateral thigh flap with infraorbital implant	Assess volume lost and needed for reconstruction Surgical planning for bony support design and placement Design and placement of implant
Category 4	Hard palate and maxillary alveolus Vertical buttress Infraorbital rim and floor Any amount of soft tissue	Composite fibula free flap +/− infraorbital implant	Surgical planning for bony support design and placement Assess volume lost and needed for reconstruction Design and placement of implant

debulking procedures. For this group of patients, the authors' approach is using soft tissue–based reconstruction alone with the radial forearm flap as the method of choice. The flap allows exact reconstitution of the surface and border of the defect, and the pedicle length can allow harvesting to additional soft tissue to precisely manage any volumetric deficits. Because this is a fascio-cutaneous (plus adipose derived from proximal pedicle) flap without a muscle component (limited atrophy), volumetric replacement is quite stable. The radial forearm provides the surface epithelium to close the defect and achieve the separation between the oral and sinonasal cavities. The pliability of the flap will not interfere with the soft palate movement. The additional pedicle volume can be used to provide the volume required for restoring soft tissue deficits, and the long vascular pedicle allows tension-free anastomosis of the vessels.

Although there is no bony reconstruction in this category, the authors advocate the use of 3D stereotactic models to get accurate volumetric analysis of the defect anticipated, and then plan the reconstruction accordingly to restore the volume loss resulting from the ablation procedure. To establish the volume needed, a combination of 3D planning with bone and soft tissue algorithms as well as intraoperative assessments are used.

Accurately estimating the soft tissue deficit greatly enhances results. If dental rehabilitation is a long-term goal, dental anchored bridge replacement or delayed bone grafting is feasible in the well-vascularized flap bed. A typical case is shown in **Fig. 2.**

Category 2

The structural loss in this category involves the anterior alveolus and facial buttresses. This category also typically results in the loss of critical anterior dentition as well as loss of the premaxillary support structure to the nose. The functional and aesthetic implications of this are far greater than those seen in category 1 defects. The structural support mechanisms must be reconstituted in the skeletal framework to reconstruct these patients appropriately. This is consequently best reconstructed with a composite fibula free flap. The bony fibula will serve as the replacement of the maxillary alveolus and will provide the support that was lost after the resection. It will also allow dental rehabilitation if desired. A skin pedicle serves to line the hard palate defect. Multiple osteotomies can be performed to contour the bone appropriately, and this can be planned stereotactically using a computer-generated model

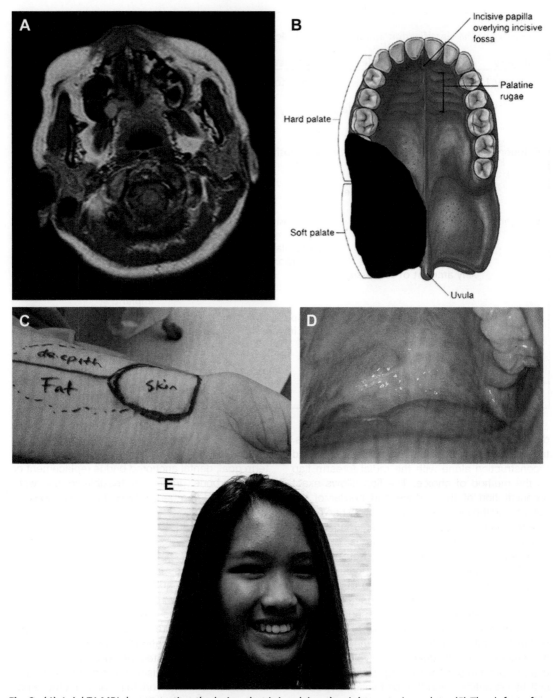

Fig. 2. (*A*) Axial T1 MRI demonstrating the lesion that is involving the right posterior palate. (*B*) The defect after the resection. (*C*) The design of the radial forearm flap, taking into consideration the volume required to fill up different segments of the reconstruction area. (*D*) Postoperative intraoral image showing the radial forearm flap in place. (*E*) The patient 7 months postoperatively.

and cutting guides to achieve a precise and accurate placement of the flap. Once more, the authors think that the use of 3D stereotactic models is invaluable as it allows the surgeon to plan the bony reconstruction and also allows accurate calculation of flap volume and design to restore volume loss. Nonanatomical placement of the bone and excess soft tissue transfer are the most common reasons for suboptimal outcomes in this type of reconstruction. Although preoperative planning is useful to define the basic framework of the reconstruction, the authors often create models to use intraoperatively to define the desired end point anatomy instead of premade guides and cutting templates. In oncological resections, the margins are unpredictable and the use of premade cutting guides can lead to malpositioned reconstructions if the tumor cuts vary from the preplanned locations. On the other hand, a preoperatively planned normal construct can serve as a reconstructive guide regardless of the extent of the ablative defect. For example, if more bone is resected, the normal model can still be used as a reference point to

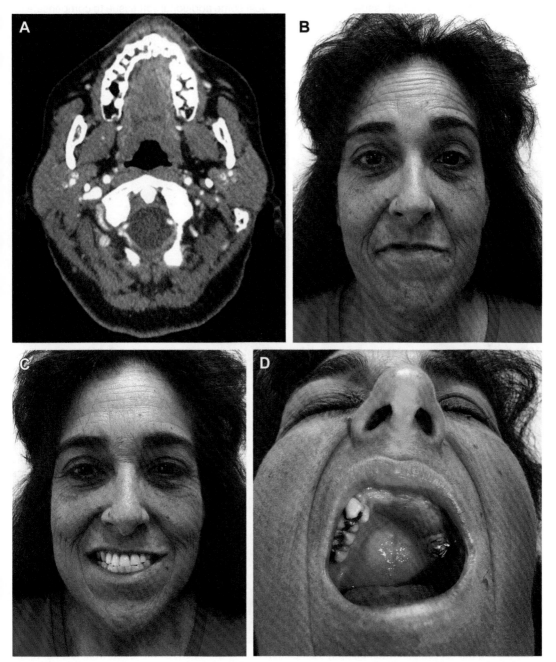

Fig. 3. (A) Axial computed tomography scan of the patient demonstrating the ill-defined lesion in the left anterior part of the palate, with the visible erosion into the maxillary alveolus. (B, C) Showing the patient 1 year postoperatively, both at rest and while smiling (with dentures in place). (D) Showing the flap: intraoral part of the flap 1 year postoperatively.

mirror the reconstruction with. A typical case is shown in **Fig. 3**.

Category 3

In this category, the aim of the reconstruction is to restore the infraorbital rim and intraorbital volume and to establish the contour and volume of the midface. With the palate intact, separation of the oral cavity is not an issue in these operations. The fibula can provide adequate support to the orbital contents; however, getting the perfect contour of the infraorbital rim is difficult because of its native curvature. Stereotactic models can provide a great aid to improve the accuracy of the bone placement and the potential soft tissue needed to get the desired contour. This is particularly seen along the tear trough region where the linear nature of the bone along the rim causes a relative volume loss. The authors will typically harvest some additional soft tissue to compensate for this often-unavoidable bony malposition medially. The alternative approach is to use a volumetric flap, such as the anterolateral thigh (ALT) flap, to

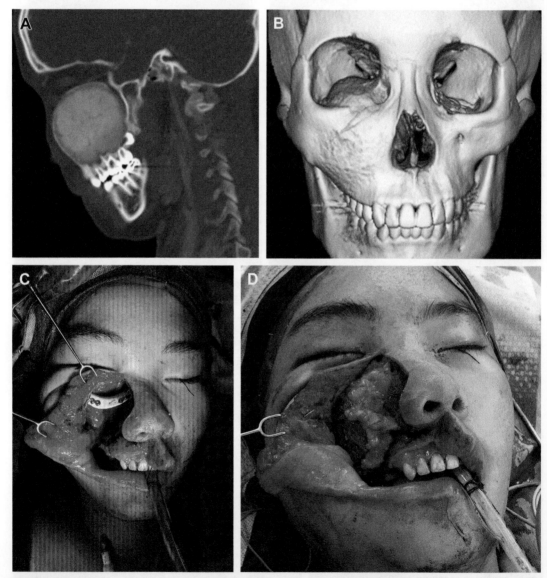

Fig. 4. (*A*) Sagittal-cut computed tomography scan demonstrating the extent of the lesion from just above the palate all the way up to the infraorbital rim. (*B*) 3D reconstruction image of the patient's facial skeleton showing the disruption of the infraorbital volume and the remodeling and expansion of the anterior vertical buttress and face of the maxilla. (*C*) Placement of the infraorbital rim PEEK implant. (*D*) Placement of the ALT flap to fill in the volume defect.

provide the soft tissue bulk needed with a custom implant mirrored from the contralateral infraorbital rim to replace the infraorbital rim and orbital floor. The implant will allow an accurate reconstitution of the orbital anatomy but will need to be completely covered by the soft tissue flap to prevent exposure to nasal flora. Infection remains a long-term risk. The skin paddle of the flap is used to line the lateral nasal wall and separate the nasal cavity. The ALT flap is ideal because of the fat content in the flap. Unlike a rectus abdominis, latissimus dorsi, or other muscle-based volumetric flaps, long-term retention is more predictable. When planning the reconstruction, overcorrection of the transferred muscle volume should be accounted for because this component will atrophy. Potential revision debulking procedures are also often needed to optimize final outcomes. A representative case showing a customized polyetheretherketone (PEEK) implant along with an ALT flap is shown in **Fig. 4.**

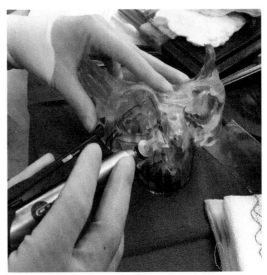

Fig. 5. Mirror-imaged 3D stereotactic model, being cut intraoperatively.

Category 4

These defects involve both the superior and inferior portions of the maxilla. As these defects are more extensive, they have a more profound impact on the midface structures and the various functions of the maxilla. There is typically a need to restore the maxillary alveolus and the hard palate, the anterior facial buttress, the infraorbital rim, as well as the soft tissue volume loss caused by the resection. The greatest intraoperative challenge in these cases is to accurately understand the normal 3D framework of the face as so much of the structure is missing. A useful clinical tool in this case is virtual planning with a stereotactic model that is a mirrored image of the normal side of the face. An example of this is shown in **Fig. 5.** This tool provides the surgeon a palpable structural reference to design the reconstruction with. Often, the authors will also model the normal side's soft tissue envelope to allow predictive planning of the volumetric components of the reconstruction. As in category 2 defects, the fibula osteocutaneous free flap provides a very good platform to reconstruct the alveolus with the skin paddle used to close the hard palate defect. The infraorbital rim is then reconstructed by making multiple osteotomies in the fibula with the orbital floor managed by an implant. The 3D modeling is critical to align all of these components. Preoperative planning is combined with normal model constructs actually used during the real-time surgery by cutting of the segment that will represent the defect from the model and then trimming it in an incremental fashion until it fits perfectly in patients'

postablation defect. This defect-matched model serves as the template to create the flap reconstruction, which is visually shown in **Fig. 6.**

Although many investigators have advocated specific design constructs and flap shapes for orbito-malar resections, the authors think that there is not any one prescriptive design that is uniformly useful to accomplish these reconstructions. In fact, a cookbook approach often limits outcomes. The authors would prefer to think of the defects as individual reconstructive problems whereby patient-specific protocols directed by detailed 3D analyses of the bony and soft tissue deficits are needed. The flap is in essence tailored to the planned reconstruction. The closer we can come to this ideal, the better the patients' outcome.

Although intuitively obvious, this concept is often underutilized in midface reconstruction. Detailed stereotactic modeling is time consuming and often expensive. The surgery with this approach is often much more complex. The willingness to make numerous osteotomies and flap modifications at the time of transfer is something an inexperienced surgeon may avoid in concern for jeopardizing flap viability. The authors recognize these are valid counterarguments to this aggressive approach to microvascular midface reconstruction and this has limited its use. Despite these concerns, the authors strongly advocate these approaches. In the end, almost normal is not normal and being cured of cancer is not being cured of your treatment. Leaving patients with significant recognizable deformity in the central face is an unforgiving end point. The functional and

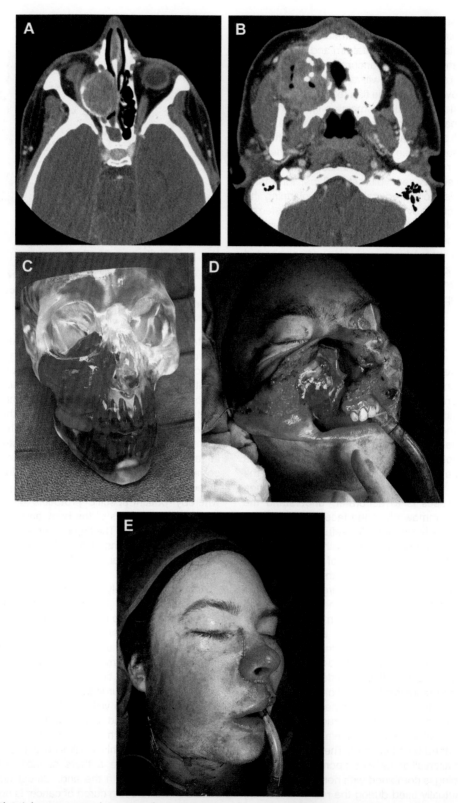

Fig. 6. (*A*) Axial-cut computed tomography scan showing the extent of the disease, which extends all the way up to the orbit involving the infraorbital rim superiorly. (*B*) Involving the hard palate and maxillary alveolus inferiorly. (*C*) 3D model reconstructed as part of the surgical planning demonstrating the lesion. (*D*) Model fitting in the postablative defect after it was incrementally trimmed. (*E*) Immediate postoperative picture.

psychosocial impact remains. The validity of the authors' argument only lies in the quality of its outcomes. The additional steps to approximate normal, while time consuming and in inexperienced hands potentially risky, are warranted for the ultimate value they bring to patients.

REFERENCES

1. Aramany. 1978.

2. McGregor, McGregor. 1986.

3. Wells MD, Luce EA. Reconstruction of midfacial defects after surgical resection of malignancies. Clin Plast Surg 1995;22:79–89.

4. Cordeiro PG, Santamaria E. A classification system and algorithm for reconstruction of maxillectomy and midfacial defects. Plast Reconstr Surg 2000; 105(7):2331–46; discussion 2347-8.

5. Costa H, Zenha H, Sequeira H, et al. Microsurgical reconstruction of the maxilla. Algorithm and concepts 2015;68(5):e89–104.

6. Spiro RH, Strong EW, Shah JP. Maxillectomy and its classification. Head Neck 1997;19(4):309–14.

7. Davison SP, Sherris DA, Meland NB. An algorithm for maxillectomy defect reconstruction. Laryngoscope 1998;108(2):215–9.

8. Kornblith AB, Zlotolow IM, Gooen J, et al. Quality of life of maxillectomy patients using an obturator prosthesis. Head Neck 1996;18(4):323–34.

9. Rogers SN, Lowe D, McNally D, et al. Health-related quality of life after maxillectomy: a comparison between prosthetic obturation and free flap. J Oral Maxillofac Surg 2003;61(2):174–81.

10. Umino S, Masuda G, Ono S, et al. Speech intelligibility following maxillectomy with and without a prosthesis: an analysis of 54 cases. J Oral Rehabil 1998; 25:153–8.

11. Brown JS, Rogers SN, McNally DN, et al. A modified classification for the maxillectomy defect. Head Neck 2000;22(1):17–26.

12. Triana RJ, Uglesic V, Virag M, et al. Microvascular free flap reconstructive options in patients with partial and total maxillectomy defects. Arch Facial Plast Surg 2000;2:91–101.

13. Cordeiro PG, Santamaria E. A classification system and algorithm for reconstruction of maxillectomy and midfacial defects. Plast Reconstr Surg 2000; 105(7):2331–46 [discussion: 2347–8].

14. Okay DJ, Genden E, Buchbinder D, et al. Prosthodontic guidelines for surgical reconstruction of the maxilla: a classification system of defects. J Prosthet Dent 2001;86:352–63.

15. Yamamoto Y, Kawashima K, Sugihara T, et al. Surgical management of maxillectomy defects based on the concept of buttress reconstruction. Head Neck 2004;26:247–56.

16. Futran ND, Mendez E. Developments in reconstruction of midface and maxilla. Lancet Oncol 2006;7(3): 249–58.

17. Rodriguez ED, Martin M, Bluebond-Langner R, et al. Microsurgical reconstruction of posttraumatic high-energy maxillary defects: establishing the effectiveness of early reconstruction. Plast Reconstr Surg 2007;120:103S–17S.

18. Akinmoladun VI, Dosumu OO, Olusanya AA, et al. Maxillectomy defects: a suggested classification scheme. Afr J Med Med Sci 2013;42(2):171–5.

19. Abu-Serriaha M, Wongb L, Richardsonb S, et al. The SECONDI MAPZ© system: new approach for the classification of oncological defects of the midface. Br J Oral Maxillofac Surg 2016;54(4):422–9.

20. Brown JS, Shaw RJ. Reconstruction of the maxilla and midface: introducing a new classification. Lancet Oncol 2010;11(10):1001–8.

21. Aggarwal, 2012.

22. Bidra AS, Jacob RF, Taylor TD. Classification of maxillectomy defects: a systematic review and criteria necessary for a universal description. J Prosthet Dent 2012;107(4):261–70.

23. Costa H, Zenha H, Sequeira H, et al. Microsurgical reconstruction of the maxilla: algorithm and concepts. J Plast Reconstr Aesthet Surg 2015;68(5): e89–104.

Craniomaxillofacial Trauma

 CrossMark

Sven-Olrik Streubel, MD, MBA[a],*, David M. Mirsky, MD[b]

KEYWORDS

- Craniomaxillofacial trauma • Advanced Trauma Life Support • Fracture • Soft tissue injury

KEY POINTS

- Facial trauma is a significant cause of morbidity in the United States.
- With injuries varying widely in fracture location, severity, and wound contamination, the clinical benefits of antibiotics use in facial fracture treatment are not easily determined.
- The pediatric population is predisposed to craniofacial trauma more so than the adult population secondary to their increased cranial mass to body ratio.
- Every patient with a traumatic injury should be assessed according to the Advanced Trauma Life Support protocol.

EPIDEMIOLOGY

Facial trauma is a significant cause of morbidity in the United States. Estimated annual costs due to emergency department visits alone approach $1 billion per year.[1] Trauma care is associated with low reimbursement by federal agencies, placing an economic burden on major trauma centers in the United States.[2] Erdmann and colleagues[3] reported on operative facial fracture management at a single academic medical center and the financial impact on the health system. The presented data confirmed a lower professional collection rate for operatively managed facial trauma in a representative US tertiary medical center compared with overall professional collection rates by the Division of Plastic and Reconstructive Surgery, Duke University Medical Center (33%) and compared with the overall collection rates for orthopedic surgery, including skeletal trauma management (32%).

National data from 2004 confirm that approximately 70% of patients with facial and skull fractures are managed in teaching institutions (http://hcup.ahrq.gov/HCUPnet.asp). VandeGriend and colleagues[4] recently published a retrospective review of all nonpediatric inpatient and outpatient facilities of the Detroit Medical Center (DMC) from 1990 to 2011 and weighted national inpatient estimates from 1993 to 2010 using the National Inpatient Survey. DMC records identified 30,260 adult facial fractures. These included nasal (30.1%), mandible (22.7%), malar-maxillary (15.4%), orbital floor (15.7%), and other (16.1%) fractures. A total of 8528 fracture repairs were performed, including nasal (17.1%), mandible (41.6%), malar (15.2%), maxillary (6.4%), and other (19.6%). Overall, from 1990 to 2011, fractures increased. Scaled and unscaled national data were very similar and showed no significant differences in trend. In an epidemiologic study of facial injuries by Walker and colleagues,[5] men were more often injured than women (68% compared with 32%). Half of all patients were between 15 and 45 years old. Falls (39%) and sport activities (29%) were the most common causes. Fractures accounted for 25% of presentations. Fractures of the nose

a Pediatric Otolaryngology and Craniomaxillofacial Surgery, Department of Otolaryngology, Children's Hospital Colorado, University of Colorado School of Medicine, 13123 East 16th Avenue, B455, Aurora, CO 80045, USA; b Pediatric Neuroradiology Fellowship, Children's Hospital Colorado, University of Colorado School of Medicine, 13123 East 16th Avenue, Box B125, Aurora, CO 80045, USA
* Corresponding author.
E-mail address: sven.streubel@childrenscolorado.org

Facial Plast Surg Clin N Am 24 (2016) 605–617
http://dx.doi.org/10.1016/j.fsc.2016.06.014
1064-7406/16/© 2016 Elsevier Inc. All rights reserved.

(50%), mandible (25%), and zygoma (12%) were the most common sites of injury.

Van Hout reported on 394 patients with facial fractures requiring an operation in a Dutch trauma center.[6] Intoxication was documented in 15% of patients, usually with alcohol (91%). The male-to-female ratio was 3:1 with a peak incidence in young men (35% of fractures). Motor vehicle accidents (MVAs) accounted for 42%. Interpersonal violence and sports led to more injuries in men than in women, and mandible and zygomatic fractures accounted for more than 80% of the total. O'Meara and colleagues[7] found that patients with facial fractures were more likely to need an operation if they had consumed alcohol within the preceding 8 hours or were victims of interpersonal violence. McAllister and colleagues[8] found that 47% of those admitted for facial injuries had evidence of illegal drugs in their urine. Cannabinoids and benzodiazepines were most often detected. Both alcohol and drugs were found in 17% of cases, although 72% of patients with positive toxicology results denied substance abuse. An unreliable substance abuse history naturally has implications for general anesthesia and analgesia. Patients with facial injuries often have associated head and extremity injuries that can prolong their hospital stay.[6,9] In a review of the management of traumatic brain injuries, Tsang and Whitfield[10] reported that 24% of patients with craniofacial fractures also had fractures in the base of the skull, which were complicated by the leakage of cerebrospinal fluid in 20%.

Children account for approximately 14% of all facial fractures.[11] Although facial fractures are less common in the pediatric population than in adults, they are still known to be a substantial source of morbidity, mortality, and resource utilization.[12] Imahara and colleagues[12] reported that children with facial fractures have more severe head and chest injuries, longer lengths of hospital and intensive care unit stays, higher hospital charges, and higher mortality rates compared with other pediatric trauma patients without facial fractures. Soleimani and colleagues[13] analyzed fractures in 21,533 pediatric patients. They found that for all age groups, the top 3 trauma mechanisms of pediatric facial fractures that resulted in hospitalization were MVA, intentional trauma (IT), and falls (43%,17%, and 11% of patients, respectively). MVA was the most frequent mechanism for all age groups. For patients younger than 10 years old, falls were more common than IT; whereas for patients 10 years and older, IT injuries were more common than falls. The incidence of inpatient facial fractures due to MVA and IT increased with age. The incidence of inpatient pediatric facial fractures

due to MVA in the United States decreased from 5.7 to 4.4 per 100,000 from 2000 to 2009. This decrease may indicate that vehicle restraints may be keeping children safer or that parents are more compliant with child vehicle restraint laws. Use of safety devices, including seatbelts and airbags, is associated with a decreased incidence of facial fractures.[14] There was a significant increase in the number of inpatient pediatric facial fractures due to IT and fall with most patients being male (70%). African American and Hispanic patients accounted for most patients in the IT group and came from the poorest neighborhoods. Most of the patients were admitted to large (68%), urban (94%), and teaching (75%) hospitals. The mandible was the most commonly fractured bone (32.2%). Multiple facial fractures were seen in 24% of patients. Nasal, zygomatic, and maxillary, and orbital floor fractures occurred in 13.8%, 6.3%, and 8.3% of patients, respectively. Concomitant injuries occurred in 58.8% of patients. Intracranial injuries and/or skull fractures (45.1%), cervical spine (2.2%), thoracic (15%), abdominopelvic (10.9%), and extremity (20.3%) injuries were all associated with facial fractures. The overall mortality rate was 2%.

PERIOPERATIVE ANTIBIOTIC AND STEROID PROPHYLAXIS

The role of antibiotics in facial fracture treatment remains controversial. With injuries varying widely in fracture location, severity, and wound contamination, the clinical benefits of antibiotics use are not easily determined. The literature has tried to distinguish between antibiotic use in mandible fractures and antibiotics with other facial fractures, including isolated condylar fractures. Surgeons agree on the need for antibiotics with infected wounds and most routinely administer antibiotics in the perioperative setting.

In 2006, Andreasen and colleagues[15] conducted a systematic review. The reviewers concluded that prophylactic antibiotics are beneficial in the treatment of mandible fractures but, because of a low risk of postoperative infection, prophylactic antibiotics were not indicated for other facial fracture sites. No benefit of prophylactic antibiotics in maxillofacial fractures, including mandible fractures, was found by Kyzas,[16] Miles and colleagues,[17] Shridharani and colleagues,[18] and Knepil and Loukota.[19] Morris and Kellman[20] summarized the available literature and recommended that antibiotics should only be given for mandible fractures from injury until completion of the perioperative course but not postoperatively. There are insufficient data to assess prophylactic antibiotics in nonmandible fractures and isolated condyle fractures but existing evidence demonstrates no benefit to postoperative antibiotics.

There is controversy about whether antibiotics should be routinely given to patients with skull base fractures in an effort to prevent infectious complications, including meningitis. In 2015, Ratilal and colleagues[21] published a Cochrane review of randomized controlled trials (RCTs), as well as non-RCTS, concerning antibiotics and skull base fractures. There was insufficient evidence for prophylactic antibiotic use in patients with skull base fractures with or without a cerebrospinal fluid leak. Until better evidence becomes available, the routine use of antibiotics in these cases should be avoided.

Glucocorticoids are often used to reduce airway edema, although evidence for this benefit is largely limited to children postextubation.[22] The Corticosteroid Randomization After Significant Head injury (CRASH) study identified an excess mortality in the presence of head injury if high-dose methylprednisolone is administered[23]; therefore, it should be avoided. This may have implications in the management of some vision threatening injuries. Similarly, the routine administration of high doses of steroids for early spinal cord injury is controversial and, despite having been advocated by Advanced Trauma Life Support (ATLS) protocol, has been questioned based on its lack of efficacy and significant complications.[24]

PEDIATRIC TRAUMA

The pediatric population is predisposed to craniofacial trauma more so than the adult population secondary to their increased cranial mass to body ratio. This translates to higher energy insults to the pediatric craniofacial skeleton.[25] Though the relatively increased size of the pediatric cranium is a larger target, it also provides several protective features. The pediatric skeleton is more flexible because of its immaturity and incomplete calcification.[25] The presence of tooth buds increases the tooth to bone ratio and contributes to the mandibular and maxillary flexibility and stability.[26,27] The cranium to face ratio of the pediatric patient is 8:1 compared with 2:1 in adults.[28] This increased cranial to face ratio decreases the risk of maxillofacial injury.[26,28] The facial fat pads confer additional protection to that age group.[26,27,29]

The frontal bone is prone to fracture in children because of its relative size. Orbital roof fractures are more common in children younger than 7 years of age before frontal sinus pneumatization.[30] After 7 years of age, orbital fractures more often involve the walls and floor.[25,30,31] The midface becomes more susceptible to fracture as it enlarges and becomes more protrusive with age.[25] These fractures are often the result of significant force. Mandible fractures are common in children and often are incomplete (Greenstick fractures). Le Fort fractures are complex fracture patterns that result from high-energy insults and are fortunately uncommon. Fracture location, complexity of injury, associated injuries, as well as patient's age and time since injury determine fracture management. The pediatric facial skeleton has increased osteogenic potential. This translates into a more rapid rate of healing necessitating earlier intervention and shorter duration of immobilization.[25,31,32]

In the past, the concern for interference with the growth and development of the pediatric facial skeleton prompted a minimalist approach in the management of pediatric facial fractures. Closed reduction and maxillomandibular fixation (MMF) were initially the treatment method of choice for all displaced facial fractures.[31] Now, open reduction and internal fixation (ORIF) is the preferred treatment of most facial fractures in pediatric patients with mixed and permanent dentition. ORIF allows fixation in 3 dimensions. No or less time is spent in MMF, thus decreasing airway risk and improving nutrition and tolerance.[25] Unfortunately, disruption of the periosteum and the vascular supply, as well as the creation of scars, may interfere with future growth of the affected area.

EVALUATION OF FACIAL TRAUMA

Every patient with a traumatic injury should be assessed according to the ATLS protocol. After life-threatening conditions are stabilized, the patient is cleaned and the face is examined. The face is assessed in thirds for neurovascular integrity, fractures, and lacerations. A screening eye examination should be performed (pupillary light reflex, extraocular movements, globe position, and visual acuity). An intranasal examination should eliminate a septal hematoma. Changes in occlusion should be noted. Attention is then directed to the examination of the scalp, ears, and neck (lacerations, hematoma, foreign body). Imaging is directed by the primary survey, mechanism of injury, and suspected injuries. Facial fractures are evaluated by computed tomography (CT) scan, and 3-dimensional CT reconstructions may be helpful. In case of suspected vascular injuries in penetrating neck injuries in zones I and III, CT angiography is recommended.[33]

SOFT TISSUE INJURIES AND MANAGEMENT
Lacerations and Avulsions

Wounds should be irrigated thoroughly with sterile saline or antibiotic solution, have debris removed, and be closed primarily. Debridement should be very conservative. Large soft tissue defects not amenable to primary closure should be dressed with a wound vacuum-assisted closure (VAC) dressing to promote healing by secondary intention. Avulsed tissue may be beneficial at its native site, either as viable tissue that heals primarily or as temporary biological dressing. Application of a moisturizing ointment, applied twice daily for 1 to 2 weeks, promotes wound healing. Permanent sutures should be removed within 5 to 7 days. Aesthetically unacceptable scars can be revised in 6 to 9 months.

The Facial Nerve and Parotid Duct

Facial nerve function should be assessed and documented according to the House-Brackmann grading scale.[34] Most penetrating injuries in the distribution of the facial nerve with incomplete facial paralysis do not require surgical intervention. Injuries lateral to the lateral canthus with complete facial paralysis should be explored. In blunt and blast injuries with associated facial paralysis, the temporal bone should be evaluated. Facial lacerations with facial nerve paralysis should be explored within 72 hours of injury because the distal nerve segment can still be identified through electrical stimulation with a probe. If the nerve is transected, the proximal and distal ends of the nerve should be mobilized to allow for a tension-free epineural repair. Nerve interposition grafts may be necessary. Neurotrophins and neurokinins, such as resveratrol and oxytocin, may add in facial nerve regeneration.[35]

Blood at the orifice of the parotid duct (Stenson duct) should prompt cannulation of the duct with a lacrimal probe to assess duct integrity. If injury to the duct is identified, the duct is closed over a silicone elastomer stent. The stent may be left in place for several weeks to divert saliva and prevent stenosis of the duct. If there is injury to the more distal duct it should be reimplanted into the papilla or into the buccal mucosa at a more posterior location. A drain should be placed in the wound bed to evacuate residual blood or saliva and prevent sialocele formation.

Bites: Human and Canine

Bite wounds should be washed out and primarily closed if possible. Antibiotics administered should cover Staphylococcus aureus, Streptococci, Pasteurella multocida, Eikenella corrodens, Corynebacterium spp, and other anaerobes. The rabies status of the animal should be determined and the patient immunized if indicated. Human bites are associated with increased pathogenicity and potential for transmission of infection. Hepatitis B and C, herpes simplex virus, syphilis, tuberculosis,

tetanus, and human immunodeficiency virus are transmissible through human bite injuries.[36]

FRACTURES
Frontal Sinus Fractures

Because of the low incidence, management of these fractures has not been investigated by prospective clinical trials. Thus there is no consensus for surgical indications, surgery timing, method of repair, or postoperative surveillance for frontal sinus fractures. Frontal sinus fractures are traditionally treated with observation for minimally displaced anterior table fractures. They are explored and reduced for more displaced fractures of the anterior table. Frontal sinus obliteration is reserved for fractures involving the nasofrontal duct, whereas frontal sinus cranialization is performed for fractures of the anterior table with cerebrospinal fluid leakage or significantly displaced or comminuted posterior table fractures. Typically, an existing laceration or a bicoronal incision is used to gain access to the frontal sinus. The traditional obliteration and cranialization techniques are increasingly replaced by endoscopic surgery techniques with less morbidity[37,38] (Fig. 1).

Naso-Orbito-Ethmoidal Fractures

Naso-orbito-ethmoidal (NOE) fractures are usually the result of a high-impact blunt trauma to the midface. They occur when the nasal root is hit hard enough to move it posteriorly. It is forced between the orbits, collapsing the ethmoids. The bones holding the medial canthal ligaments are released, allowing the lids to move laterally. This leads to telecanthus or pseudohypertelorism.[39] NOE fractures can occur in isolation but usually are part of panfacial fractures. They are classified based on the extent of bony comminution and condition of the medial canthal tendon.[40] Physical examination should include palpation of the nasal bones, visual acuity check, evaluation of eyelid and globe condition and position, and intranasal inspection. A CT scan of the face allows for assessment of the fracture degree. Patients present with telecanthus, enophthalmos, epiphora, nasal airway obstruction, and epistaxis. The treatment of NOE fractures should reestablish the intercanthal distance, nasal projection, and internal orbital structures. This includes fracture reduction and stabilization with miniplates and sutures, and bone grafting, as well as canthal tendon reconstruction with transnasal wiring (Fig. 2).

Orbital Fractures

The goal of orbital fracture repair is to restore orbital contour and volume. Assessment should

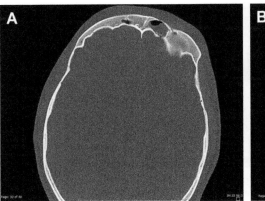
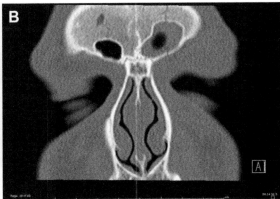

Fig. 1. (A) Axial CT image demonstrates fractures of the outer and inner tables of the left frontal sinus with presence of internal fluid. (B) Coronal reformatted CT image illustrates the vertical component of the fracture.

include palpation of the orbital rims, evaluation of eyelid and globe condition and position, visual acuity check with extraocular muscle function, and evaluation of forehead and midface sensation. Ophthalmology should be consulted for any vision symptoms or orbital injury. Surgical access for orbital fractures is obtained through a lateral eyebrow, subtarsal, subciliary, transconjunctival, transcaruncular, or bicoronal incision. Eyelid complications are increased with subciliary approaches to the orbit compared with the transconjunctival approach.[41] The decision of whether a fracture should be surgically repaired depends on the fracture's impact on vision, ocular motility, diplopia, and cosmesis. The evidence for timing and size of fracture repair, as well as repair material, is insufficient.[42,43] It is also unclear if the benefits of preoperative planning and intraoperative imaging and navigation into the management

of orbital fracture repair warrant the increased cost.[44] According to a retrospective study by Kunz and colleagues,[44] fractures of the orbital wall may be treated conservatively if the defect is small (less than 3 cm^2), with little enophthalmos (less than 2 mm), and if there is no entrapment of periorbital tissue. In children, 45% to 56% of all facial fractures are orbital fractures.[45] The orbital roof is more likely to fracture than the floor in children younger than 7 years because of the protuberance of the frontal bone. Muscle entrapment with orbital floor fractures is more common in patients younger than 16 years because of bony plasticity, which allows the floor to hinge rather than break.[46] Nausea and vomiting suggests entrapment and should prompt repair within 24 to 48 hours (white-eye blowout fracture).[45] The white-eyed blowout fracture is an orbital injury in children that is commonly initially

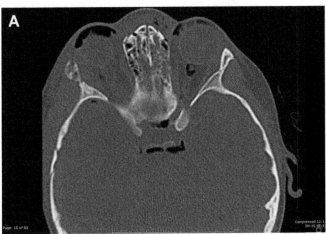
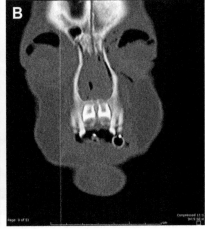

Fig. 2. (A) Axial CT image reveals comminuted fractures of the naso-orbital-ethmoidal regions. (B) Coronal reformatted CT image demonstrates involvement of the medial canthal regions.

misdiagnosed as a head injury because of predominant autonomic features (nausea, vomiting, bradycardia, and syncope) and lack of soft-tissue signs (periorbital hematoma, enophthalmos, dystopia, and subconjunctival ecchymosis). It can manifest as a linear or hinge-like trapdoor deformity. The elasticity of pediatric bone, incomplete fused suture lines, thicker periosteum, and increased soft tissue padding over the malar eminence allow the pediatric orbital bone to absorb energy yet sustain minimal bony structural damage. Hundepool and colleagues[47] found that endoscopic fracture reduction of the orbital floor improved enophthalmos and diplopia when compared with controls because it allowed visualization of the entire defect (**Figs. 3** and **4**).

Zygomatico-Maxillary Complex Fractures

Zygomatico-maxillary complex (ZMC) fractures involve fractures of the lateral orbital wall, orbital floor, inferior orbital rim, anterior maxillary sinus wall, lateral maxillary sinus wall, and zygomatic arch. They can cause significant aesthetic deformity because the malar eminence of the zygoma is the most anterior projection of the lateral midface and the zygomatic arch is the most lateral projection of the midface. The goal of treatment of a ZMC fracture is to restore the bone to its preinjury location and maintain orbital volume, thereby enhancing both the functional and cosmetic outcome.[48] ZMC fractures are evaluated by palpation of the zygoma, intraoral and intranasal examination, mouth opening, visual acuity check with extraocular muscle function, and midface sensation. Ophthalmology should be consulted for any vision symptoms or orbital injury. A CT scan of the face is the standard radiographic imaging study. Patients with ZMC fractures may experience epistaxis, vision changes, midface and dental numbness, malar depression, enophthalmos, trismus, and malocclusion. A

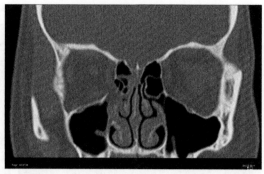

Fig. 4. Coronal reformatted CT image illustrates a fracture of the right medial orbital wall with extension of orbital fat and partial herniation of medial rectus muscle through the defect.

combination of surgical approaches helps in fracture exposure and reduction: upper gingivobuccal (sublabial), lateral upper blepharoplasty, transconjunctival, subciliary, or Gilles. Extraocular muscle entrapment during fracture reduction should be excluded by forced duction testing. Fixation is recommended at a minimum of 2 fracture points with plates and screws. Rana and colleagues[49] noted better malar projection, less vertical dystopia, and greater stability after 3-point fixation. Isolated zygomatic arch fractures may need to be reduced if the fracture produces a depression over the lateral face or if the fracture segments impinge on the temporalis muscle, leading to trismus or masticatory dysfunction. Maxillary sinus fractures in isolation without other associated ZMC fractures rarely require intervention (**Fig. 5**).

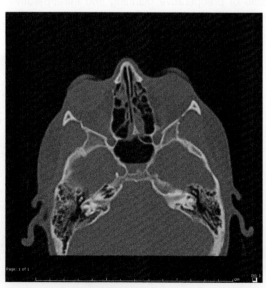

Fig. 5. Axial CT image reveals a partially displaced fracture of the right lateral orbital wall.

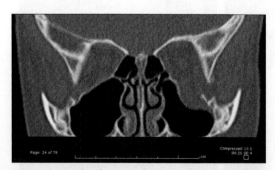

Fig. 3. Coronal reformatted CT image shows a fracture of the left orbital floor with herniation of orbital fat and inferior rectus muscle into the subjacent maxillary sinus.

Le Fort Fractures

Le Fort type I is a horizontal fracture through the maxilla superior to the maxillary dentition. Type II is a pyramidal fracture through the maxilla, orbit, and nasal radix. Type III is a fracture separating the facial bones from the skull through the nasal radix and lateral orbital rims. All Le Fort fractures have bilateral pterygoid plate and nasal septal fractures. These fractures are usually caused by high impact trauma. Assessment should include manipulation of the hard palate relative to the skull, facial sensation, visual acuity check with extraocular muscle function, and intraoral and intranasal examination. CT scan of the facial bones and sinuses is a critical portion of the assessment of Le Fort fractures. Signs and symptoms include facial anesthesia, epistaxis, vision changes, and malocclusion. The treatment of Le Fort fractures should reestablish the continuity of the facial bones with the cranium and the preinjury occlusion. Initial MMF maintains proper occlusion and provides a stable foundation for the remainder of the repair. Type I injuries can be approached through an upper gingivobuccal (sublabial) incision. Type II and III injuries usually require the addition of eyelid incisions or a coronal approach (**Figs. 6–8**).

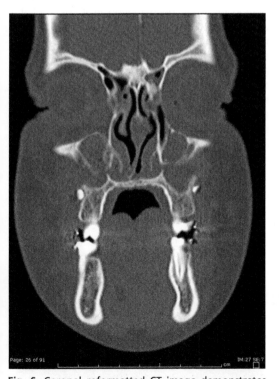

Fig. 6. Coronal reformatted CT image demonstrates fractures of the inferior medial and lateral maxillary buttresses.

Nasal Fractures

Nasal bone fractures are the most common facial fractures.[1] The nasal bones should be assessed by palpation and an intranasal examination should be performed to rule out a septal hematoma or fracture. Radiographic imaging in isolated nasal bone fractures is of little benefit. Signs and symptoms may include epistaxis, nasal airway obstruction, change in olfaction and deformity. Nasal fracture management should reestablish nasal airway patency and nasal contour. Nasal fractures can be treated with closed or open reduction. Closed reduction consists of mobilizing the displaced nasal bones and cartilages usually with a blunt elevating instrument. Rapid healing of these fractures requires surgical intervention within 7 to 10 days of the injury. After reduction of the nasal fracture, external fixation is applied with a nasal splint. A septal hematoma should be drained as soon as possible because it may lead to septal cartilage necrosis, septal perforation, and potential saddle nose deformity.

Although nasal fractures are commonly managed with closed reduction, the efficacy of this procedure is not established. No prospective RCT has been conducted to directly compare open and closed techniques. In 2002, Staffel[50] examined the effectiveness of closed nasal reduction by reviewing several studies in the literature and proposing a treatment algorithm to improve outcomes. General anesthesia, sedation, and local anesthesia can all be effective and are well tolerated by patients undergoing nasal reduction.[51–53] Al-Moraissi and Ellis[54] reviewed the choice of anesthesia for closed nasal fracture reduction and reported that patient satisfaction was higher with general anesthesia (**Fig. 9**).

Mandible Fractures

Mandible fractures are the second most common facial fracture.[1] Mandible fractures are classified according to the location of the fracture: symphysis-parasymphysis, body, angle, ramus, coronoid process, and condyle. The most common sites of fracture are the angle and body, followed by the symphysis-parasymphysis.[55] Evaluation of mandible fractures should include palpation of the mandible, inspection of the mandibular and maxillary dentition or occlusion, and inferior alveolar nerve function. CT scan of the face is standard to evaluate the extent of injury. Patients with a mandible fracture may present with trismus, malocclusion, numbness, and loose or missing teeth. The repair of mandible fractures should restore the preinjury occlusion and bony union after reduction of the fracture segments. It should

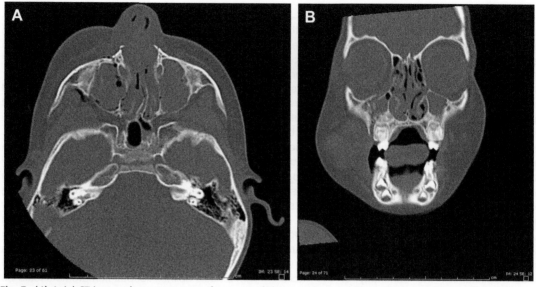

Fig. 7. (*A*) Axial CT image shows numerous fractures of the superior medial maxillary buttresses. (*B*) Coronal reformatted CT image illustrates fractures of the inferior lateral maxillary buttress and right orbital floor (transverse maxillary buttress).

preserve facial contour and height. The surgical approach is based on the location and type of mandible fracture. Nondisplaced ramus and subcondylar fractures in adults without malocclusion can be treated with soft diet alone.

MMF is required in patients who cannot spontaneously bring their teeth to their preinjury occlusion. Arch bars are applied to the maxillary and mandibular gingiva and tightly secured to the underlying dentition with loops of 24-gauge and 26-gauge wire. The maxillary and mandibular arch bars are then fastened, locking the patient into rigid fixation and, ideally, the preinjury occlusion. Elastic bands instead of rigid fixation may be

sufficient in some instances. In adults, MMF should be maintained for approximately 6 weeks. The potential risk of aspiration and airway compromise in patients with MMF who may not be capable of removing it requires supervision by a person who has been trained in it. Beyond the airway risks, MMF is associated with poor dental hygiene and enamel loss, discomfort, and speech and articulation difficulties. The inability to chew and the lack of solid food consumption for 6 weeks can result in weight loss. Prolonged and significant morbidities, advancements in plating systems and a better understanding of the biomechanics of the mandible have led to the increased use of open

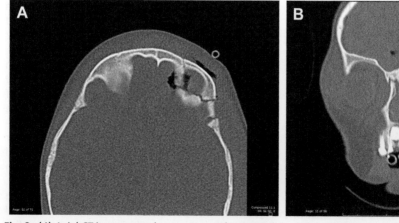

Fig. 8. (*A*) Axial CT image reveals a transverse fracture of the left orbital roof. (*B*) Coronal reformatted CT image demonstrates fractures of the bilateral superior medial maxillary buttresses.

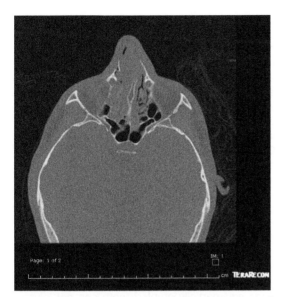

Fig. 9. Axial CT image shows a displaced fracture of the right nasal bone.

approaches with permanent rigid internal fixation for mandible fracture repair.

Condylar fractures are unique because of the complexities with surgical approach and the difficulties with plating at this location. They can be managed with a closed approach (with or without MMF) or an open approach. The closed approach without MMF can be used in patients with good spontaneous occlusion. These patients are encouraged to exercise a full range of motion while maintaining a soft diet. The closed approach with MMF can also be used but a greater concern exists for subsequent temporomandibular joint (TMJ) dysfunction because of the inflammatory response at the TMJ in condylar fractures. The open approach, either transoral or transcervical, involves plating across the fractured condylar segments with or without the assistance of endoscopic instrumentation. The indications for open repair of condylar fractures are displacement into the middle cranial fossa, poor occlusion with closed reduction, lateral extracapsular displacement of the condyle, presence of a foreign body, and open fracture with potential for fibrosis.[56] Most high ramus and nondisplaced angle fractures do not warrant the morbidity of an open approach and can be treated with a closed approach with or without MMF. Isolated coronoid process fractures are rare and usually do not require treatment (**Fig. 10**).

Fractures of the mandibular angle

The presence of third molars and thin cortices of bone make the mandibular angle among the most common sites of fracture. Angle fractures have been investigated with several RCTs. Noncomminuted angle fractures can be repaired with a standard Champy plate alone[57] or 1 miniplate.[58,59]

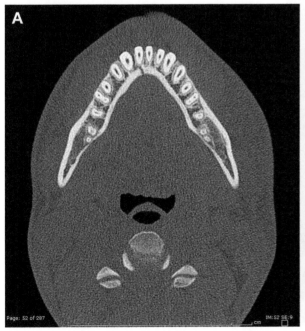
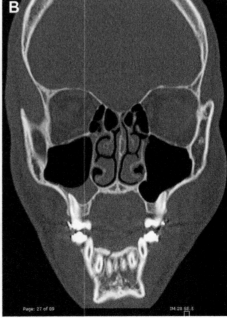

Fig. 10. (A) Axial CT image illustrates a right parasymphyseal mandibular fracture. (B) Coronal reformatted CT image demonstrates the oblique component of the mandibular fracture.

There is only limited lower level evidence to determine an optimal length of MMF. Adeyemi and colleagues[60] compared 4 to 6 weeks of MMF with a treatment group receiving only 2 weeks. Both groups healed their fractures but recovery of full mouth opening was more rapid with a shorter period of MMF. Kaplan and colleagues[61] compared mandible fractures repaired with miniplates plus 2 weeks of postoperative MMF with fractures repaired with no postoperative MMF. They found no differences between the groups in terms of weight loss, trismus, dental hygiene, or wound complications. These studies suggest that in the appropriate fractures, a brief period of MMF or no MMF improves outcomes and patient satisfaction. Dorri and colleagues[62] performed a Cochrane review regarding the use of resorbable plates in mandible fractures and concluded that, based on the increased costs and technical difficulties of these fixation systems for mandible fractures, their use is not supported by the current literature (**Fig. 11**).

Condylar fractures

Several recent prospective RCTs suggest improved outcomes with open repair of displaced condylar fractures.[63–67] Closed management of condylar fractures requires early mobilization and aggressive physiotherapy. Even then, the condyle is not in its normal position and there is diminished ramus height. To minimize facial nerve injury and maximize the benefits of ORIF of condylar fractures, the endoscopic approach has received more interest. Schmelzeisen and colleagues[68] compared endoscopically-assisted fixation with standard open technique and reported longer operative times in the endoscopic group but equivalent function. Computer-aided design using reformatted CT can simulate the reduction of a fracture and guide the length and placement of screws[69–71] (**Fig. 12**).

The management of mandible fractures in children is tailored to minimal disruption of growth. Bone fragments in children fuse partially by day 4, necessitating early treatment. The mandibular cortex is thinner and less dense than in adults. Tooth buds are present throughout the body of the mandible. Therefore, the developing tooth buds and partially erupted teeth can get injured by screws or intraosseous wires during ORIF. The shape and height of deciduous crowns make it more difficult to place circumdental wires and arch bars. Most body and symphysis fractures in children are nondisplaced without malocclusion and can be managed by close observation, soft diet, and limited physical activity. Closed reduction and immobilization is recommended for

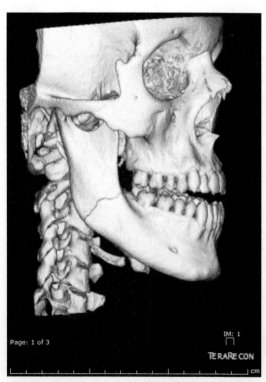

Fig. 11. Three-dimensional reconstructed CT image shows a fracture of the right angle of the mandible.

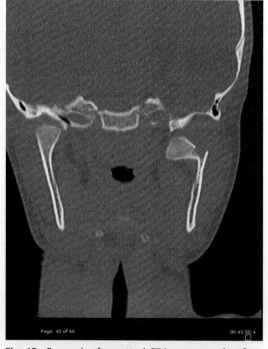

Fig. 12. Coronal reformatted CT image reveals a fracture of the left mandibular condylar neck with medial displacement and angulation of the condylar head.

displaced body and symphyseal fractures. The dental age of the child dictates the method of immobilization. In children younger than 2 years of age a lingual splint is placed with circummandibular wires for 3 weeks. If MMF is required, piriform or zygoma wires can be placed. In children with mixed dentition, arch bars can be an option and the jaw is immobilized with elastics. If possible, a monocortical plate can be applied to the inferior border of the mandible. Fractures of the angle in children require closed reduction and MMF for 3 weeks. The treatment of condylar fractures in children is based on the degree of interincisal opening, dental age, occlusion, and pain level. ORIF is not indicated in children unless the displaced fragment causes a mechanical obstruction. Because of the potential for ankylosis in children with intracapsular condylar fractures or crush injuries, mandibular exercises and jaw stretching should be initiated early. Children with primary or mixed dentition and unilateral subcondylar fractures can be treated with soft diet and analgesics for 7 days. Significant pain and severe malocclusion may require immobilization for 7 days, potentially followed by training elastics. Children with bilateral subcondylar fractures, relatively normal opening, and occlusion can be managed with soft diet and analgesics. Children with primary and mixed dentition with bilateral subcondylar fractures and open-bite malocclusion need MMF for 7 days, followed by guiding elastics for 7 more days. Children with permanent dentition who sustained unilateral or bilateral condylar fractures, underwent intermaxillary fixation for 7 days, and have persistent malocclusion should be considered for open reduction to restore ramus length.

REFERENCES

1. Allareddy V, Allareddy V, Nalliah RP. Epidemiology of facial fracture injuries. J Oral Maxillofac Surg 2011; 69:2613–8.
2. Lanzarotti S, Cook CS, Porter JM, et al. The cost of trauma. Am Surg 2003;69:766–70.
3. Erdmann D, Price K, Reed S, et al. A financial analysis of operative facial fracture management. Plast Reconstr Surg 2008;121:1323–7.
4. VandeGriend ZP, Hashemi A, Shkoukani M. Changing trends in adult facial trauma epidemiology. J Craniofac Surg 2015;26:108–12.
5. Walker TW, Byrne S, Donnellan J, et al. West of Ireland facial injury study. Part 1. Br J Oral Maxillofac Surg 2012;50:631–5.
6. Van Hout WMMT, Van Cann EM, Abbink JH, et al. An epidemiological study of maxillofacial fractures requiring surgical treatment at a tertiary trauma centre between 2005 and 2010. Br J Oral Maxillofac Surg 2013;51:416–20.
7. O'Meara C, Witherspoon R, Hapangama N, et al. Mandible fracture severity may be increased by alcohol and interpersonal violence. Aust Dent J 2011;56:166–70.
8. McAllister P, Jenner S, Laverick S. Toxicology screening in oral and maxillofacial trauma patients. Br J Oral Maxillofac Surg 2013;51:773–8.
9. Walker TWM, Donnellan J, Byrne S, et al. West of Ireland facial injury study. Part 2. Br J Oral Maxillofac Surg 2012;50:e99–103.
10. Tsang KK-T, Whitfield PC. Traumatic brain injury: review of current management strategies. Br J Oral Maxillofac Surg 2012;50:298–308.
11. Vyas RM, Dickinson BP, Wasson KL, et al. Pediatric facial fractures: current national incidence, distribution, and health care resource use. J Craniofac Surg 2008;19:339–49 [discussion: 350].
12. Imahara SD, Hopper RA, Wang J, et al. Patterns and outcomes of pediatric facial fractures in the united states: a survey of the National Trauma Data Bank. J Am Coll Surg 2008;207:710–6.
13. Soleimani T, Greathouse ST, Bell TM, et al. Epidemiology and cause-specific outcomes of facial fracture in hospitalized children. J Craniomaxillofac Surg 2015;43:1979–85.
14. Stacey DH, Doyle JF, Gutowski KA. Safety device use affects the incidence patterns of facial trauma in motor vehicle collisions: an analysis of the National Trauma Database from 2000 to 2004. Plast Reconstr Surg 2008;121:2057–64.
15. Andreasen JO, Jensen SS, Schwartz O, et al. A systematic review of prophylactic antibiotics in the surgical treatment of maxillofacial fractures. J Oral Maxillofac Surg 2006;64:1664–8.
16. Kyzas PA. Use of antibiotics in the treatment of mandible fractures: a systematic review. J Oral Maxillofac Surg 2011;69:1129–45.
17. Miles BA, Potter JK, Ellis E. The efficacy of postoperative antibiotic regimens in the open treatment of mandibular fractures: a prospective randomized trial. J Oral Maxillofac Surg 2006;64:576–82.
18. Shridharani SM, Berli J, Manson PN, et al. The role of postoperative antibiotics in mandible fractures: a systematic review of the literature. Ann Plast Surg 2015;75:353–7.
19. Knepil GJ, Loukota RA. Outcomes of prophylactic antibiotics following surgery for zygomatic bone fractures. J Craniomaxillofac Surg 2010;38:131–3.
20. Morris LM, Kellman RM. Are prophylactic antibiotics useful in the management of facial fractures? Laryngoscope 2014;124:1282–4.
21. Ratilal BO, Costa J, Pappamikail L, et al. Antibiotic prophylaxis for preventing meningitis in patients with basilar skull fractures. Cochrane Database Syst Rev 2015;(4):CD004884.

22. Khemani RG, Randolph A, Markovitz B. Corticosteroids for the prevention and treatment of post-extubation stridor in neonates, children and adults. Cochrane Database Syst Rev 2009;(3):CD001000.

23. Roberts I, Yates D, Sandercock P, et al. Effect of intravenous corticosteroids on death within 14 days in 10008 adults with clinically significant head injury (MRC CRASH trial): randomised placebo-controlled trial. Lancet 2004;364:1321–8.

24. Trauma.org | Initial Assessment of Spinal Injury. Available at: http://www.trauma.org/index.php/main/article/380/. April 1, 2002.

25. Haug RH, Foss J. Maxillofacial injuries in the pediatric patient. Oral Surg Oral Med Oral Pathol Oral Radiol Endod 2000;90:126–34.

26. Ferreira PC, Amarante JM, Silva PN, et al. Retrospective study of 1251 maxillofacial fractures in children and adolescents. Plast Reconstr Surg 2005; 115:1500–8.

27. Maniglia AJ, Kline SN. Maxillofacial trauma in the pediatric age group. Otolaryngol Clin North Am 1983; 16:717–30.

28. Munante-Cardenas JL, Olate S, Asprino L, et al. Pattern and treatment of facial trauma in pediatric and adolescent patients. J Craniofac Surg 2011; 22:1251–5.

29. Shaikh ZS, Worrall SF. Epidemiology of facial trauma in a sample of patients aged 1-18 years. Injury 2002; 33:669–71.

30. Ryan ML, Thorson CM, Otero CA, et al. Pediatric facial trauma: a review of guidelines for assessment, evaluation, and management in the emergency department. J Craniofac Surg 2011;22:1183–9.

31. Zimmermann CE, Troulis MJ, Kaban LB. Pediatric facial fractures: recent advances in prevention, diagnosis and management. Int J Oral Maxillofac Surg 2005;34:823–33.

32. Siy RW, Brown RH, Koshy JC, et al. General management considerations in pediatric facial fractures. J Craniofac Surg 2011;22:1190–5.

33. Bell RB, Osborn T, Dierks EJ, et al. Management of penetrating neck injuries: a new paradigm for civilian trauma. J Oral Maxillofac Surg 2007;65: 691–705.

34. House JW, Brackmann DE. Facial nerve grading system. Otolaryngol Head Neck Surg 1985;93: 146–7.

35. Tanyeri G, Celik O, Erbas O, et al. The effectiveness of different neuroprotective agents in facial nerve injury: an experimental study. Laryngoscope 2015; 125:E356–64.

36. Harrison M. A 4-year review of human bite injuries presenting to emergency medicine and proposed evidence-based guidelines. Injury 2009;40:826–30.

37. Guy WM, Brissett AE. Contemporary management of traumatic fractures of the frontal sinus. Otolaryngol Clin North Am 2013;46:733–48.

38. Pawar SS, Rhee JS. Frontal sinus and naso-orbital-ethmoid fractures. JAMA Facial Plast Surg 2014; 16:284–9.

39. Stotland MA, Do NK. Pediatric orbital fractures. J Craniofac Surg 2011;22:1230–5.

40. Rosenberger E, Kriet JD, Humphrey C. Management of nasoethmoid fractures. Curr Opin Otolaryngol Head Neck Surg 2013;21:410–6.

41. Ridgway EB, Chen C, Colakoglu S, et al. The incidence of lower eyelid malposition after facial fracture repair: a retrospective study and meta-analysis comparing subtarsal, subciliary, and trans-conjunctival incisions. Plast Reconstr Surg 2009; 124:1578–86.

42. Dubois L, Steenen SA, Gooris PJJ, et al. Controversies in orbital reconstruction - I. Defect-driven orbital reconstruction: a systematic review. Int J Oral Maxillofac Surg 2015;44:308–15.

43. Dubois L, Steenen SA, Gooris PJJ, et al. Controversies in orbital reconstruction - II. Timing of post-traumatic orbital reconstruction: a systematic review. Int J Oral Maxillofac Surg 2015;44:433–40.

44. Kunz C, Sigron GR, Jaquiéry C. Functional outcome after non-surgical management of orbital fractures-the bias of decision-making according to size of defect: critical review of 48 patients. Br J Oral Maxillofac Surg 2013;51:486–92.

45. Cobb ARM, Jeelani NO, Ayliffe PR. Orbital fractures in children. Br J Oral Maxillofac Surg 2013;51:41–6.

46. Gerber B, Kiwanuka P, Dhariwal D. Orbital fractures in children: a review of outcomes. Br J Oral Maxillofac Surg 2013;51:789–93.

47. Hundepool AC, Willemsen MAP, Koudstaal MJ, et al. Open reduction versus endoscopically controlled reconstruction of orbital floor fractures: a retrospective analysis. Int J Oral Maxillofac Surg 2012;41:489–93.

48. Ellstrom CL, Evans GR. Evidence-based medicine: zygoma fractures. Plast Reconstr Surg 2013;132: 1649–57.

49. Rana M, Warraich R, Tahir S, et al. Surgical treatment of zygomatic bone fracture using two points fixation versus three point fixation-a randomised prospective clinical trial. Trials 2012;13:36.

50. Staffel JG. Optimizing treatment of nasal fractures. Laryngoscope 2002;112:1709–19.

51. Khwaja S, Pahade AV, Luff D, et al. Nasal fracture reduction: local versus general anaesthesia. Rhinology 2007;45:83–8.

52. Chadha NK, Repanos C, Carswell AJ. Local anaesthesia for manipulation of nasal fractures: systematic review. J Laryngol Otol 2009;123:830–6.

53. Atighechi S, Baradaranfar MH, Akbari SA. Reduction of nasal bone fractures: a comparative study of general, local, and topical anesthesia techniques. J Craniofac Surg 2009;20:382–4.

54. Al-Moraissi EA, Ellis E. Local versus general anesthesia for the management of nasal bone fractures: a

systematic review and meta-analysis. J Oral Maxillofac Surg 2015;73:606–15.

55. Ogundare BO, Bonnick A, Bayley N. Pattern of mandibular fractures in an urban major trauma center. J Oral Maxillofac Surg 2003;61:713–8.

56. Zide MF, Kent JN. Indications for open reduction of mandibular condyle fractures. J Oral Maxillofac Surg 1983;41:89–98.

57. Danda AK. Comparison of a single noncompression miniplate versus 2 noncompression miniplates in the treatment of mandibular angle fractures: a prospective, randomized clinical trial. J Oral Maxillofac Surg 2010;68:1565–7.

58. Siddiqui A, Markose G, Moos KF, et al. One miniplate versus two in the management of mandibular angle fractures: a prospective randomised study. Br J Oral Maxillofac Surg 2007;45:223–5.

59. Laverick S, Siddappa P, Wong H, et al. Intraoral external oblique ridge compared with transbuccal lateral cortical plate fixation for the treatment of fractures of the mandibular angle: prospective randomised trial. Br J Oral Maxillofac Surg 2012;50:344–9.

60. Adeyemi MF, Adeyemo WL, Ogunlewe MO, et al. Is healing outcome of 2 weeks intermaxillary fixation different from that of 4 to 6 weeks intermaxillary fixation in the treatment of mandibular fractures? J Oral Maxillofac Surg 2012;70:1896–902.

61. Kaplan BA, Hoard MA, Park SS. Immediate mobilization following fixation of mandible fractures: a prospective, randomized study. Laryngoscope 2001; 111:1520–4.

62. Dorri M, Nasser M, Oliver R. Resorbable versus titanium plates for facial fractures. Cochrane Database Syst Rev 2009;(1):CD007158.

63. Eckelt U, Schneider M, Erasmus F, et al. Open versus closed treatment of fractures of the mandibular condylar process-a prospective randomized multi-centre study. J Craniomaxillofac Surg 2006; 34:306–14.

64. Singh V, Bhagol A, Goel M, et al. Outcomes of open versus closed treatment of mandibular subcondylar fractures: a prospective randomized study. J Oral Maxillofac Surg 2010;68:1304–9.

65. Danda AK, Muthusekhar MR, Narayanan V, et al. Open versus closed treatment of unilateral subcondylar and condylar neck fractures: a prospective, randomized clinical study. J Oral Maxillofac Surg 2010;68:1238–41.

66. Kotrashetti SM, Lingaraj JB, Khurana V. A comparative study of closed versus open reduction and internal fixation (using retromandibular approach) in the management of subcondylar fracture. Oral Surg Oral Med Oral Pathol Oral Radiol 2013;115:e7–11.

67. Liu Y, Bai N, Song G, et al. Open versus closed treatment of unilateral moderately displaced mandibular condylar fractures: a meta-analysis of randomized controlled trials. Oral Surg Oral Med Oral Pathol Oral Radiol 2013;116:169–73.

68. Schmelzeisen R, Cienfuegos-Monroy R, Schön R, et al. Patient benefit from endoscopically assisted fixation of condylar neck fractures-a randomized controlled trial. J Oral Maxillofac Surg 2009;67: 147–58.

69. Yang ML, Zhang B, Zhou Q, et al. Minimally-invasive open reduction of intracapsular condylar fractures with preoperative simulation using computer-aided design. Br J Oral Maxillofac Surg 2013;51:e29–33.

70. Iwai T, Yajima Y, Matsui Y, et al. Computer-assisted preoperative simulation for screw fixation of fractures of the condylar head. Br J Oral Maxillofac Surg 2013;51:176–7.

71. Wang WH, Li M, Xia B, et al. Computer-assisted virtual technology in intracapsular condylar fracture with two resorbable long-screws. Br J Oral Maxillofac Surg 2013;51:138–43.

Index

Note: Page numbers of article titles are in **boldface** type.

facialplastic.theclinics.com

UNITED STATES POSTAL SERVICE ® Statement of Ownership, Management, and Circulation (All Periodicals Publications Except Requester Publications)

1. Publication Title	2. Publication Number	3. Filing Date
FACIAL PLASTIC SURGERY CLINICS OF NORTH AMERICA	013 – 122	9/18/2016

4. Issue Frequency	5. Number of Issues Published Annually	6. Annual Subscription Price
FEB, MAY, AUG, NOV	4	$373.00

7. Complete Mailing Address of Known Office of Publication (Not printer) (Street, city, county, state, and ZIP+4®)

ELSEVIER INC.
360 PARK AVENUE SOUTH
NEW YORK, NY 10010-1710

Contact Person
STEPHEN R. BUSHING

Telephone (Include area code)
215-239-3688

8. Complete Mailing Address of Headquarters or General Business Office of Publisher (Not printer)

ELSEVIER INC.
360 PARK AVENUE SOUTH
NEW YORK, NY 10010-1710

9. Full Names and Complete Mailing Addresses of Publisher, Editor, and Managing Editor (Do not leave blank)

Publisher (Name and complete mailing address)

ADRIANNE BRIGIDO, ELSEVIER INC.
1600 JOHN F KENNEDY BLVD. SUITE 1800
PHILADELPHIA, PA 19103-2899

Editor (Name and complete mailing address)

JESSICA MCCOOL, ELSEVIER INC.
1600 JOHN F KENNEDY BLVD. SUITE 1800
PHILADELPHIA, PA 19103-2899

Managing Editor (Name and complete mailing address)

PATRICK MANLEY, ELSEVIER INC.
1600 JOHN F KENNEDY BLVD. SUITE 1800
PHILADELPHIA, PA 19103-2899

10. Owner (Do not leave blank. If the publication is owned by a corporation, give the name and address of the corporation immediately followed by the names and addresses of all stockholders owning or holding 1 percent or more of the total amount of stock. If not owned by a corporation, give the names and addresses of the individual owners. If owned by a partnership or other unincorporated firm, give its name and address as well as those of each individual owner. If the publication is published by a nonprofit organization, give its name and address.)

Full Name	Complete Mailing Address
WHOLLY OWNED SUBSIDIARY OF REED/ELSEVIER, US HOLDINGS	1600 JOHN F KENNEDY BLVD. SUITE 1800 PHILADELPHIA, PA 19103-2899

11. Known Bondholders, Mortgagees, and Other Security Holders Owning or Holding 1 Percent or More of Total Amount of Bonds, Mortgages, or Other Securities. If none, check box ▶ ☐ None

Full Name	Complete Mailing Address
N/A	

12. Tax Status (For completion by nonprofit organizations authorized to mail at nonprofit rates) (Check one)
The purpose, function, and nonprofit status of this organization and the exempt status for federal income tax purposes:
☐ Has Not Changed During Preceding 12 Months
☐ Has Changed During Preceding 12 Months (Publisher must submit explanation of change with this statement)

13. Publication Title	14. Issue Date for Circulation Data Below
FACIAL PLASTIC SURGERY CLINICS OF NORTH AMERICA	AUGUST 2016

15. Extent and Nature of Circulation		Average No. Copies Each Issue During Preceding 12 Months	No. Copies of Single Issue Published Nearest to Filing Date
a. Total Number of Copies (Net press run)		307	362
b. Paid Circulation (By Mail and Outside the Mail)	(1) Mailed Outside-County Paid Subscriptions Stated on PS Form 3541 (Include paid distribution above nominal rate, advertiser's proof copies, and exchange copies)	156	192
	(2) Mailed In-County Paid Subscriptions Stated on PS Form 3541 (Include paid distribution above nominal rate, advertiser's proof copies, and exchange copies)	0	0
	(3) Paid Distribution Outside the Mails Including Sales Through Dealers and Carriers, Street Vendors, Counter Sales, and Other Paid Distribution Outside USPS®	31	42
	(4) Paid Distribution by Other Classes of Mail Through the USPS (e.g., First-Class Mail®)	0	0
c. Total Paid Distribution (Sum of 15b (1), (2), (3), and (4))	▶	187	234
d. Free or Nominal Rate Distribution (By Mail and Outside the Mail)	(1) Free or Nominal Rate Outside-County Copies included on PS Form 3541	23	28
	(2) Free or Nominal Rate In-County Copies Included on PS Form 3541	0	0
	(3) Free or Nominal Rate Copies Mailed at Other Classes Through the USPS (e.g., First-Class Mail)	0	0
	(4) Free or Nominal Rate Distribution Outside the Mail (Carriers or other means)	0	0
e. Total Free or Nominal Rate Distribution (Sum of 15d (1), (2), (3) and (4))	▶	23	28
f. Total Distribution (Sum of 15c and 15e)	▶	210	262
g. Copies not Distributed (See Instructions to Publishers #4 (page #3))	▶	97	100
h. Total (Sum of 15f and g)	▶	307	362
i. Percent Paid (15c divided by 15f times 100)		89%	89%

* If you are claiming electronic copies, go to line 16 on page 3. If you are not claiming electronic copies, skip to line 17 on page 3.

16. Electronic Copy Circulation	Average No. Copies Each Issue During Preceding 12 Months	No. Copies of Single Issue Published Nearest to Filing Date
a. Paid Electronic Copies ▶	0	0
b. Total Paid Print Copies (Line 15c) + Paid Electronic Copies (Line 16a) ▶	187	234
c. Total Print Distribution (Line 15f) + Paid Electronic Copies (Line 16a) ▶	210	262
d. Percent Paid (Both Print & Electronic Copies) (16b divided by 16c × 100) ▶	89%	89%

☒ I certify that 50% of all my distributed copies (electronic and print) are paid above a nominal price.

17. Publication of Statement of Ownership
☒ If the publication is a general publication, publication of this statement is required. Will be printed ☐ Publication not required.
in the NOVEMBER 2016 issue of this publication.

18. Signature and Title of Editor, Publisher, Business Manager, or Owner

STEPHEN R. BUSHING - INVENTORY DISTRIBUTION CONTROL MANAGER

Stephen R. Bushing   Date 9/18/2016

I certify that all information furnished on this form is true and complete. I understand that anyone who furnishes false or misleading information on this form or who omits material or information requested on the form may be subject to criminal sanctions (including fines and imprisonment) and/or civil sanctions (including civil penalties).

PS Form 3526, July 2014 [Page 3 of 4] PSN: 7530-01-000-9931   PRIVACY NOTICE: See our privacy policy on www.usps.com.

PS Form 3526, July 2014 (Page 1 of 4 (see instructions page 4)) PSN: 7530-01-000-9931   PRIVACY NOTICE: See our privacy policy on www.usps.com.

Moving?

Make sure your subscription moves with you!

To notify us of your new address, find your **Clinics Account Number** (located on your mailing label above your name), and contact customer service at:

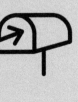

Email: journalscustomerservice-usa@elsevier.com

800-654-2452 (subscribers in the U.S. & Canada)
314-447-8871 (subscribers outside of the U.S. & Canada)

Fax number: 314-447-8029

Elsevier Health Sciences Division
Subscription Customer Service
3251 Riverport Lane
Maryland Heights, MO 63043

ELSEVIER

Printed and bound by CPI Group (UK) Ltd, Croydon, CR0 4YY

08/05/2025

01864693-0003